ANTIEPILEPTIC DRUG INTERACTIONS

Antiepileptic Drug Interactions

Editor

William H. Pitlick, Ph.D.

Research Training and Research Resources Officer
Office of the Director
National Institutes of Health
Bethesda, Maryland, U.S.A.

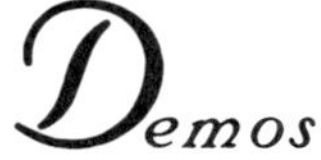

Demos Publications, 156 Fifth Avenue, New York, New York 10010

Made in the United States of America

Great care has been taken to maintain the accuracy of the information contained in this volume. However, neither the editor nor Demos Publications can be held responsible for errors or for any consequences arising from the use of the information contained herein.

ISBN: 0-939957-14-0
LC: 88-71752

Preface

One of the major problems encountered in the development of new antiepileptic drugs is the number and intensity of drug interactions that can occur when a new drug is added to standard therapy. Further development and use of antiepileptic drug therapy could benefit greatly from quantitative as well as qualitative knowledge of the mechanism and predictability of drug interactions. For example, a priori estimation of interaction potential could shorten and conceivably improve methods for clinical testing of a new drug. Such estimates may be developed by application of relevant concepts in the areas of medicinal chemistry and biochemical pharmacology and analysis of data from carefully designed animal pharmacology and toxicology studies.

Over the last decade, a very large body of knowledge and experience has been accumulated relative to the interactions of antiepileptic drugs. Many people in the scientific community agreed it would be timely to discuss and publish the accumulated data, so that we may more efficiently predict, characterize, and compensate for drug interactions in clinical testing and use of antiepileptic drugs.

It has been over 10 years since the last comprehensive text on interactions of antiepileptic drugs was published. Since that time, many new drugs have entered clinical testing and the presence of interactions of these new drugs with existing therapies has been daunting.

There are four sections in the book. The first focuses on interaction problems and their solution for the practicing neurologist. The second section is devoted to the implications of interactions of antiepileptic drugs in clinical testing, including the detection and characterization of drug interactions in epileptic patients, the design of efficacy studies involving drugs that interact, and statistical problems in study design when drugs interact. The third and fourth sections are devoted to basic mechanisms of drug interactions, including discussions of how enzyme inhibition and induction occur, how drug interactions occur in distribution of drugs, the effects of protein binding on free drug clearance, and a small portion devoted to pharmacodynamic drug interactions. These sections also discuss in vivo and in vitro models that can be used to study and predict drug interactions as well as extrapolate data from animal studies to human studies.

This volume will be of interest to all clinicians who manage patients with epilepsy and to pharmacologists and other researchers involved in the development and testing of antiepileptic drugs.

Contents

Contributors

Blaise F. D. Bourgeois, M.D., Staff Neurologist, Department of Neurology, Section of Epilepsy and Clinical Neurophysiology, The Cleveland Clinic Foundation, Cleveland, Ohio, U.S.A.

Thomas R. Browne, M.D., Assistant Chief of Neurology, Veterans Administration Medical Center, Boston, Massachusetts, U.S.A.

Richard A. Carchman, Ph.D., Professor of Pharmacology and Toxicology, Biostatistics, Medical College of Virginia/Virginia Commonwealth University, Richmond, Virginia, U.S.A.

Walter H. Carter, Jr., Ph.D., Professor and Chairman, Biostatistics, Professor of Biostatistics, Medical College of Virginia/Virginia Commonwealth University, Richmond, Virginia, U.S.A.

Joyce A. Cramer, B.S., Project Director, Epilepsy Center, Veterans Administration Medical Center, West Haven, Connecticut, U.S.A.

W. Edwin Dodson, M.D., Professor of Pediatrics and Neurology, The Mallinckrodt Department of Pediatrics and Department of Neurology and Neurological Surgery (Neurology), Washington University School of Medicine, St. Louis Children's Hospital, St. Louis, Missouri, U.S.A.

Barbara A. Evans, Mass Spectrometry Laboratory, Eunice Kennedy Shriver Center, Waltham, Massachusetts, U.S.A.

James E. Evans, Director, Mass Spectrometry Laboratory, Eunice Kennedy Shriver Center, Waltham, Massachusetts, U.S.A.

Michael R. Franklin, Ph.D., Professor of Pharmacology and Toxicology, Department of Pharmacology and Toxicology, University of Utah, Salt Lake City, Utah, U.S.A.

Chris Gennings, Ph.D., Assistant Professor, Biostatistics, Medical College of Virginia/Virginia Commonwealth University, Richmond, Virginia, U.S.A.

Nina M. Graves, Pharm.D., Assistant Professor, Department of Pharmacy Practice, College of Pharmacy, University of Minnesota, Minneapolis, Minnesota, U.S.A.

David J. Greenblatt, M.D., Professor of Pharmacology and Psychiatry, Tufts University School of Medicine; Chief, Clinical Pharmacology Laboratory, Tufts New England Medical Center, Boston, Massachusetts, U.S.A.

James P. Hubbell, Ph.D., Senior Research Scientist, Division of Medicinal Biochemistry, The Wellcome Research Laboratories, Research Triangle Park, North Carolina, U.S.A.

Nancy C. James, Pharm.D., Clinical Research Scientist, Clinical Pharmacokinetics/Dynamics Section, Burroughs Wellcome Co., Research Triangle Park, North Carolina, U.S.A.

Bradley M. Kerr, Ph.D., Department of Pharmaceutics, University of Washington, Seattle, Washington, U.S.A.

Alvin N. Kotake, Ph.D., Director of Clinical Biology, CIBA-GEIGY Corp., Summit, New Jersey, U.S.A.

Harvey J. Kupferberg, Ph.D., Chief, Preclinical Pharmacology Section, Epilepsy Branch, Division of Convulsive, Developmental and Neuromuscular Disorders, National Institutes of Neurological Disorders and Stroke, National Institutes of Health, Bethesda, Maryland, U.S.A.

Henn Kutt, M.D., Associate Professor of Neurology and Pharmacology, Department of Neurology and Pharmacology, Cornell University Medical College, New York, New York, U.S.A.

Steven K. Kuwahara, Ph.D., Research Associate, Department of Clinical Pharmacology, Johns Hopkins Hospital, Baltimore, Maryland, U.S.A.

Allen A. Lai, Ph.D., Head, Department of Clinical Development, Burroughs Wellcome Co., Research Triangle Park, North Carolina, U.S.A.

George H. Lambert, M.D., Associate Professor, Department of Pediatrics, Loyola University, Maywood, Illinois, U.S.A.

Ilo E. Leppik, M.D., Professor of Neurology, Comprehensive Epilepsy Program, University of Minnesota, Minneapolis, Minnesota, U.S.A.

René H. Levy, Ph.D., Chairman, Department of Pharmaceutics, School of Pharmacy, University of Washington, Seattle, Washington, U.S.A.

Pierre Loiseau, M.D., Professor of Neurology, University Hospital, Bordeaux, France.

Richard H. Mattson, M.D., Professor of Neurology, Yale University, School of Medicine, New Haven, Connecticut, U.S.A.

Xianzhong Meng, Head, Department of Experimental Pathology, Kashan Disease Institute, Harbin Medical College, Harbin, Peoples Republic of China.

Derrick N. Parsons, Ph.D., Head, Drug Metabolism and Radiochemistry, Wellcome Research Laboratories, Beckenham, Kent, U.K.

Robert J. Perchalsky, Ph.D., Research Chemist, FBI Academy, Forensic Science Research and Training Center, Quantico, Virginia, U.S.A.

Emilio Perucca, M.D., Ph.D., Associate Professor of Clinical Pharmacology, Division of Clinical Pharmacology, Department of Internal Medicine and Therapeutics, University of Pavia, Pavia, Italy.

Charles E. Pippenger, Ph.D., Head, Section of Applied Clinical Pharmacology, Department of Biochemistry, The Cleveland Clinic Foundation, Cleveland, Ohio, U.S.A.

Gordon W. Pledger, Ph.D., Chief, Technical Information Section, Epilepsy Branch, Division of Convulsive, Developmental and Neuromuscular Disorders, National Institute of Neurological Disorders and Stroke, National Institutes of Health, Bethesda, Maryland, U.S.A.

Roger J. Porter, M.D., Deputy Director, National Institute of Neurological Disorders and Stroke, National Institutes of Health, Bethesda, Maryland, U.S.A.

Richard J. Pylilo, Research Clinical Chemist, Neuropharmacology Laboratory, Boston Veterans Administration Medical Center, Boston, Massachusetts, U.S.A.

Rogelio J. Rangel, M.D., Post-Doctoral Fellow in Neurology, Veterans Administration Medical Center and University of Florida College of Medicine, Gainesville, Florida, U.S.A.

Rory P. Remmel, Ph.D., Assistant Professor, Department of Medicinal Chemistry, College of Pharmacy, University of Minnesota, Minneapolis, Minnesota, U.S.A.

Alan Richens, M.B., B.S., B.Sc., Ph.D., F.R.C.P., Professor of Pharmacology and Therapeutics, Department of Pharmacology and Therapeutics, University of Wales College of Medicine, Heath Park, Cardiff, South Wales, U.K.

Dale A. Schoeller, Ph.D., Research Associate (Professor), Department of Medicine, University of Chicago, Chicago, Illinois, U.S.A.

Gerald E. Schumacher, Pharm.D., Ph.D., Professor of Pharmacy, Northeastern University, Boston, Massachusetts, U.S.A.

Ewart A. Swinyard, Ph.D., Emeritus Professor of Pharmacology, Department of Pharmacology and Toxicology, College of Pharmacy, University of Utah, Salt Lake City, Utah, U.S.A.

George K. Szabo, M.T. (A.S.C.P.), Clinical Instructor in Neurology, Boston University School of Medicine; Technical Director, Neuropharmacology Laboratory, Boston Veterans Administration Medical Center, Boston, Massachusetts, U.S.A.

Jack Tor, M.D., Director of Chemical Research, Laboratoires Biocodex, Montrouge, France.

William F. Trager, Ph.D., Professor, Department of Medicinal Chemistry, University of Washington, Seattle, Washington, U.S.A.

David M. Treiman, M.D., Associate Professor of Neurology, University of California at Los Angeles, School of Medicine, Reed Neurological Research Center, Los Angeles, California, U.S.A.

Frederick Van Lente, Ph.D., Chairman, Department of Biochemistry, The Cleveland Clinic Foundation, Cleveland, Ohio, U.S.A.

Richard M. Welch, Ph.D., Assistant Division Director, Division of Medicinal Biochemistry, The Wellcome Research Laboratories, Research Triangle Park, North Carolina, U.S.A.

B. J. Wilder, M.D., Chief, Neurology Service, Veterans Administration Medical Center, University of Florida College of Medicine, Gainesville, Florida, U.S.A.

Harold H. Wolf, Ph.D., Professor of Pharmacology, Department of Pharmacology and Toxicology, College of Pharmacy, University of Utah, Salt Lake City, Utah, U.S.A.

Jose H. Woodhead, B.S., Senior Research Specialist, Department of Pharmacology and Toxicology, College of Pharmacy, University of Utah, Salt Lake City, Utah, U.S.A.

I. Clinical Relevance of Drug Interactions

1

Comparison of Methods for Determination of Pharmacokinetic Drug Interactions and Proposals for New Methods

Thomas R. Browne, David J. Greenblatt, Gerald E. Schumacher, George K. Szabo, James E. Evans, Barbara A. Evans, Robert J. Perchalski, and Richard J. Pylilo

Departments of Neurology and Pharmacology and Experimental Therapeutics, Boston University School of Medicine and Boston Veterans Administration Medical Center, Departments of Psychiatry and Medicine, Tufts University School of Medicine, and College of Pharmacy and Allied Health Professions, Northeastern University, Boston, Massachusetts; Mass Spectrometry Laboratory, Eunice Kennedy Shriver Center, Waltham, Massachusetts; and FBI Academy, Quantico, Virginia, U.S.A.

Pharmacokinetic drug interactions are those resulting from alterations in absorption, distribution, biotransformation, or excretion of a drug as a consequence of co-administration of one or more additional drugs (1). Clinically significant drug interactions may occur when addition of a second drug has one or more of the following effects on the first drug: (a) decreased or increased absorption rate and/or extent, (b) alteration of tissue binding (especially plasma protein binding), and/or (c) decreased or increased rate of biotransformation and/or excretion. Pharmacokinetic drug interactions may be bidirectional (i.e., the pharmacokinetics of both drugs are affected by the presence of the other drug), and one drug may have more than one type of pharmacokinetic drug interaction with the other drug (1).

Methods for studying the pharmacokinetic drug interactions fall into three categories: (a) studies of absorption, (b) studies of distribution, and (c) studies of biotransformation and/or excretion. Each method has its own set of procedures, assumptions, advantages, and disadvantages, and these will be reviewed in this chapter. Studies of biotransformation and excretion will be emphasized since this is where the majority of work on pharmacokinetic drug interactions has been performed. The lists of examples and references cited are illustrative but not comprehensive. Conclusions regarding the relative merits of the methods in each of the three categories of method will be drawn. Finally, some new methods will be proposed that do not have certain limitations of existing methods.

GENERAL COMMENTS

Paradigms

In studying pharmacokinetic drug interactions, two paradigms are usually possible: (a) pharmacokinetic values for Drug 1 are determined before and after addition of Drug 2, or (b) pharmacokinetic values for Drug 2 are determined in the presence of Drug 1 and after removal of Drug 1. Unless otherwise stated, the methods described in this chapter can be utilized with either paradigm and have similar procedures, assumptions, advantages, and disadvantages with either paradigm. Only paradigm 1 will be illustrated for most methods.

Analytical Methodology

Most methods of studying pharmacokinetic drug interactions require analytic determinations of drug concentrations in biological fluids. The commonly employed analytical methods are gas chromatography (GC), gas chromatographic–mass spectrometry (GC–MS), high-pressure liquid chromatography (HPLC), and competitive protein assays such as radioimmunoassay (RIA), fluorescence polarization immunoassay (FPIA), and enzyme multiplied immunoassay technique (R) [EMIT (R)]. These methods are subject to between-method and, for the same method, between-laboratory, between-day, and within-day variations. Between-method variability may exceed 10% coefficient of variation (CV) for repeated determinations of the same sample, and, even worse, may introduce systematic, nonrandom error. Between-laboratory variability has not been extensively studied but probably has the potential to exceed 10% CV. Typical within-day and between-CV values are: GC–MS = <5% for research; GC, HPLC, RIA, FPIA = <5% for research; GC, HPLC, RIA, FPIA < 10% for clinical use; EMIT (R) = 15% for research or clinical use. Note that most clinical laboratories accept a CV of 10% as satisfactory for routine clinical use and that the manufacturer of EMIT (R) does not guarantee a within-day or between-day CV of less than 15%.

Random variability introduced by analytical methodology reduces the ability of statistical tests to demonstrate significant difference or equivalence of values obtained before and after addition of Drug 2 to Drug 1. This diminishes the value of results and requires study of a larger number of subjects in order to show statistical significance. In order to minimize analytical method variability: (a) all determinations should be performed at the same center, (b) only one analytical method should be used, and (c) all determinations for a given subject should be performed on the same day.

METHODS FOR STUDYING DRUG ABSORPTION

Measurement of Drug Plasma Concentration

Procedures. Mean steady-state plasma concentration of Drug 1 is determined before and after addition of Drug 2. Fraction of drug absorbed *(FA)* is calculated using the equation:

$$FA = \frac{\bar{C}_{ss} \times CL}{DP \times FT} \tag{1}$$

where $\bar{C}_{ss}$ is the mean steady-state plasma concentration, CL is the drug clearance, DP is the prescribed dosing rate, and FT is the fraction of prescribed dosing rate actually taken. $\bar{C}_{ss}$ and DP can be measured for each subject. The value for CL must be an assumed population value. FT is usually assumed to be 1.0.

Assumptions. This method assumes: (a) all subjects have been completely compliant in taking their medications, or degree of noncompliance is known, (b) $\bar{C}_{ss}$ value employed represents *mean* (not trough, maximum, or random) plasma concentration, (c) $\bar{C}_{ss}$ value employed represents steady-state value, (d) clearance value of all subjects is the population mean value, and (e) clearance value is the same before and after addition of second drug.

Assumptions a–c are difficult to achieve in practice and often are violated (see below). Clearance of many drugs varies widely among individuals (e.g., assumption b) and may be altered by addition of a second drug (e.g., assumption c).

Advantages. This method is rapid, simple, inexpensive, and minimally inconvenient to the subject.

Disadvantages. This method is based on five assumptions, four of which often are not validated in the course of performance of the study. Unless all assumptions are validated, this method yields suspect results (see below). Also, this method measures extent of, and not rate of, absorption.

Measurement of Total Drug Excreted

Procedure. Total amount of Drug 1 excreted as parent drug and metabolites per unit time is measured before and after addition of Drug 2. Excreta (urine, feces, etc.) are collected for a unit of time (e.g., 24 h), and volume is measured. Concentration of drug or metabolite in excreta is determined by GC, HPLC, and so on, and amount of drug or metabolite excreted is obtained by multiplying volume of excreta times concentration of drug or metabolite.

Assumptions. This method is based on the principle that, at steady state, the amount of drug excreted per unit time *(DE)* is equal to *DP* per unit time times *FT* times *FA*.

$$DE = DP \times FT \times FA \tag{2}$$

Solving for *FA:*

$$FA = \frac{DE}{DP \times FT} \tag{3}$$

This method assumes: (a) drug compliance has been complete or is known, (b) steady state has been attained at the time determinations are performed, and (c) all of the excreted drug and drug metabolites can be obtained and quantitated. Drug-taking compliance is difficult to assure, but methods for assurance do exist. The time required to attain steady state is known for many drugs, making compliance with assumption b possible. Assumption (c) can be validated for drugs with 100% oral bioavailability (measured *DE* should equal *DA* $\times$ *FT* $\times$ *FA*) or drugs that can be administered intravenously.

Advantages. This method has the following advantages: (a) it is based on assumptions that can be validated, (b) it yields definitive results, and (c) it is minimally inconvenient to subjects. Depending on complexity of drug routes of elimination and necessary analytical methodology, this method may be relatively simple or difficult to carry out. Note that demonstration of absence of change in amount of drug and metabolite excreted per unit time before and after adding Drug 2 can be very helpful in demonstrating that an observed change in steady-state plasma concentration is *not* due to a change in fraction of drug absorbed or to a change in patient compliance (3) (e.g., Eq. 2 and Table 1-1).

Disadvantages. This method measures extent but not rate of absorption. The assumption that all of an administered dose of drug can be recovered and measured in excreta cannot be met for many drugs.

Tracer Methods

Procedures. Labeled (stable or radioactive) tracer doses of Drug 1 are administered by the oral route before and after administration of Drug 2 is begun (4). Tracer-dose plasma concentration versus time relationships are used to calculate absorption rate constant and absorption half-life as

Table 1-1.   Phenytoin Pharmacokinetic Values Before 4 and 12 Weeks After Adding Carbamazepine in Six Subjects

	Before Wk 0	Wk 4	Wk 12	Significance[a]
Mean steady-state serum concentration (μg/ml)	13.2[b] ±6.6	13.4 ±5.6	17.8 ±7.1	0.00025
Clearance (ml/min/kg)	0.271 ±0.148	0.246 ±0.150	0.172 ±0.074	0.025
Elimination half-life (h)	37.7 ±19.3	41.8 ±23.1	50.3 ±27.3	0.005
Volume of distribution (L/kg)	0.65 ±0.08	0.69 ±0.09	0.63 ±0.08	NS
48-h urinary excretion of phenytoin, p-hydroxyphenyl-phenylhydantoin, and phenytoin dihydrodiol (mg)	580.2 ±146.0	ND	597.8 ±79.0	NS

ND, not determined; NS, not significant.
Reproduced with permission from Browne et al. (3).
[a]By analysis of variance.
[b]Mean ± SD.

measurements of *rate* of drug absorption. The area under the serum concentration versus time curve (AUC) measures the *relative extent* of drug absorption. Also, measurement of the amount of labeled metabolites excreted measures *absolute extent* of drug absorbed.

Assumptions. This method assumes: (a) the absorption, distribution, biotransformation, and excretion of labeled drug are the same as unlabeled drug, (b) there is an absence of deep pool effect (see below), and (c) all of the excreted labeled drug and labeled metabolites can be obtained and quantitated. Methods exist for validation of assumptions a and b (see below). Assumption c can be validated for drugs with 100% oral bioavailability or drugs that can be administered intravenously.

Advantages. This method has the following advantages: (a) it is based on three assumptions that can be validated, and (b) *rate and relative extent* of changes in absorption can be measured accurately in all subjects. Depending on complexity of drug routes of elimination and necessary analytical methodology, determination of absolute extent of absorption may be relatively simple or difficult.

Disadvantages. This method has the following disadvantages: (a) methodology required is often relatively complex and expensive, (b) there is relatively high subject inconvenience (frequent blood and urine collections), (c) absolute extent of absorption can be measured only if all of excreted labeled drug and metabolites can be obtained and quantitated, and (d) if radioactive tracers are used, a special set of problems is introduced (see below).

Conclusions

The "measurement of total drug excreted" method provides an accurate and convenient method (for subject) to determine *extent* of drug absorption if all of excreted drug and metabolites can be collected and quantitated. Tracer methods provide accurate data, usually at greater cost and subject inconvenience, whenever data on *rate and extent* of absorption are required or when it is impossible to collect and quantitate all of the drug and metabolites excreted. The measurement of drug plasma concentration method yields suspect results unless five assumptions are validated (seldom done in practice).

METHODS FOR STUDYING DRUG DISTRIBUTION

In Vitro and In Vivo Plasma Protein Binding

Procedures. The extent of plasma protein binding at therapeutic plasma concentrations of Drug 1 is determined in vitro or in vivo alone and in the presence of Drug 2 (5,6) (Table 1-2).

Assumptions. This method assumes: (a) a given plasma concentration of Drug 2 has the same effect on protein binding of Drug 1 in vivo or in vitro (in vitro method), and (b) errors introduced in separating free-drug from protein-bound drug are minimal. Assumption (a) is not always true, and the methodology involved in separating free from protein-bound drug can be problematic (5).

Advantages. This method is rapid, inexpensive, and minimally inconvenient to subjects.

Table 1-2. Phenytoin Protein Binding Following Valproic Acid Administration

	Valproic acid dose (mg/day)		
	0	900	1,350
Number of patients	25	11	9
Mean percent free phenytoin	10.9	16.1	20.0

Reproduced with permission from Mattson et al. (6).

Table 1-3. Phenytoin Pharmacokinetic Values Before and 4 and 12 Weeks After Adding Phenobarbital in Six Subjects

	Before Wk 0	Wk 4	Wk 12	Significance[a]
Mean steady-state serum concentration (μg/ml)	13.2[b] ±5.4	13.2 ±5.7	15.0 ±5.6	0.51
Clearance (ml/min/kg)	0.29 ±0.18	0.31 ±0.19	0.29 ±0.20	0.43[c]
Elimination half-life (h)	34.3 ±16.4	29.6 ±12.5	32.5 ±17.2	0.53
Volume of distribution (L/kg)	0.69 ±0.06	0.64 ±0.09	0.60 ±0.05	0.10

Reproduced with permission from Browne et al. (7).
[a]By analysis of variance.
[b]Mean ± SD.
[c]Probability of missing a truly significant change of 20% or greater (Type II or beta error) = 0.01.

Disadvantages. This method has the following disadvantages: (a) assumptions are not always met, and (b) only distribution to protein binding sites is measured.

Measurement of Distribution Half-Life and Volume of Distribution with Tracer Studies

Procedures. Intravenous (i.v.) labeled (stable or radioactive) tracer doses of Drug 1 are administered before and after addition of Drug 2. Labeled drug plasma concentration versus time relationships are used to calculate distribution half-life and volume of distribution (3,7) (e.g., Tables 1-1 and 1-3).

Assumptions. This method assumes: (a) absorption and distribution of labeled drug are the same as unlabeled drug, and (b) tracer drug can be given by i.v. route. Methods exist to verify assumption (a) for a given labeled form of drug (see below).

Advantages. This method has the following advantages: (a) assumptions can be verified, and (b) accurate measurement of *rate and extent* of distribution is possible.

Disadvantages. This method is relatively complex and expensive. An i.v. formulation of tracer dose must be available. Data is not obtained on the rate and extent of drug entry into specific target organs.

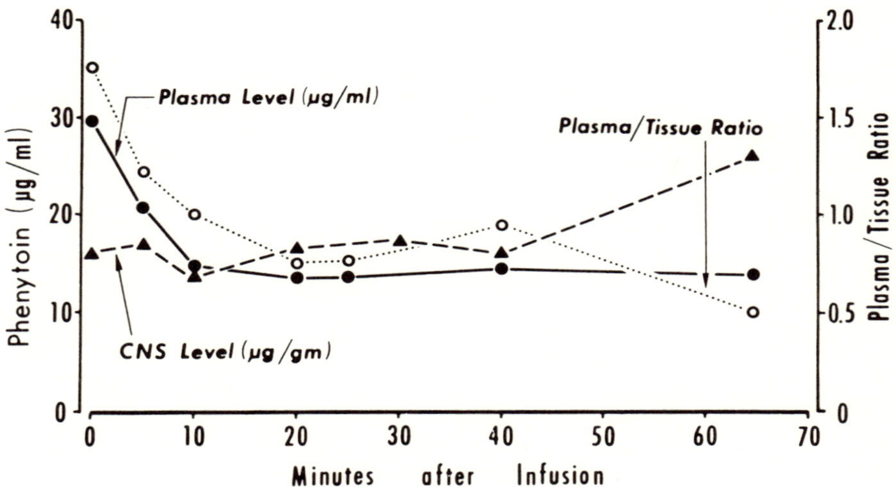

FIG. 1-1. Mean phenytoin concentration values after i.v. infusion (13 mg/kg) in plasma (solid line) and brain (dashed line) in three patients and the corresponding plasma/tissue ratio (dotted line). [Reproduced from Wilder et al. (8) with permission.]

Measurement of Rate of Entry of Drug into Tissues Other Than Blood

Procedures. Serial samples of tissue [e.g., brain, cerebrospinal fluid (CSF), liver] are obtained after Drug 1 is administered (8) (e.g., Fig. 1-1). Alternatively, serial injections of Drug 1 with different labels can be administered at predetermined times prior to collection of a single tissue specimen (staggered stable isotope technique) (9) (Fig. 1-2). Drug–tissue entry rate constant and entry half-life are determined from tissue concentration versus time relationships. Procedure is repeated after addition of Drug 2.

Assumptions. This method assumes: (a) the experimental methods (e.g., CSF collection, biopsy) employed do not alter distribution, and (b) the staggered stable isotope technique yields similar results to the conventional multiple-specimen collection technique. The second assumption has been verified (9).

Advantages. Rate of entry of drug into a specific tissue can be determined.

Disadvantages. This method is invasive and inconvenient to subject (less so if staggered stable isotope method is used) and subject to all of the disadvantages of tracer studies listed below.

Conclusions

Intravenous tracer dose methods can measure accurately the rate and extent of total body drug distribution before and after addition of a sec-

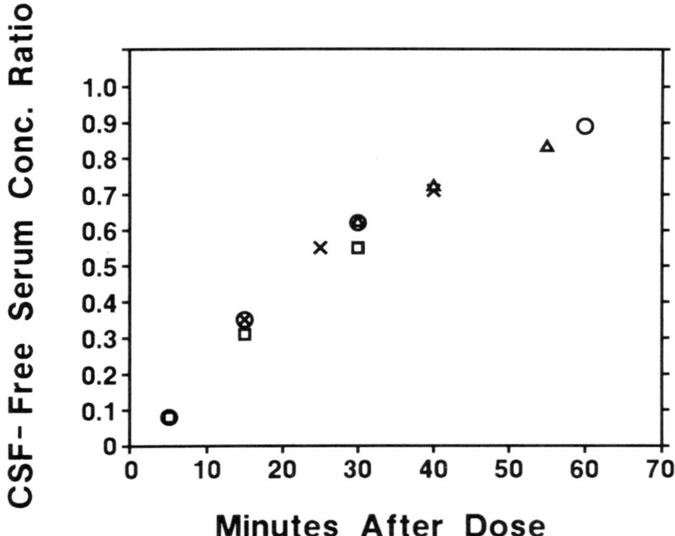

FIG. 1-2. Phenobarbital (PB) cerebrospinal fluid (CSF)-free serum concentration ratio versus time data points from a staggered stable isotope administration study in a dog. (○) from four sets of specimens collected 5, 15, 30, and 60 min after infusion of +0 PB. (□) from single set of serum and CSF specimens collected 5 min after infusion of +0 PB, 15 min after infusion of +3 PB, and 30 min after infusion of +5 PB. (X) from single set of specimens collected 15 min after infusion of +0 PB, 25 min after infusion of +3 PB, and 40 min after infusion of +5 PB. (△) from single set of specimens collected 30 min after infusion of +0 PB, 40 min after infusion of +3 PB, and 55 min after infusion of +5 PB. [Reproduced from Evans et al. (9) with permission.]

ond drug, but they are relatively costly and inconvenient to subjects. Drug plasma protein binding can be measured relatively easily before and after addition of a second drug. Measurement of the rate and extent of entry of drug into tissues other than plasma is possible, but logistically it is difficult, expensive, and inconvenient to subjects.

METHODS FOR STUDYING DRUG BIOTRANSFORMATION AND EXCRETION

Measurement of Drug Plasma Concentration

Procedures. Mean steady-state plasma concentration of Drug 1 is determined before and after addition of Drug 2. Mean steady-state plasma concentration values are compared directly.

Drug 1 clearance is calculated using the equation:

$$CL = \frac{DP \times FT \times FA}{\overline{C}_{ss}} \qquad (4)$$

Drug 1 elimination half-life ($t_{1/2}$) is calculated using the equation:

$$t_{1/2} = \frac{0.693 \times V}{CL} \qquad (5)$$

where V is the volume of distribution.

It is also possible to calculate V_{max} (maximum velocity) and K_m (Michaelis constant) for the enzyme system metabolizing Drug 1 if: (a) Drug 1 is metabolized by a single enzyme system, (b) $\overline{C}_{ss}$ and DP vary in a nonlinear manner, and (c) $\overline{C}_{ss}$ is determined at two different values for DP before adding Drug 2 and after adding Drug 2 (10,11). The following equations are used (10):

$$k = \frac{CL}{V} \qquad (6)$$

where k = elimination rate constant;

$$K_m = \frac{k_2 \times \overline{C}_{ss2} - k_1 \times \overline{C}_{ss1}}{k_1 - k_2} \qquad (7)$$

where subscripts 1 and 2 represent values at first and second dosing rate of Drug 1 before adding Drug 2.

$$V_{max} = k_1 \times (K_m + \overline{C}_{ss1}) = k_2 \times (K_m + \overline{C}_{ss2}) \qquad (8)$$

Note values for k_1, k_2, $\overline{C}_{ss1}$, and $\overline{C}_{ss2}$ must be determined again at two dosing rates of Drug 1 after adding Drug 2 to obtain values of K_m and V_{max} after adding Drug 2.

Assumptions. This method assumes: (a) all subjects have been completely compliant in taking their medications, or degree of noncompliance is known, (b) $\overline{C}_{ss}$ value employed represents *mean* value (not trough, maximum, or random), (c) $\overline{C}_{ss}$ employed represents steady-state value, (d) fraction of drug absorbed for each subject is exactly the same as a mean population value or is known for each subject, (e) fraction of Drug 1 absorbed does not change in the presence of Drug 2, (f) volume of distribution of each subject is exactly the same as population mean, or value is known for each subject (for calculation of elimination half-life), and (g) volume of distribution of Drug 1 does not change in the presence of Drug 2.

Of typical outpatients, 25–50% do not take medication as directed (12).

Table 1-4.   Effects of Assumptions on Calculated[a] Values for Clearance and Elimination Half-life of Phenytoin in Study of 15 Subjects

Assumptions	Assumed value utilized in calculation	Values that would result in significant differences[b] in calculated value for CL or $t_{1/2}$	Range of possible values
Compliance = 100%	100%	91% or 109%	0–100% (usually 50%–75%)[a]
Fraction absorbed = mean population value	86%	78% or 94%	58%–100%[b]
Random serum concentration value = mean serum concentration value	Random value	Mean value ± 9%	Mean value ± 25%[c]
Trough serum concentration value = mean serum concentration value	Trough value	Mean value −9%	Mean value −4% to mean value −44%
Volumes of distribution = mean population value (L/kg)	0.78	0.71–0.85	0.54–0.90 (2,3,7)

[a]Clearance = Dosing rate × compliance × fraction absorbed/mean steady-state plasma concentration; elimination half-life = 0.693 × volume of distribution/clearance.

[b]Clearance and elimination half-life were calculated in 15 subjects in which assumptions (see text) were validated (13). Then the deviation from assumed value of each variable necessary to produce a statistically significant change ($p < 0.05$) in clearance and elimination half-life was calculated with the paired student's t test.

[c]If dosing interval = 1 elimination half-life.

This amount of deviation from the assumed value for compliance ($FT = 1.0$) can significantly alter pharmacokinetic values calculated by this method (Table 1-4).

The value for $\overline{C}_{ss}$ frequently employed in this type of study is a single trough or random value; mean value can be determined only by multiple determinations performed over one or more complete trough-peak-trough cycles. The error introduced by assuming that a trough, peak, or random plasma concentration value equals the mean value can significantly alter pharmacokinetic values calculated by this method (13) (Table 1-4). Some studies have focused on only measuring clearance calculated using trough plasma concentration as an indicator of pharmacokinetic changes. This method is of limited value. Clearance calculated using trough plasma con-

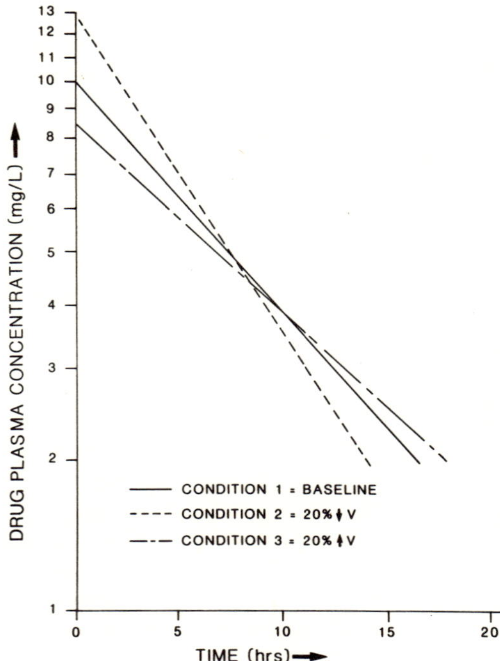

FIG. 1-3. Drug plasma concentration versus time relationships following an intravenous injection of 10 mg/kg of a drug with a clearance rate of 0.1 L/kg/h at three different values of volume of distribution (V) (condition 1, V = 1.0 L/kg; condition 2, V = 0.8 L/kg; condition 3, V = 1.2 L/kg). Elimination half-life was calculated using Eq. 5; time = 0 intercept was calculated as dose/V. Note that elimination half-life, maximum plasma concentration, and minimum plasma concentration (at any predetermined time after dose) are different for each value of V, whereas clearance remains unchanged.

centration values can differ significantly from clearance values calculated using mean plasma concentration values. In a study of 15 patients on phenytoin, clearance values calculated with trough plasma concentration values differed by 33% (p<0.01) from clearance values calculated with mean plasma concentration values (13). A change in only the volume of distribution of Drug 1 after Drug 2 is added will change fasting plasma concentration, whereas mean plasma concentration and clearance remain unchanged (14) (Eq. 5, Fig. 1-3). Fasting plasma concentration of Drug 1 may increase, decrease, or remain unchanged with either an increase or a decrease in volume of distribution (Fig. 1-3).

It is possible to know when steady-state serum concentration has been obtained. However, this can be problematic for drugs with nonlinear pharmacokinetics (15,16) or drugs in early phases of development whose time to attain steady-state plasma concentration has not been extensively studied.

The fraction of drug absorbed and drug volume of distribution may vary among individuals. This is especially true for the non-water soluble, lipid soluble drugs used to treat neurological disease (e.g., phenytoin, carbamazepine). Furthermore, addition of Drug 2 may change the fraction absorbed or volume of distribution of Drug 1 (5). The error introduced by assuming that all individuals have average values for fraction of drug absorbed or volume of distribution or by assuming that Drug 2 does not alter the volume of distribution of Drug 1 can significantly alter pharmacokinetic values calculated by this method (Table 1-4). It is possible to measure the fraction of drug absorbed and the volume of distribution for each subject using i.v. drug administration and the plasma concentration at multiple times after i.v. drug administration (see above). However, this would make the study extraordinarily complex and expensive.

Despite all of these negatives, sometimes it is possible to obtain relatively reliable results with this method *if assumptions a-c are verified* (13). This can be done with moderate difficulty. Verifying assumptions d-g is very laborious and has seldom been done.

Advantages. This method is simple, inexpensive, and minimally inconvenient to subjects if assumptions are *not* verified. It is possible sometimes to calculate changes in values for K_m and V_{max}.

Disadvantages. This method is dependent on seven assumptions, six of which are often untrue, are seldom verified, and have the potential to introduce significant errors in derived pharmacokinetic values. If all assumptions are verified, the method can yield accurate results but becomes extraordinarily complex, expensive, and inconvenient to subjects. In particular, verification of assumptions d-g requires i.v. studies and multiple specimen collections. If one is going to do i.v. studies, one might as well do an i.v. tracer study whose assumptions are easier to verify (see below).

Tracer Methods

Procedures. Labeled (stable or radioactive) tracer doses of Drug 1 are administered by the i.v. route before and after addition of Drug 2 (3,7). Labeled drug plasma concentration versus time relationships are used to calculate clearance, $t_{1/2}$, volume of distribution, elimination rate constant, and AUC (2). Mean plasma concentration of Drug 1 over each study interval can be determined from values of total (labeled and unlabeled) Drug 1 plasma concentration determined at multiple times and analyzed by the trapezoidal method (2). If tracer studies of Drug 1 are performed at two different plasma concentrations of Drug 1 before adding Drug 2 and again after adding Drug 2, differences in K_m and V_{max} can be determined using values of elimination rate constant and mean plasma concentration (10) (Eqs. 7 and 8). If desired, the rate of appearance of labeled drug and/or metabolites in plasma and/or urine can also be determined (2).

If tracer doses are administered orally, it is possible to measure directly absorption half-life, $t_{1/2}$, and AUC. Clearance cannot be measured directly and must be computed using Eq. 5 and an assumed value for volume of distribution.

Assumptions. The tracer dose method assumes: (a) the volume of distribution and the rate of metabolic biotransformation of isotope labeled drug is the same as unlabeled drug (i.e., absence of isotope effect), (b) the tracer label employed poses no risk to the subject or to the environment, and (c) absence of deep pool effect (see below). There is a large body of literature demonstrating that metabolic isotope effect can be avoided by placing an appropriate stable isotope at an appropriate location on a molecule (17). Similarity of V and rates of biotransformation of labeled and unlabeled drug can be demonstrated by simultaneous administration of both forms of drug and simultaneous measurement of V and rates of biotransformation and metabolite formation (18). There is overwhelming scientific evidence that the amount of stable isotope label (deuterium, ^{13}C, ^{15}N, etc.) administered in a tracer dose of drug poses no risks to humans or to the environment (19).

If a portion of chronically administered drug is distributed to a deep peripheral compartment, the drug's actual $t_{1/2}$ during the terminal exponential phase of elimination may be longer than determined by single-dose tracer studies if the single-dose studies are not carried out for a sufficient length of time to detect the deep compartment (usually due to insufficient assay sensitivity to detect low plasma concentrations of tracer drug at later times after administration) (20). This has been called deep pool effect and could lead to an overestimation of actual clearance in single-dose tracer studies because of factitiously small values for apparent $t_{1/2}$ and plasma concentration-time AUC (20). We have reported a method of checking for deep pool effect that requires only data routinely obtained in the course of performing tracer studies (20). Methods for independent investigation of deep pool effect have been reported (20), and at the end of this chapter we will propose another. Thus, the i.v. stable isotope method is dependent on three assumptions, all of which can be validated.

When tracer doses of drug are administered by the oral route, special problems arise. The $t_{1/2}$ can be measured directly, but clearance must be calculated using measured $t_{1/2}$ and an assumed value for volume of distribution (Eq. 5). If addition of Drug 2 changes only the volume of distribution of Drug 1, $t_{1/2}$ will change significantly. However, clearance, mean steady state-state plasma concentration, and dosing rate to maintain a given mean steady-state plasma concentration will not change (14) (Eq. 5 and Fig. 1-3). Even worse, if volume of distribution and clearance change in the same direction (decrease or increase), $t_{1/2}$ may not change significantly despite significant changes in clearance, mean steady-state plasma concentration, and dosing rate needed to maintain a given mean steady-state plasma concentration (Eqs. 4 and 5 and Fig. 1-4). The only certain value of knowing $t_{1/2}$ is that changes in $t_{1/2}$ may necessitate changes in dosing interval (but not dosing rate).

Radioactive tracers present some additional problems. Typically, the amount of radioactivity used in a drug tracer study is relatively small and, in many cases, can be shown by careful scientific logic to pose minimal

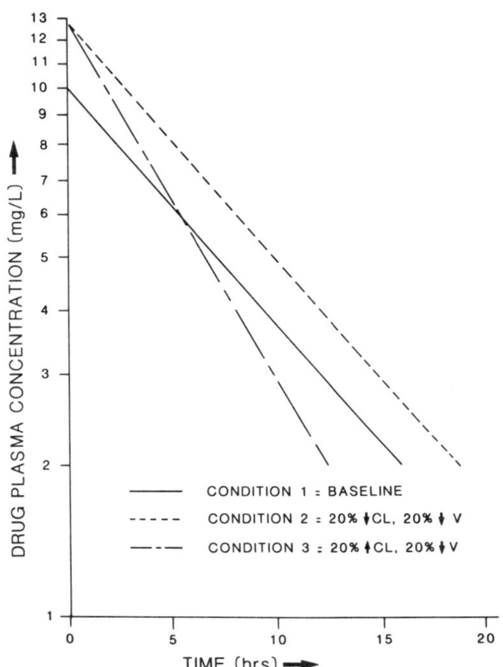

FIG. 1-4. Drug plasma concentration versus time relationships following an intravenous injection of 10 mg/kg of drug under three conditions. Under condition 1 (baseline), Drug 1 has a clearance (CL) of 0.1 L/kg/h, volume of distribution (V) of 1.0 L/kg, and an elimination half-life of 6.93 h (Eq. 5). Under condition 2, a similar *decrease in both* CL and V occurs. Note that Drug 1 elimination half-life remains unchanged under these conditions. Under condition 3, a *20% increase* in CL and a *20% decrease* in V occurs. Note that, depending on time interval selected, trough plasma concentration under condition 3 may be the same, higher, or lower than under condition 1.

risk to subjects or, if accidentally spilled, to the environment. Nevertheless, the word "radioactive" causes difficulty in obtaining approval to perform studies from some institutional review boards. Additionally, extensive regulatory requirements regarding handling, storing, and disposing of radioactive specimens make use of radioactive tracers difficult or impossible in some institutions. Finally, if counting of radioactivity is to be used as the analytical method, it must be established that the radioactivity being counted is due only to the compound being studied (usually Drug 1) and not to metabolites. This may require special preparation (e.g., chemical extraction, preparative HPLC) to isolate the compound(s) of interest.

Advantages. Intravenous stable isotope tracer methods offer the following advantages: (a) they are based on assumptions that generally are true and can be validated as part of the study, (b) the high precision and accuracy of GC–MS analytical methodology and the absence of random noise due to assumed values for compliance, fraction absorbed, volume of distribution, and mean steady-state plasma concentration reduce statistical variance and the number of subjects required to obtain statistical significance (presence or absence of a change in clearance can often be established with six subjects) (3,7) (Tables 2-1 and 2-3), (c) the methods allow direct and accurate measurement of drug clearance and volume of distribution, (d) measurement of rate of appearance of metabolites in plasma and urine is possible, (e) measurement of K_m and V_{max} is possible, and (f) safety to subjects concerning tracer compounds employed is unquestionable. Radioactive tracer methods enjoy advantages a–e.

Disadvantages. Stable and radioactive isotope tracer methods require expensive and sophisticated equipment and pose inconvenience to subjects. Tracer doses must be given intravenously to calculate clearance and volume of distribution and to eliminate the potential problems of analyses based only on $t_{1/2}$ data. Radioactive tracer methods may pose additional problems related to subject safety and handling of radioactive materials.

Stopping Drug Administration

Procedures. Administration of Drug 1 is stopped for a period of time. Serial plasma specimens are obtained after stopping Drug 1. The $t_{1/2}$ of Drug 1 is determined from plasma concentration versus time relationships. Clearance is calculated using measured $t_{1/2}$, an assumed value for volume of distribution, and Eq. 5. The procedure is repeated after Drug 2 has been added to Drug 1.

Assumptions. This method assumes: (a) it is safe to discontinue abruptly administration of Drug 1, (b) the addition of Drug 2 does not alter the V of Drug 1, (c) Drug 1 has linear pharmacokinetic properties, and (d) plasma concentration versus time relationships for Drug 1 are followed for sufficient time to detect the terminal exponential phase of elimination (i.e., absence of deep pool effect as defined above).

It is known that abruptly stopping administration of antiepileptic drugs in patients with epilepsy may precipitate seizures and/or status epilepticus (21–23). This applies even to drugs with very long $t_{1/2}$ such as phenobarbital or clonazepam (22,23). It is this reviewer's opinion that the risk to patients with epilepsy of suddenly stopping an antiepileptic drug present at therapeutic plasma concentration to study drug pharmacokinetics is seldom justifiable. It is, however, possible to measure the $t_{1/2}$ of the last dose of drug given to a patient being tapered off Drug 2 for a good medical reason, such as lack of efficacy or unacceptable toxicity (24). This situation typically arises when Drug 2 is added and then must be discontinued. The $t_{1/2}$ value for Drug 2 thus obtained can be helpful in selecting a dosing interval for Drug 2 when given in combination with Drug 1 (24) (Table 1-5).

As discussed above, measurement of $t_{1/2}$ only and not volume of distribution may yield misleading results. The $t_{1/2}$ of Drug 1 may change significantly with no changes in Drug 1 clearance, mean steady-state plasma concentration, or dosing rate needed to maintain a given mean steady-state plasma concentration if Drug 2 alters only the volume of distribution

Table 1-5. Elimination Half-life of Last Tapering Dose of Zonisamide After 91–165 Days of Administration to Seven Patients Taking Phenytoin and Carbamazepine

Elimination half-life values (h)
  14.3, 15.8, 25.9, 26.4, 27.1, 27.4, 35.4

Conclusions
  Zonisamide has an elimination half-life of at least 14 h after chronic administration in the presence of phenytoin and carbamazepine.
  Zonisamide needs to be given at a frequency no greater than twice daily in the presence of phenytoin and carbamazepine.

Reproduced with permission from Browne et al. (24).

of Drug 1 (14) (Eq. 5 and Fig. 1-3). Even worse, the $t_{1/2}$ of Drug 1 may not change significantly despite significant changes in clearance, volume of distribution, mean steady-state plasma concentration, and dosing rate necessary to maintain a given mean steady-state plasma concentration if volume of distribution and clearance of Drug 1 change in the same direction after addition of Drug 2 (Eqs. 4 and 5 and Fig. 1-4). Changes in $t_{1/2}$ are useful only in guiding changes in dosing interval.

The portion of the plasma concentration versus time curve used to calculate $t_{1/2}$ is that terminal portion that is semi-log linear. For drugs with linear pharmacokinetics, the portion of the curve after absorption and distribution that are complete will be semi-log linear unless deep compartments are present (20). For drugs with nonlinear pharmacokinetics, only the portion of the curve occurring after drug serum concentration has fallen below the K_m value for the drug will be semi-log linear. The $t_{1/2}$ measured at this low value for plasma concentration may be significantly less than the $t_{1/2}$ at higher (including therapeutics range) plasma concentrations (2,25). It is sometimes possible to estimate $t_{1/2}$ at therapeutic plasma concentration of a drug with nonlinear pharmacokinetics using all of the obtained plasma concentration versus time data and a Baysian correction (26). However, this method requires assuming the subject has values for V_{max} and K_m similar to population values. Interindividual variation in values for K_m and V_{max} may be considerable (10,11).

Advantages. This method is simple and inexpensive.

Disadvantages. The risks of this method seldom are justified by the benefits in persons with epilepsy. The $t_{1/2}$ data can yield misleading information when utilized to make inferences regarding clearance, mean steady-state plasma concentration, or dosing rate. Use of this method for drugs with nonlinear pharmacokinetics is problematic. Unless plasma concentration is followed down to zero, the $t_{1/2}$ value obtained may be too small due to deep pool effect (20).

Single Dose of Drug 2 Method

Procedure. A single dose of Drug 2 is given (usually by the oral route) in the presence of a therapeutic plasma concentration of Drug 1. The $t_{1/2}$ of Drug 2 is calculated from plasma concentration versus time relationships. The $t_{1/2}$ of Drug 2 in the presence of Drug 1 is compared with $t_{1/2}$ of Drug 2 when administered alone (usually a literature value).

Assumptions. This method assumes: (a) the volume of distribution of Drug 2 is the same alone or in the presence of Drug 1, (b) Drug 2 does not possess dose-dependent or time-dependent pharmacokinetics, and (c) plasma concentration versus time relationships for Drug 2 are followed for sufficient time to detect the terminal exponential phase of elimination (i.e., absence of deep pool effect as defined above).

If the volume of distribution of Drug 2 is changed by Drug 1, the $t_{1/2}$ data obtained in the presence of Drug 1 (whether similar or dissimilar to values obtained in the absence of Drug 1) may be misleading when utilized to make inferences regarding clearance, mean steady-state plasma concentration, or dosing rate necessary to obtain a given mean steady-state plasma concentration (14) (Eqs. 4 and 5 and Figs. 1-3 and 1-4). If Drug 2 possesses dose-dependent or time-dependent pharmacokinetics, values for $t_{1/2}$ and clearance of Drug 2 during chronic administration at therapeutic plasma concentration will be different from values obtained in single-dose studies, regardless of the presence or absence of Drug 1 (2,27).

Advantages. This method is relatively simple and inexpensive.

Disadvantages. This method is based on three assumptions that may not be true for a given drug and are not validated in the performance of the study. If any of the assumptions are not met, the $t_{1/2}$ data obtained will yield misleading information when utilized to predict Drug 2 clearance at steady-state plasma concentration or dosing rate necessary to achieve a given mean steady-state plasma concentration.

Conclusions

Intravenous stable isotope tracer methods allow for a complete and accurate assessment of the changes in pharmacokinetics of Drug 1 after addition of Drug 2. All assumptions utilized by the method can be validated. Sources of random variance are minimized, and statistically significant results (presence or absence of change) can often be demonstrated with a small number of subjects (e.g., six subjects). The safety of stable isotope tracers is established. The stable isotope tracer method is the method of choice for studying changes in volume of distribution, biotransformation, and excretion due to pharmacokinetic drug interactions provided that: (a) the tracer dose of drug can be administered by the i.v. route, and (b) resources for GC–MS studies are available.

Radioactive tracer studies are hampered by safety and regulatory considerations. These considerations make such studies difficult or impossible at many institutions.

Oral tracer dose studies, stopping drug administration, and administration of a single dose of Drug 2 all suffer the disadvantage of allowing only measurement of $t_{1/2}$. The $t_{1/2}$ data in the absence of data on volume of distribution can yield misleading results when used to make inferences regarding clearance, mean steady-state serum plasma concentration, or dosing rate necessary to obtain a given mean steady-state plasma concentration. In addition, the stopping drug administration method has severe ethical drawbacks, and the administration of a single dose of Drug 2 method must assume Drug 2 does not have dose-dependent or time-dependent pharmacokinetic properties.

The measurement of drug plasma concentration method is based on assumptions that often are untrue, are seldom verified, and can introduce significant errors. If all assumptions are verified, the method can yield accurate results. However, verification of all assumptions is extraordinarily difficult and expensive.

PROPOSALS FOR NEW METHODS

A comprehensive review of existing methods for study of pharmacokinetic drug interactions reveals two major needs: (a) a method with the accuracy and safety of stable isotope tracer methods that does not require expensive and scarce GC–MS equipment, and (b) a method for determining mean steady-state plasma, for use in computations, that does not require obtaining multiple drug plasma concentration determinations. We propose below two methods for performing serial pharmacokinetic studies with stable isotope (deuterium) labeled drug using HPLC with ultraviolet (UV) detection rather than GC–MS analytical methodology. We also propose a method for conversion of a single trough drug steady-state plasma concentration value into an accurate estimate of mean drug steady-state plasma concentration.

The first two methods to be proposed rely on the observation that a heavily deuterated analogue of drug can be separated from its unlabeled analogue using high-resolution HPLC columns. Both analogues can then be quantitated using a conventional UV detector. We have demonstrated baseline resolution of a mixture of D_{10} carbamazepine, carbamazepine, d_{10}-phenytoin, phenytoin, and an internal standard (10,11-dihydrocarbamazepine) under the following HPLC conditions: column, BAS phase II 5μm ODS 3.9 mm I.D. $\times 250$ mm (Bioanalytical Systems); mobile phase,

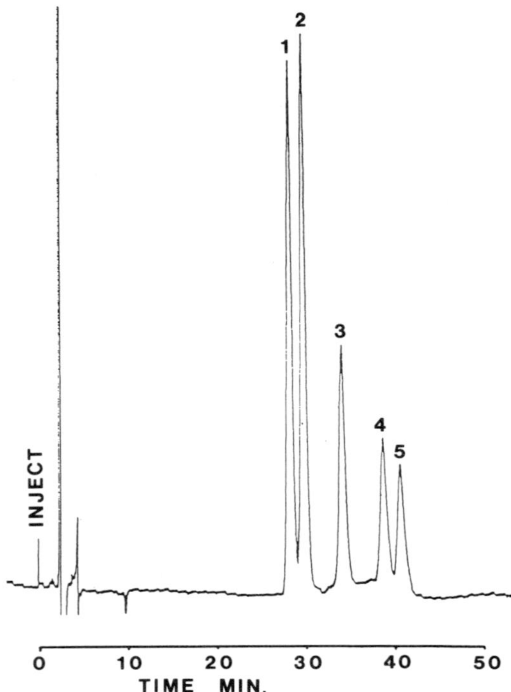

FIG. 1-5. High-pressure liquid chromatograph of 10-μ1 injections of: (1) d_{10}-carbamazepine, 10 μg/ml; (2) carbamazepine, 10 μg/ml; (3) 10,11-dihydrocarbamazepine, 10 μg/ml (internal standard); (4) d_{10}-phenytoin, 10 μg/ml; (5) phenytoin, 10 μg/ml.

acetonitrile and tetrahydrafuran with H_2O (16:4:80 v.v.); flow rate, 1.0 ml/min; temperature, 55°C; wavelength monitored, 214 μm (Fig. 1-5). With this method, serum standard curves were linear ($r^2 < 0.99$) over a range of 0.5–20 μg/ml for phenytoin and d_{10}-phenytoin and 0.5–12 μg/ml for carbamazepine and d_{10}-carbamazepine.

Methods for Performing Stable Isotope Studies Using HPLC/UV Rather than GC–MS Analytical Methods

Deuterium-labeled tracer dose method. A deuterium-labeled tracer dose of drug is administered and serial plasma specimens are collected in classic tracer-dose fashion. Labeled and unlabeled drug are separated by high-resolution HPLC and quantitated with a UV detector. Tracer-dose pharmacokinetic values are calculated in the usual fashion.

This method has the following advantages: (a) GC–MS is not required, (b) reliability and safety of stable isotope tracer studies with GC–MS are retained, (c) method requires only a small amount of isotope, and (d) i.v. administration is possible, allowing measurement of V. This method has the following disadvantages: (a) one must quantitate small tracer drug concentrations with HPLC, (b) stable isotope-labeled drug must be synthesized and shown not to possess isotope effect or deep pool effect (see above).

Labeled drug substitution method. Labeled drug is substituted for unlabeled drug for a period of time to maintain the patient's usual steady-state plasma concentration of drug. Serial plasma specimens are obtained. Labeled and unlabeled drug are separated by high-resolution HPLC and quantitated with a UV detector. The washout of unlabeled drug is followed over the course of the study. Note that this method allows following the elimination of unlabeled, chronically administered drug for a prolonged period of time and thus can be used also as a test for deep pool effect (defined above).

This method has the following advantages: (a) GC–MS is not required, (b) reliability and safety of stable isotope tracer studies with GC–MS are retained, and (c) drug concentrations to be quantitated by HPLC are higher than with the deuterium-labeled tracer method. This method has the following disadvantages: (a) it requires large amounts of isotope, (b) it is not possible to measure V because drug is not given intravenously, and (c) stable isotope-labeled drug must be synthesized and shown not to possess isotope effect or deep pool effect (see below).

Estimation of Mean Steady-State Plasma Concentration from Trough Steady-State Plasma Concentration

Trough plasma concentration is the one plasma concentration value that can be determined consistently with a single determination. However, many pharmacokinetic computations require a value for mean steady-state plasma concentration, which requires multiple plasma concentration determinations over one or more dosing intervals. Substitution of trough steady-state plasma concentration values for mean steady-state plasma concentration values on Eqs. 4 and 5 can result in significant differences in computed clearance and $t_{1/2}$ values (13). Elsewhere (13), we have recently shown that an accurate estimate of mean steady-state plasma concentration value $(\bar{C}_{ss})$ can be calculated from a trough steady-state plasma concentration value $(C_{\min})$ as follows:

$$\bar{C}_{ss} = \frac{C_{\min} \times (1 - e^{\beta T})}{B \times T \times (e^{-\beta T})} \tag{9}$$

where $T =$ dosing interval and $\beta = \ln 2/t_{1/2}$ (estimated using $C_{\min}$, dosing rate, assumed fraction absorbed and Eqs. 4 and 5). Thus, one can estimate $\bar{C}_{ss}$ with Eqs. 4, 5, and 9, using only $C_{\min}$, dosing interval, dosing rate, and assumed values for fraction absorbed and volume of distribution. In a study of 15 patients on phenytoin monotherapy, phenytoin $\bar{C}_{ss}$ estimated with Eq. 9 and $C_{\min}$ did not differ significantly from measured (with multiple determinations) values for $\bar{C}_{ss}$ (13). When put into Eqs. 4 and 5, the estimated $\bar{C}_{ss}$ values produced values for clearance and $t_{1/2}$ that did not differ significantly from values calculated with $\bar{C}_{ss}$ values. Use of estimated $\bar{C}_{ss}$ (with Eq. 9) to calculate clearance and $t_{1/2}$ (using Eqs. 4 and 5) of Drug 1 before and after addition of Drug 2 assumes Drug 2 does not alter the volume of distribution or fraction absorbed of Drug 1.

Acknowledgment: We gratefully acknowledge Errol Baker, Ph.D., for assistance with statistical analysis, and Carol Walsh, Ph.D., and J. Worth Estes, M.D., for critical review of this manuscript. This chapter was supported in part by the Veterans Administration and by USPHS Grants NIH-HD-05515-13, NIH-HD-4147-14, and MH-34223.

REFERENCES

1. Browne TR. Pharmacologic principles of antiepileptic drug administration. In: Browne TR, Feldman RG, eds. *Epilepsy: Diagnosis and Management*. Boston: Little, Brown, 1983:145–60.
2. Browne TR, Evans JE, Szabo GK, Evans BA, Greenblatt DJ, Schumacher GE. Studies with stable isotopes. I: Changes in phenytoin pharmacokinetics and biotransformation during monotherapy. *J Clin Pharmacol* 1985;25:43–50.
3. Browne TR, Szabo GK, Evans BA, Greenblatt DJ. Carbamazepine increases phenytoin serum concentration and reduces phenytoin clearance. *Neurology* 1988;38:1146–50.
4. Wolen RL. Absorption: applications of stable isotope studies of drug bioavailability and bioequivalence. *J Clin Pharmacol* 1986;26:419–24.
5. Cramer JA. Practical considerations and techniques used to monitor free drug levels. In: Porter RJ, et al., eds. *Advances in Epileptology: XVth Epilepsy International Symposium*. New York: Raven Press, 1985:143–8.
6. Mattson RH, Cramer JA, Williamson PD. Valproic acid in epilepsy: clinical and pharmacologic effects. *Ann Neurol* 1978;3:20–5.
7. Browne TR, Szabo GK, Evans JE, Evans BA, Greenblatt DJ. Phenobarbital does not alter phenytoin steady state serum concentrations or pharmacokinetics. *Neurology* 1988;38:639–42.
8. Wilder BJ, Ramsay RE, Willmore LJ, Feassner GH, Perchalski RJ, Schumate JB. Efficacy of intravenous phenytoin in treatment of status epilepticus: kinetics of central nervous system penetration. *Ann Neurol* 1977;1:511–7.
9. Evans JE, Browne TR, Kasdon DL, Szabo GK, Evans BA, Greenblatt DJ. Staggered stable isotope technique for study of drug distribution. *J Clin Pharmacol* 1985;25:309–12.
10. Browne TR, Greenblatt DJ, Evans JE, Evans BA, Szabo GK, Schumacher GE. Determination of a drug's in vivo K_m and V_{max} with tracer studies. *J Clin Pharmacol* 1987;27:321–4.
11. Leppik IE, Pepin SM, Jacobi J, Miller KW. Effect of carbamazepine on Michaelis-Meten parameters of phenytoin. In: Levy RH, Pitlick WH, Eichelbaum M, Meijer J, eds. *Metabolism of Antiepileptic Drugs*. New York: Raven Press, 1984:217–22.

12. Browne TR, Cramer JA. Antiepileptic drug serum concentration determinations ("blood levels"). In: Browne TR, Feldman RG, eds. *Epilepsy: Diagnosis and Management*. Boston: Little, Brown, 1983:161–74.

13. Browne TR, Greenblatt DJ, Szabo GK, Evans JE, Evans BA. Mean versus trough serum concentrations for calculation of clearance and half-life. Submitted to *Clin Pharmacol Ther*.

14. Oie S. Drug distribution and binding. *J Clin Pharmacol* 1986;26:583–6.

15. Theodore WH, Wu ZP, Tsay, et al. Phenytoin: the pseudo-steady-state phenomenon. *Clin Pharmacol Ther* 1984;35:822–5.

16. Wagner JG. Time to reach steady state and prediction of steady-state concentration for drugs obeying Michaelis-Menten elimination kinetics. *J Pharmacokinet Biopharm* 1978;6:209–25.

17. Van Langenhove A. Isotope effects: definitions and consequences for pharmacologic studies. *J Clin Pharmacol* 1986;26:383–9.

18. Browne TR, Van Langenhove A, Costello CE, et al. Kinetic equivalence of stable-isotope-labeled and unlabeled phenytoin. *Clin Pharmacol Ther* 29:511–5.

19. Klein PD, Klein ER. Stable isotopes: origins and safety. *J Clin Pharmacol* 1986;26:378–82.

20. Browne TR, Greenblatt DJ, Schumacher GE, Szabo GK, Evans JE, Evans BA. Clearance of stable isotope labeled tracer drug versus unlabeled chronically administered drug. Submitted to *J Clin Pharmacol*.

21. Browne TR. Benzodiazepines. In: Browne TR, Feldman RG, eds. *Epilepsy: Diagnosis and Management*. Boston: Little, Brown, 1983:235–45.

22. Spencer SS, Spencer DD, Williamson PD, Mattson RH. Ictal effects of anticonvulsant medication withdrawal in epileptic patients. *Epilepsia* 1981;21:297–308.

23. Theodore WH, Porter RJ, Ranbertas RF. Seizures during barbiturate withdrawal: relation to blood levels. *Ann Neurol* 1987;22:644–7.

24. Browne TR, Szabo GK, Kres J. Elimination half-life of zonisamide (CI-912) after chronic administration (abstract). *J Clin Pharmacol* 1986;26:555.

25. Browne TR, Greenblatt DJ, Evans JE, Szabo GK, Evans BA, Schumacher GE. Estimation of a drug's elimination half-life at any serum concentration when the drug's K_m and V_{max} are known: calculations and validation with phenytoin. *J Clin Pharmacol* 1987;27:318–20.

26. Schumacher GE. Using pharmacokinetics in drug therapy: comparing methods for dealing with non-linear drugs like phenytoin. *Am J Hosp Pharm* 1980;37:128–32.

27. Bertilsson L, Thomson T, Tybring G. Pharmacokinetics: time dependent changes: autoinduction of carbamazepine epoxidation. *J Clin Pharmacol* 1986;26:459–62.

2

Interactions Between Drugs Used in the Treatment of Epilepsy

Alan Richens and [1]Emilio Perucca

Department of Pharmacology and Therapeutics, University of Wales College of Medicine, Heath Park, Cardiff, U.K.; and [1]Division of Clinical Pharmacology, Department of Internal Medicine and Therapeutics, University of Pavia, Pavia, Italy

Although most patients with epilepsy can be satisfactorily controlled on a single drug, there are some in whom combination drug therapy is necessary for the control of seizures. When two or more drugs are prescribed together, there is a risk of interaction, i.e., effects may occur that are not seen when each of these compounds is given alone.

Classically, a distinction is made between pharmacokinetic and pharmacodynamic drug interactions. The former involve a modification of the absorption, distribution, and/or elimination of the affected drug, whereas the latter consist of synergistic or antagonistic effects at the site of action. The number of pharmacokinetic interactions leading to altered serum drug concentrations is large. Pharmacodynamic interactions are more difficult to document objectively, but they may be just as important.

Although in clinical practice anticonvulsant drug interactions are a common occurrence, it must be acknowledged that in most situations their importance is probably small. Unfortunately, only for a limited number of examples is it possible to distinguish beforehand between those interactions that are clinically significant and those that are not. In most other cases, the clinical consequences of the interaction (if any) vary greatly depending on the dosage of the interacting drugs and the characteristics of the host. Since it is impractical for the clinician to memorize endless lists of potentially interfering compounds, the best approach to the prevention of potentially harmful effects of drug interactions is to remember those that are most obviously important, to understand the underlying mechanisms, and to monitor the patient carefully whenever a drug combination is introduced. A knowledge of the mechanisms of interaction is useful because it may allow anticipation of the observed effects; for example, if a patient is taking an enzyme-inducing agent such as phenobarbital, the elimination of a concurrently administered drug known to be metabolized by the hepatic microsomal enzymes may be enhanced, and its effects could consequently be reduced (1).

Several comprehensive reviews of antiepileptic drug interactions have been published in recent years (2–7). This chapter discusses some relevant examples for each of the main mechanisms involved. Although references are given for the most recently reported interactions, the reader is referred to the aforementioned reviews for a more comprehensive list and for a source of older references.

PHARMACOKINETIC INTERACTIONS

Interaction by Induction of Hepatic Metabolism

Phenobarbital, primidone, phenytoin, and carbamazepine are potent inducers of the hepatic drug-metabolizing enzymes (8) and have been shown to increase significantly the metabolic clearance of each other as well as of other concurrently used antiepileptic drugs (Table 2-1) (Fig. 2-1). Usually, these interactions result in decreased serum levels and decreased clinical efficacy of "standard doses" of the affected drug. If the latter is converted to active metabolites, however, the situation may be more complex, and paradoxically, potentiation of therapeutic and/or toxic effects may occur. A possible example of the latter is provided by the observation that patients receiving concurrent therapy with enzyme-inducing anticonvulsants

Table 2-1. Some Antiepileptic Drugs Whose Metabolism May Be Stimulated by Enzyme Induction

Drug	Active metabolite	Reference
Benzodiazepines		
Clobazam	N-desmethylclobazam	9
Clonazepam		10
Diazepam	N-desmethyldiazepam	11
Carbamazepine	10,11-epoxide	12
Ethosuximide		13
Lamotrigine		14
Phenobarbital		15
Phenytoin		15
Primidone	Phenobarbital, PEMA	16
Valproate		17

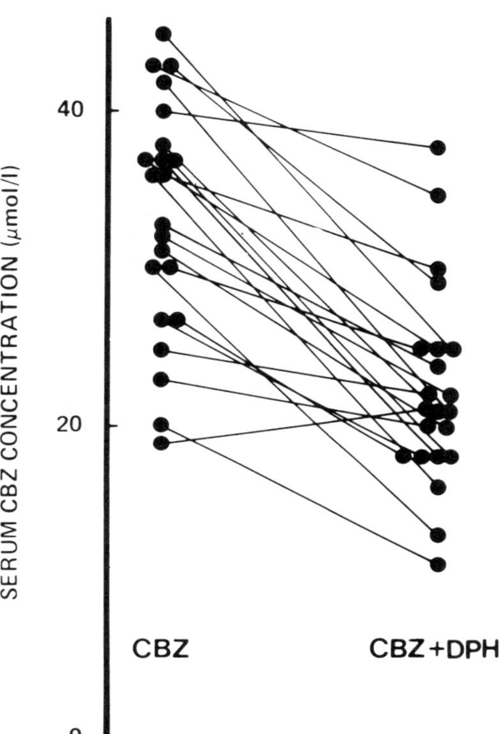

FIG. 2-1. Steady-state serum carbamazepine concentration in 22 pairs of patients receiving chronic treatment with carbamazepine (CBZ) alone and in combination with phenytoin (CBZ + DPH). Patients were matched for carbamazepine dosage. Note the depressing effect of phenytoin on serum carbamazepine. [Reproduced from Perucca and Richens (19) with permission.]

are more liable to develop hyperammonemia and liver toxicity from valproic acid, possibly due to enhanced production of toxic metabolites (18). Conversely, induction of the oxidation of primidone to its metabolites phenobarbital and phenylethylmalonamide (PEMA) may prevent the initial intolerance that is often seen on starting primidone therapy, an effect thought to be due to high concentrations of the parent drug. It is well known that the phenobarbital–primidone concentration ratio is increased (i.e., primidone levels decreased) by concurrent administration of inducing antiepileptic drugs (16).

When enzyme-inducing agents are prescribed in combination, their inducing effects may be additive, resulting in reciprocal stimulation of metabolism. The most important example of such an occurrence is the increase in carbamazepine clearance by phenytoin and barbiturates (Fig. 2-1). As a result of this interaction, the dosage of carbamazepine required to achieve a given serum level is higher in patients receiving other inducers in combination than in monotherapy patients (12,19). However, one advantage of this interaction is that water intoxication resulting from carbamazepine is less likely to occur because of the lower serum levels (19). Nevertheless, the 10,11-epoxide metabolite of carbamazepine has anti-

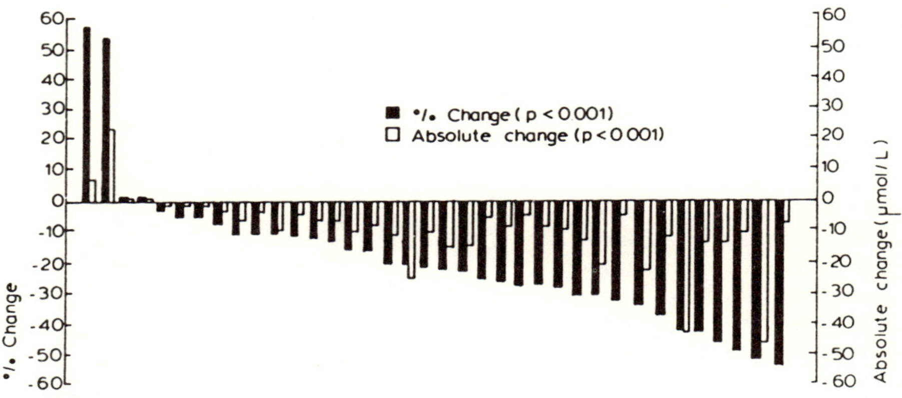

FIG. 2-2. Absolute and percent change in steady-state serum phenytoin concentration following administration of folic acid (30 mg/day for 3 months) to 41 patients on a stable phenytoin dose. [Reproduced from Perucca and Richens (5) with permission.]

epileptic activity, and a relative increase in its plasma concentration compared to the parent drug may compensate in part for loss of activity. The same is true for other drugs with active metabolites, such as diazepam and clobazam.

As far as the effect of carbamazepine on phenytoin metabolism is concerned, conflicting data have been reported (20,21), and this interaction is in any case less consistent and of much smaller clinical significance. The interaction between phenytoin and phenobarbital is complex; it has been suggested that phenobarbital can induce and inhibit phenytoin metabolism at the same time, and therefore the occurrence (and direction) of an interaction depends on whether either of these effects will prevail in an individual patient (15). As far as the reciprocal interaction is concerned, phenytoin tends to raise serum phenobarbital levels, probably because in this case inhibition prevails over the induction (22).

Folic acid administration to folate-deficient epileptic patients can also stimulate the metabolism of phenytoin and phenobarbital (Fig. 2-2). This is an unusual example of an enzyme-inducing drug inhibiting its own metabolism, or metabolism of related drugs, by causing a deficiency of folate in the blood. This vitamin is required as a co-factor for drug metabolism, and therefore its deficiency causes a slowing of drug elimination. Replacement therapy will stimulate it once again, causing a fall in steady-state drug levels (23).

Interactions Leading to Inhibition of Metabolism

The metabolism of virtually all major anticonvulsants is vulnerable to inhibition by concurrently administered agents (Table 2-2). Many of these

Table 2-2. Inhibition of the Metabolism of Phenytoin, Phenobarbitone, and Carbamazepine by Other Antiepileptic Drugs

Drug affected	Inhibiting drug	Reference
Phenytoin	Sulthiame	24
	Phenobarbitone	15
	Valproate	25
	Methsuximide	26
	Denzimol	27
	Nafimidone	28
Phenobarbitone	Valproate	29
	Phenytoin	30
	Sulthiame	31
	Methsuximide	26
	Pheneturide	32
Carbamazepine	Valpromide	33–36
	Valproate	37
	Diltiazem	39
	Verapamil	38
	Denzimol	27
	Nafimidone	28

interactions are clinically important, because the consequent increase in serum drug concentration can easily result in clinical signs of toxicity.

One of the prototypes of these interactions is that occurring between phenytoin and sulthiame, a drug that has now been withdrawn from the United Kingdom market. Sulthiame is a potent metabolic inhibitor, and its antiepileptic effects and toxic potential were likely to be mediated mainly by its capacity to elevate serum levels of phenytoin and other anticonvulsants (24). There was frequently a delay of 1–3 weeks between the onset of sulthiame therapy and the rise in serum phenytoin concentration (Fig. 2-3), suggesting that the mechanism of inhibition may have been noncompetitive. The list of non-antiepileptic drugs that have also been reported to inhibit phenytoin metabolism and to cause phenytoin intoxication is impressive (7), but the only antiepileptic drugs that have been shown to have this effect are phenobarbitone (transiently) (15), valproic acid (inconsistently) (25), methsuximide (26), denzimol (27), and nafimidone (28)— the latter two being compounds that have recently been tested as potential antiepileptic drugs (see below).

An increase in serum phenobarbital levels, probably due to inhibition of metabolism, may be caused by valproic acid (29), phenytoin (30), sulthiame (31), methsuximide (26), and pheneturide (32). Probably the most important among these interactions is that involving valproic acid. If valproate is given to patients stabilized on phenobarbital, serum phenobar-

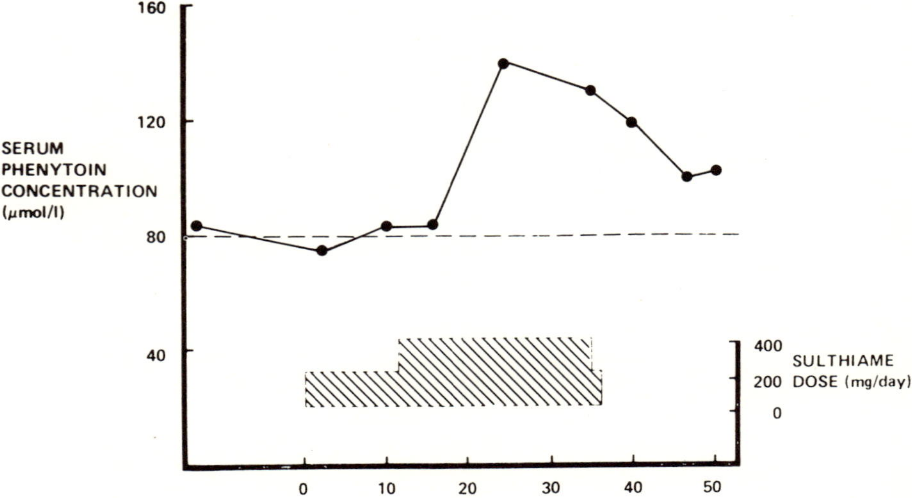

FIG. 2-3. Changes in serum phenytoin levels after adding sulthiame to the therapeutic regimen of a patient stabilized on a constant dosage of phenytoin. The horizontal broken line indicates the upper limit of the commonly accepted optimal range of serum phenytoin. [Reproduced from Perucca and Richens (5) with permission.]

bital levels will rise 25–50% (3). If barbiturate dosage is not reduced, sedation and other signs of toxicity may ensue.

In recent years, the list of interactions leading to impaired carbamazepine metabolism has been increasing steadily. Examples of drugs that have been shown to increase serum carbamazepine levels include many non-antiepileptic drugs, but also several established or potential antiepileptic drugs may have this effect. Meijer and co-workers (33) first described the occurrence of carbamazepine toxicity in patients in whom sodium valproate was replaced by valpromide, the amide derivative of valproic acid. Surprisingly, the interaction was not associated with any major changes in serum carbamazepine levels, but a striking elevation of serum carbamazepine-10,11-epoxide was observed. Subsequent studies have confirmed the clinical relevance of the elevating effect of valpromide on serum carbamazepine-10,11-epoxide levels (Fig. 2-4) and demonstrated that the interaction is due to inhibition of the catabolism of the metabolite through inhibition of epoxide hydrolase (34–36) (Fig. 2-5). Interestingly, sodium valproate also has an elevating effect on serum carbamazepine-10,11-epoxide levels (37), but this is much less marked than that caused by equivalent doses of valpromide. Since epoxide hydrolases play a crucial role in the detoxication of various reactive intermediates, the inhibitory effect of valpromide (and to a lesser extent, valproic acid) may have implications far beyond the interaction with carbamazepine (35).

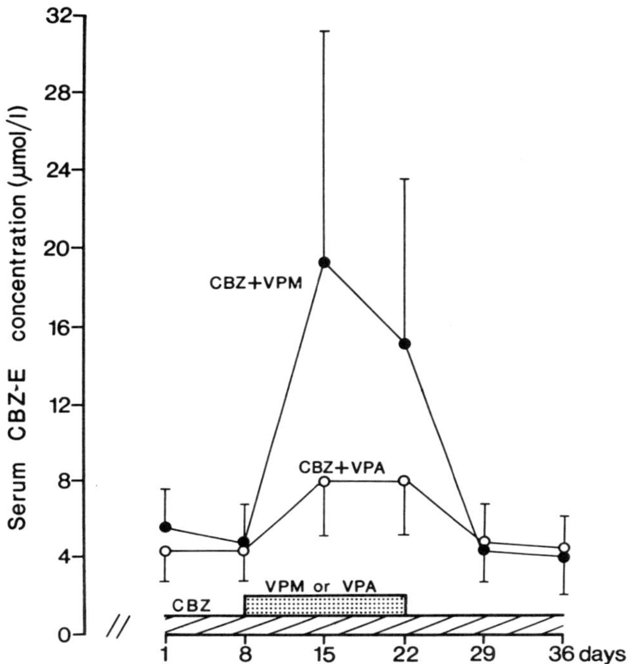

FIG. 2-4. Changes in serum carbamazepine-10,11-epoxide (CBZ-E) levels after addition of bioequivalent doses of valpromide (VPM) (1,200 mg/day) and sodium valproate (VPA) (1,100 mg/day) for 2 weeks to the therapeutic regimen of patients stabilized on a constant dosage of carbamazepine (CBZ). Values are means ± SD (n = 6 for each group). Serum carbamazepine levels were not affected by the interaction. The apparent moderate decrease in CBZ-E levels on day 22 in the valpromide group is due to exclusion of two patients with very high CBZ-E concentrations who required early discontinuation of valpromide because of intolerable side-effects. [Reproduced from Pisani et al. (34) with permission.]

Other drugs that have recently been reported to inhibit carbamazepine metabolism are the two imidazole compounds denzimol (27) and nafimidone (28) and the two calcium antagonists verapamil (38) and diltiazem (but not nifedipine) (39). In two of these studies the plasma concentration of the 10,11-epoxide was measured also; denzimol increased the concentration of the metabolite as well as the parent drug (27), presumably by concurrent inhibition of epoxide hydrolase, whereas verapamil reduced the epoxide–carbamazepine ratio (38). Denzimol and nafimidone are both substituted imidazol compounds, related to metronidazole, clotrimazole, and cimetidine. As this group of compounds has been shown to inhibit drug metabolism by an effect on microsomal P_{450} (28), it is not surprising that the two new agents have this effect. The degree of inhibition, how-

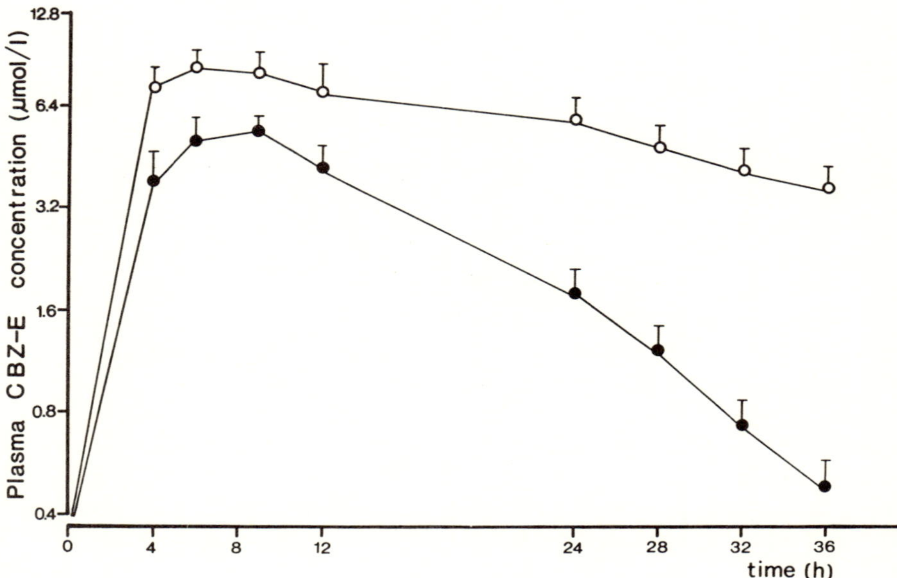

FIG. 2-5. Plasma levels of carbamazepine-10,11-epoxide (CBZ-E) (mean ± SD) in six subjects after administration of a single dose of CBZ-E (100 mg) in a control session (●) and during co-administration of valpromide (600 mg daily for one week) (○). Note the marked inhibitory effect of valpromide on CBZ-E elimination. [Reproduced from Pisani et al. (36) with permission.]

ever, appears to be greater than with any other antiepileptic drug interaction; the dose of carbamazepine had to be reduced to less than 50% on addition of nafimidone in the study of Treiman and Ben-Menachem (28). One problem created by such a major interaction is how to evaluate the antiepileptic potential of the new drug when the conventional approach is to start with add-on trials. It is almost impossible to separate the effect of the new drug itself from its effect by elevating plasma levels of existing drugs. Perhaps such compounds should not be developed further when the interaction reveals itself, because their clinical use would be hazardous in the hands of the average prescriber.

As discussed above, valproic acid inhibits the metabolism of carbamazepine, phenobarbital, and (inconsistently) phenytoin. The metabolism of two other antiepileptic drugs, ethosuximide (40) and lamotrigine (14,41), are inhibited by this drug. The elimination half-life of lamotrigine is 30 ± 10 h in patients on valproate compared with 24 ± 6 in healthy volunteers (and 14 ± 7 h in enzyme-induced patients) (14), and this has required a dosing schedule in clinical trials that takes into account the patient's background therapy.

Interactions Involving Altered Plasma Protein Binding

Valproic acid has been shown to displace phenytoin from plasma protein binding sites (25,42,43). Phenytoin is a low clearance compound, and the displaced drug molecules partly redistribute into large tissue stores and partly become metabolized. Therefore, the interaction results in decreased serum levels of the protein-bound drug, whereas the levels of free, pharmacologically active drug remain practically unmodified (7). The total (free plus bound) drug level will therefore fall. Under these conditions, the main implication of the interaction is a change in the relationship between the total level of the displaced drug and clinical effect; in the presence of associated valproic acid therapy, phenytoin toxicity may occur at concentrations of total phenytoin lower than usual.

A significant alteration in clinical response after administration of a displacing agent is usually due to an additional mechanism of interaction. Valproic acid, for instance, may cause phenytoin intoxication by additionally inhibiting its metabolism (44,45). The interactions may not be easily recognized by serum level monitoring because, due to the displacing effect, the rise in free phenytoin may not be associated with appreciable changes in total drug concentration (44).

Valproic acid also displaces carbamazepine (46) and diazepam (47) from their protein binding sites.

Other Mechanisms of Action

Alkalinization of the urine enhances the urinary excretion of phenobarbital by increasing the degree of ionization of this drug in the renal tubules. Acetazolamide, a carbonic anhydrase inhibitor with both diuretic and antiepileptic activity, has this effect.

The new antiepileptic drug vigabatrin (γ-vinyl GABA) has been shown to reduce steady-state plasma concentrations of phenytoin when added on to existing therapy in a clinical trial (48). A subsequent study confirmed this effect, but the fall in plasma phenytoin concentrations did not occur until the fourth week of vigabatrin therapy, and there was no evidence that the plasma protein binding of phenytoin was altered or its metabolism stimulated (49). The mechanism of this interaction still needs to be elucidated.

PHARMACODYNAMIC DRUG INTERACTIONS

Pharmacodynamic interactions affecting the response to antiepileptic drugs are probably common, but their objective documentation is usually difficult. These interactions may be either adverse or beneficial. Examples of adverse interactions may include the increased risk of valproic acid-induced coma and stupor in patients also receiving barbiturates and, more generally, the reciprocal potentiation of adverse effects by concomitantly administered antiepileptics. A clinically beneficial interaction, probably pharmacodynamic in nature, occurs between ethosuximide and valproic acid. These two drugs may exert synergistic (or at least additive) therapeutic effects, since patients with absence seizures refractory to either agent may respond favorably to their combination (50).

Acknowledgment: We thank Barbara Cantoni for her skillful help in the preparation of the artwork and Sue Forster for typing the manuscript.

REFERENCES

1. Perucca E. Clinical implications of hepatic microsomal enzyme induction by antiepileptic drugs. *Pharmacol Ther* 1987;33:139–44.
2. Baciewicz AM. Carbamazepine drug interactions. *Ther Drug Monit* 1986;8:305–17.
3. Levy RH, Koch KM. Drug interactions with valproic acid. *Drugs* 1982;24:543–56.
4. Perucca E. Pharmacokinetic interactions with antiepileptic drugs. *Clin Pharmacokinet* 1982;7:57–84.
5. Perucca E, Richens A. Drug interactions with phenytoin. *Drugs* 1981;21:230–7.
6. Perucca E, Richens A. Drug interactions involving drugs used in the treatment of epilepsy. In: Petrie JC, ed. *Clinically Important Adverse Drug Interactions: Nervous System, Endocrine System and Infusion Therapy*. Amsterdam: Elsevier, 1984:99–145.
7. Perucca E, Richens A. Antiepileptic drug interactions. In: Frey H-H, Janz D, eds. *Antiepileptic Drugs. Handbook of Experimental Pharmacology Vol. 74* Berlin: Springer-Verlag, 1985:831–55.
8. Perucca E, Hedges A, Makki KA, Ruprah M, Wilson JF, Richens A. A comparative study of the enzyme inducing properties of anticonvulsant drugs in epileptic patients. *Br J Clin Pharmacol* 1984;18:401–10.
9. Jawad S, Richens A, Oxley J. Single dose pharmacokinetic study of clobazam in normal volunteer 8 and epileptic patients. *Br J Clin Pharmacol* 1984;18:873–77.
10. Sjö O, Hvidberg EF, Naestoft J, Lund M. Pharmacokinetics and side effects of clonazepam and its 7-amino metabolite in man. *Eur J Clin Pharmacol* 1975;8:249–54.
11. Dhillon S, Richens A. Pharmacokinetics of diazepam in epileptic patients and normal volunteers following intravenous administration. *Br J Clin Pharmacol* 1981;12:591–2.
12. Eichelbaum M, Kothe KW, Hoffmann F, Von Unruh GE. Kinetics and metabolism of carbamazepine during combined antiepileptic therapy. *Clin Pharmacol Ther* 1979;26:367–71.
13. Warren JW, Benmaman JD, Braxton B, Wannamaker BB, Levy RH. Kinetics of a carbamazepine-ethosuximide interaction. *Clin Pharmacol Ther* 1980;28:646–51.

14. Jawad S, Yuen WC, Peck AW, Hamilton MJ, Oxley JR, Richens A. Lamotrigine: single dose pharmacokinetics and initial one week experience in refractory epilepsy. *Epilepsy Res* 1987;1:194–201.
15. Kutt H. Interactions between anticonvulsants and other commonly prescribed drugs. *Epilepsia* 1984;25(suppl 2):S118–S131.
16. Fincham RW, Schottelius DD, Sahs AL. The influence of diphenylhydantoin on primidone metabolism. *Arch Neurol* 1974;30:259–62.
17. Bowdle TA, Levy RH, Cutler RE. Effect of carbamazepine on valproic acid kinetics in normal subjects. *Clin Pharmacol Ther* 1979;26:629–34.
18. Zaccara G, Paganini M, Campostrini R, et al. Effect of associated antiepileptic treatment on valproate-induced hyperammonaemia. *Ther Drug Monit* 1985;7:185–90.
19. Perucca E, Richens A. Reversal by phenytoin of carbamazepine-induced water intoxication: a pharmacokinetic interaction. *J Neurol Neurosurg Psychiatry* 1980;43:540–5.
20. Hansen JM, Siersbaek-Nielsen K, Skovsted K. Carbamazepine-induced acceleration of diphenylhydantoin and warfarin metabolism in man. *Clin Pharmacol Ther* 1971;12:539–43.
21. Browne TR, Evans JE, Szabo GK. Effect of carbamazepine on phenytoin pharmacokinetics determined by a stable isotope technique. *Neurology* 1984;35(suppl 1):284.
22. Pisani F, Fazio A, Artesi C, et al. An epidemiological study of the clinical impact of pharmacokinetic anticonvulsant drug interactions based on serum drug level analysis. *Ital J Neurol Sci* 1987;8:135–42.
23. Makki KA, Perucca E, Richens A. Metabolic effects of folic acid replacement therapy in folate-deficient epileptic patients. In: Johanessen SI, Morselli PL, Pippenger CE, Richens A, Schmidt D, Meinardi H, eds. *Antiepileptic Therapy. Advances in Drug Monitoring* New York: Raven, 1980:391–6.
24. Houghton GW, Richens A. Inhibition of phenytoin metabolism by sulthiame in epileptic patients. *Br J Clin Pharmacol* 1974;1:59–66.
25. Perucca E, Hebdige S, Gatti G, Lecchini S, Frigo GM, Crema A. Interaction between phenytoin and valproic acid: plasma protein binding and metabolic effects. *Clin Pharmacol Ther* 1980;28:779–89.
26. Rambeck B. Pharmacological interactions of methsuximide with phenobarbital and phenytoin in hospitalized epileptic patients. *Epilepsia* 1979;20:147–56.
27. Patsalos PN, Shorvon SD, Elyas AA, Smith G. The interaction of denzimol (a new anticonvulsant) with carbamazepine and phenytoin. *J Neurol Neurosurg Psychiatry* 1985;48:374–7.
28. Treiman DM, Ben-Menachem E. Inhibition of carbamazepine and phenytoin metabolism by nafimidone, a new antiepileptic drug. *Epilepsia* 1987;28:699–705.
29. Gugler R, Von Unrhuh GE. Clinical pharmacokinetics of valproic acid. *Clin Pharmacokinet* 1980;5:67–83.
30. Lambie DG, Johnson R. The effects of phenytoin on phenobarbitone and primidone metabolism. *J Neurol Neurosurg Psychiatry* 1981;44:148–51.
31. Richens A. *Drug Treatment of Epilepsy*. London: Kimpton, 1976:108–9.
32. Huisman JW, van Heycop Ten Ham MW, van Zijl CHW. Influence of ethylphenacemide on serum levels of other antiepileptic drugs. *Epilepsia* 1970;11:207–15.

33. Meijer JWA, Binnie CD, Debets RMC, Van Parys JAP, De Beer-Pawlikowski NKB. Possible hazard of valpromide-carbamazepine combination in epilepsy. *Lancet* 1984;1:802.

34. Pisani F, Fazio A, Oteri G, et al. Sodium valproate and valpromide: differential interactions with carbamazepine in epileptic patients. *Epilepsia* 1986;27:548–52.

35. Pacifici GM, Tomson T, Bertilsson L, Rane A. Valpromide/carbamazepine and risk of teratogenicity. *Lancet* 1985;2:397–8.

36. Pisani F, Fazio A, Oteri G, Spina E, Perucca E, Bertilsson L. Effect of valpromide on the pharmacokinetics of carbamazepine-10,11-epoxide. *Br J Clin Pharmacol* 1988 (in press).

37. Macphee GJA, Mitchell J, Wiseman L, et al. Effect of sodium valproate on disposition and psychomotor profile of carbamazepine in healthy subjects. *Br J Clin Pharmacol* 1988;25:59–66.

38. Macphee GJA, McInnes GT, Thompson GG, Brodie MJ. Verapamil potentiates carbamazepine neurotoxicity: a clinically important inhibitory interaction. *Lancet* 1986;1:700–3.

39. Brodie MJ, Macphee GJA. Carbamazepine neurotoxicity precipitated by diltiazem. *Br Med J* 1986;292:1170–1.

40. Pisani F, Narbone MC, Trunfio C, et al. Valproic acid-ethosuximide interaction: a pharmacokinetic study. *Epilepsia* 1984;25:229–33.

41. Binnie CD, Van Embde Boas W, Land GS, Meijer JWA, Overweg J, Van Wieringen A. Preliminary single-dose studies of a potential new antiepileptic drug, lamotrigine (BW430C), in epileptic patients. *Br J Clin Pharmacol* 1985;20:285–286P.

42. Monks A, Richens A. Effect of a single dose of sodium valproate on serum phenytoin concentration and protein binding in epileptic patients. *Clin Pharmacol Ther* 1980;27:89–95.

43. Mattson RH, Cramer JA, Williamson PC, Novelly RA. Valproic acid in epilepsy: clinical and pharmacological effects. *Ann Neurol* 1978;3:20–5.

44. Perucca E. Free level monitoring of antiepileptic drugs: clinical usefulness and case studies. *Clin Pharmacokinet* 1984;9(suppl 1):71–8.

45. Santucci M, Procaccianti G, Baruzzi A. Time-dependent interaction between phenytoin and valproic acid: diurnal changes in free phenytoin concentration and fraction. *Neurology* 1985;35:510–5.

46. Mattson GF, Mattson RH, Cramer JA. Interaction between valproic acid and carbamazepine: an in vitro study of protein binding. *Ther Drug Monit* 1982;4:181–4.

47. Dhillon S, Richens A. Valproic acid and diazepam interaction in vivo. *Br J Clin Pharmacol* 1982;13:553–60.

48. Rimmer EM, Richens A. Double-blind study of gamma-vinyl-GABA in patients with refractory epilepsy. *Lancet* 1984;1:189–90.

49. Rimmer EM, Richens A. Interaction between vigabatrin and phenytoin. *Br J Clin Pharmacol* (in press).

50. Rowan AJ, Meijer JWA, De Beer-Pawlikowski N, Van der Geest P, Meinardi H. Valproate-ethosuximide combination therapy for refractory absence seizures. *Arch Neurol* 1983;40:797–802.

3

Interactions Between Antiepileptic and Other Drugs

Henn Kutt

Cornell University Medical College, New York, New York, U.S.A.

Interactions between antiepileptic and other drugs occur frequently. For recent reviews see Perucca (1) and Kutt (2). The majority of these interactions manifest themselves in some changes of the pharmacokinetic parameters of the antiepileptic drug or the other drug. Interactions involving pharmacodynamic parameters have been assumed to take place with some drug combinations.

Pharmacokinetic interactions often become evident by the appearance of signs of antiepileptic drug intoxication in patients receiving common doses of antiepileptic drugs in combination with common doses of other drugs. Less often, the indication of an interaction is lack of effectiveness. Monitoring the drug concentrations usually shows a change in the plasma maximal concentration (C_{max}) or steady-state ($\bar{C}_{ss}$) concentration of the first drug. Further detailed studies will reveal changes in plasma clearance (Cl) and elimination half-life ($t_{1/2}$) with or without changes of the volume of distribution (V_d). Another indicator is a change of the area under curve (AUC) of concentrations of single test-doses.

The same drug in combination with an antiepileptic drug may not have the same effect in all patients. First, the extent of the interaction-related change in the drug concentration may vary among individuals. Second, the direction of the change may be up in some patients and down in others. The reasons for the variability among individuals in the magnitude or direction of the interaction are multiple. Genetic factors are important. For instance, a patient who is a slow metabolizer of phenytoin or the interacting drug is more likely to have a severe interaction. The magnitude of inducibility of hepatic drug-metabolizing enzymes is to some extent also genetically controlled, as was demonstrated in Vesell's studies (3): The induction of antipyrine metabolism by phenobarbital was nearly identical in each of the identical twin pairs but varied considerably in fraternal twin pairs. Environmental factors such as previous drug exposure can influence the extent and direction of an interaction, as does the dual effect of some drugs that cause induction of drug-metabolizing enzyme production while inhibiting its action. Individual susceptibility can vary tremendously.

Clinical significance of interactions depends on whether there is a need to adjust the drug dosages. It also depends on whether the interaction with a given drug combination is likely to occur in the majority of patients. The end result in an individual patient is also of importance. An elevation of a low antiepileptic drug level may improve seizure control; a small elevation of a nearly toxic level may cause intoxication; a marked elevation in an unusually susceptible individual with a combination that causes little changes in the majority of patients is significant in that patient.

Early reports of interactions sometimes warned against using the "reported" drug combinations. It has become clear by now that, with monitoring of plasma drug levels and adjustment of dosages, nearly all drug combinations can be used. The critical period with most drug combinations that may interact is usually the first few weeks or months. Close clinical and laboratory monitoring in that period is prudent.

MECHANISMS INVOLVED IN PHARMACOKINETIC INTERACTIONS

Pharmaceutical Interactions

Intentional modification of phenytoin absorption characteristics is practiced by the manufacturers. To that effect the USP lists "Phenytoin Prompt" (rapid maximum blood-level peak) and "Phenytoin Extended" (delayed maximum blood-level peak). To maintain the tranquility in a stabilized patient, it is best to prescribe phenytoin from the same manufacturer. An unintentional event was the "Australian Incident" of intoxication in patients whose phenytoin level rose when the filler was changed from calcium sulfate to lactose (4).

A pharmaceutical interaction is to be considered precipitation of parenteral phenytoin in a large-volume glucose-containing fluid.

Alterations of Absorption

Interactions can alter the absorption rate or the total amount absorbed or both. Several mechanisms are involved including changes of gastric pH and emptying time, and the motility of the gastrointestinal tract in general. The agents of concern in this respect are antacids. The magnesium-containing antacids primarily increase the gastric pH, which enhances the solubility of weak acids but reduces the absorption rate from the stomach as it increases the ionization of weak acids (5). Aluminum-containing antacids furthermore prolong gastric emptying time, which under these circumstances slows the rate of absorption (6). The increased gastric motility and diarrhea may add another factor in reduction of bioavailability of phenytoin by antacids.

Alteration of Protein Binding

The highly bound antiepileptic drugs, such as phenytoin (90%), valproate (90%), and to some extent carbamazepine (75%), may become displaced to some extent by other strongly binding drugs, such as tolbutamide (7), salicylates (8), and phenylbutazone (1), among others. This effects an increase in the unbound fraction of the antiepileptic drug and leads to some increase of clearance as the free drug reaches the liver. The result is some lowering of the total plasma concentration, but loss of effectiveness may not occur, since at the new lower steady state, the actual free concentration may remain relatively unchanged. If the displacing drug, however, also happens to be an inhibitor of the antiepileptic drug-metabolizing system and/or this system was nearly saturated already, the displacing drug may lead to elevation of the total plasma level.

Alterations of Biotransformation

The interactions based on inhibition or induction of biotransformation make up the largest portion of reported interactions. Those based on inhibition leading to accumulation of active parent drug are of greatest potential danger. Induction, on the other hand, leads to loss of effectiveness; rarely does an increase of toxic metabolites take place.

Sometimes a dual effect occurs: induction of enzyme production accompanied by inhibition of its action, usually from competition with the substrate. The net effect varies according to individual patient disposition.

CLINICAL INTERACTIONS IN WHICH ANTIEPILEPTIC DRUG KINETICS ARE ALTERED BY OTHER DRUGS

Analgesics and Antipyretics

Salicylates

Phenytoin. Salicylates displace phenytoin from the plasma protein-binding sites in vitro and in vivo. An increase of the unbound fraction of phenytoin from the prestudy 10% to nearly 16% and an increase of phenytoin clearance by acetylsalicylic acid was observed in a clinical study (8).

The changes were to some degree proportional to the acetylsalicylic acid dose, which ranged from 900 mg per day to 3,600 mg per day. High repeated doses of acetylsalicylic acid in epileptic patients are expected to cause a small decline of total plasma phenytoin level but a slight increase in the relative percent of free phenytoin (9). A need for dosage adjustment may not occur.

Valproate. Acetylsalicylic acid in doses of 15–30 mg/kg caused some decrease of beta oxidation and a modest increase of 4-en production in patients stabilized on valproate. There was an increase of the free fraction but not of the total concentration of valproate (10). The clinical consequences would be variable but small.

Propoxyphene

Phenytoin. In five patients a small increase of plasma phenytoin level was observed after giving the patients 65 mg of propoxyphene three times daily for 6 days (11). In another patient, large amounts (10 or more times 65 mg) of propoxyphene given for several days (2) caused phenytoin accumulation to the toxic range. In rat liver microsomal preparations, propoxyphene inhibited phenytoin metabolism (12). With the conventional use of propoxyphene, significant elevations of plasma phenytoin levels are infrequent.

Phenobarbital. In four epileptic patients stabilized on phenobarbital monotherapy administration of 65 mg dextropropoxyphene three times a day for 6 days caused a modest (10–15%) elevation of plasma phenobarbital level in all patients by the sixth day (11). A need to adjust the phenobarbital dose has not been reported.

Carbamazepine. Propoxyphene (65 mg 3 times daily) was found to elevate carbamazepine blood levels to a variable extent and was found to reduce the clearance in epileptic patients, whereas carbamazepine–epoxide concentrations declined somewhat (13). Clinical carbamazepine intoxication occurred in some patients; the elevations in others were mostly modest (14). With the usual sporadic use of propoxyphene, clinically significant carbamazepine accumulation is likely to be individually variable.

Phenylbutazone

Phenytoin. Administration of phenylbutazone (100 mg 3 times daily) had a variable effect on total phenytoin level but caused an increase of unbound phenytoin concentration (1). In other studies marked prolongation of phenytoin half-life caused by phenylbutazone was observed, and phenytoin intoxication has occurred in some epileptic patients. The major factor in this interaction is displacement of phenytoin from plasma binding sites associated with some inhibition of phenytoin metabolism (1,2). A need to adjust phenytoin dosage may occur with this drug combination.

Ibuprofen

Phenytoin. There are no reports so far of clinical interactions between antiepileptic drugs and ibuprofen. In a study of volunteers taking 600 mg ibuprofen 4 times daily for 5 days, ibuprofen had no effect on the kinetics of a 900-mg test-dose of phenytoin (15).

Anticoagulants

Phenytoin. Both bishydroxycoumarin and phenprocoumon have been reported to cause elevation of plasma phenytoin levels in some patients (16). On the other hand, warfarin and phenindione have caused no change of plasma phenytoin levels. It has been the general experience that patients taking phenytoin and anticoagulants together tolerate common doses of phenytoin well.

Antimicrobial Agents

Chloramphenicol

Phenytoin. Modest elevations of plasma phenytoin levels in some patients and marked elevations in other patients have been caused by chloramphenicol (17,18). The need to reduce phenytoin dose is likely to vary and is influenced also by the duration of chloramphenicol administration.

Phenobarbital. Elevation of phenobarbital level has been observed in a patient after addition of chloramphenicol, concomitant with a 40% reduction of phenobarbital clearance (18).

Erythromycin

Carbamazepine. Several studies report accumulation of carbamazepine after addition of erythromycin in epileptic patients (14). Elevation of carbamazepine concentration with clinical signs of intoxication occurred in some patients. In a study of eight volunteers, reduction of carbamazepine clearance without change in V_d, elimination rate constant, and absorption rate constant was observed (19). The severity of this interaction would depend also on the duration of antibiotic therapy.

Triacetyloleandomycin

Carbamazepine. Triacetyloleandomycin caused clinical intoxication and elevations of carbamazepine level in several patients, sometimes within 24 h of the onset of co-medication (14).

Oxacillin

Phenytoin. A decline of phenytoin plasma level was observed in a patient after oxacillin was started. This was thought to be caused by reduction of phenytoin absorption (1,20).

Isoniazid

Phenytoin. Isoniazid is a noncompetitive inhibitor of phenytoin metabolism demonstrable in vitro with microsomal preparations (12,21). In vitro inhibition of phenytoin metabolism occurs with isoniazid concentrations (5 μg/ml) (12) that have been measured in the plasma of slow acetylators of isoniazid. In groups of patients taking phenytoin and isoniazid together, significant phenytoin accumulation and intoxication have been reported to occur in 10–15% of the subjects (22,23), who in some studies were identified as very slow acetylators (22).

Clinical management of this interaction is handled best by frequent monitoring of plasma phenytoin levels after the onset of combined therapy with conventional doses. If the plasma phenytoin level continues to rise, as is likely in a very slow acetylator, phenytoin dose is reduced to a new maintenance dose. Prophylactic reduction of phenytoin dose is not practical unless the patient is known to be a very slow acetylator.

Carbamazepine. Isoniazid given prophylactically was found to cause signs of carbamazepine intoxication in 10 of 13 patients in an institution. In another report, isoniazid caused elevation of carbamazepine level but not phenytoin level in one patient (14). Dosage adjustments may be necessary.

Primidone. Isoniazid was reported to cause accumulation of primidone in one patient, whereas the concentration of phenobarbital and PEMA declined (1). Plasma half-life of primidone was increased.

Ethosuximide. Elevation of ethosuximide level was observed in one patient after isoniazid was added (24).

Diazepam. Clearance of diazepam was reduced in nine volunteers receiving isoniazid. This effect was counteracted by the inducing influence of rifampin in patients receiving combined medication (25).

Rifampin

Phenytoin. Rifampin lowered phenytoin levels and increased its clearance by a factor of two. The rifampin co-medication minimized the inhibitory effect of isoniazid even in slow isoniazid acetylators (26).

Sulfonamides

Phenytoin. Several bacteriostatic sulfonamides such as sulfadiazine, sulfamethizole, sulfamethoxazole, and sulfaphenazole have been reported to reduce phenytoin clearance and prolong the half-life. In some patients clinically evident phenytoin intoxication has occurred during sulfonamide therapy. The mechanism appears to be inhibition of phenytoin metabolism, and sulfaphenazole is the strongest inhibitor (27). Adjustment of phenytoin dosage may become necessary during sulfonamide therapy.

Metronidazole

Phenytoin. Unexpectedly, metronidazole caused only minor variable changes of phenytoin clearance and half-life in five volunteers despite its being a structural analog of cimetidine (28).

Antifungal Agents

Miconazole

Phenytoin. Miconazole in combination with flucytosine was found to cause elevation of phenytoin levels in an epileptic patient (29).

Antineoplastic Agents

Phenytoin. Unexpectedly low phenytoin levels relative to the dose have been observed in several patients undergoing antineoplastic therapy with vinblastine, cisplatinum, and/or bleomycin (20,30,31). The reason for this manifestation may be multifactorial. Reduced absorption is likely to play a role, and concomitant administration of steroids and antacids may also contribute.

Antiulcer Agents

Antacids

Phenytoin. Aluminum and magnesium hydroxides and calcium carbonate have been found to reduce or maintain low phenytoin blood levels in some patients but not in others (2,32,33). The complex effects of antacids on drug bioavailability affect drug dissolution, ionization, and gastrointestinal tract motility in addition to chelation (6); thus variations in their effects in different patients are expected. The antacid dose and time of ingestion also have an effect on the outcome. Generally, with small doses of antacid (10 ml every 6 h), little or no effect was seen (34,35). Higher doses (15–45 ml), however, were found to reduce phenytoin bioavailability (32). The effect is usually more noticeable if the antacid is given at the same time as, or near the time of, phenytoin ingestion. Therefore, if unexpectedly low phenytoin concentrations occur in patients who take antacids close to the time of phenytoin ingestion, a staggering of the intake times by 1–2 h may result in an increase of phenytoin levels (33,36).

Valproate. Antacids, on the other hand, may alter positively the rate of valproate absorption and may even increase the AUC (37).

Cimetidine

Phenytoin. Elevations of phenytoin concentrations caused by cimetidine have occurred (38–40). A dose of 300 mg of cimetidine given four times a day increased phenytoin blood levels in a few days in five of nine study subjects, and the elevations were more marked in patients whose precimetidine phenytoin levels were higher (38). In another study, after addition of cimetidine, phenytoin level increased in six patients, causing intoxication in two; no change or only a slight decline was seen in the remaining four patients (39). The mechanism of this interaction is inhibition of phenytoin metabolism; cimetidine has been shown to be an inhibitor of hepatic mixed-function oxidase systems. Dosage adjustments with this drug combination may be necessary during the periods of cimetidine administration guided by monitoring of phenytoin blood levels.

Carbamazepine. Cimetidine was noted to elevate carbamazepine level and cause intoxication in one patient (41). A number of controlled studies since then with volunteers, ulcer patients, and epileptic patients using single or repeated doses of carbamazepine have been reported. Single doses in nonepileptics usually show modest prolongation of half-life and reduction of clearance of carbamazepine (14,42). On the other hand, in epileptic patients long stabilized on carbamazepine, little if any change was caused by cimetidine (40). Furthermore, the inhibitory effect seen with repeated doses in volunteers disappeared after a few days (42). It appears that the modest inhibition seen in noninduced subjects can be compensated for by the several pathways of carbamazepine metabolism in stabilized patients.

Valproate. Little if any change was caused by cimetidine in the kinetics of valproate test-doses in 12 subjects (43).

Ranitidine

Phenytoin. Several studies indicate that ranitidine has little or no effect on phenytoin metabolism and blood levels (44,45).

Carbamazepine. Ranitidine has been found not to alter the kinetics of carbamazepine (43,45).

Antihistaminics

Phenyramidol

Phenytoin. Phenyramidol was noted to cause some elevation of phenytoin levels in several patients: dosage adjustment was not necessary (46).

Chlorpheniramine

Phenytoin. Modest elevation of phenytoin plasma levels occurred in some patients after addition of chlorpheniramine (47).

Other Benzodiazepines

Diazepam

Phenytoin. Diazepam effect on plasma phenytoin level varies among patients. In some studies, elevations of phenytoin levels in some patients have been reported (48), whereas in other studies and other patients the opposite has occurred (49). In the majority of patients, the commonly used diazepam doses do not seem to cause significant changes of plasma phenytoin levels.

Chlordiazepoxide

Phenytoin. Chlordiazepoxide has caused phenytoin accumulation in some patients (2,48), but this occurs as a rare exception rather than as the rule.

Cardiac Drugs

Amiodarone

Phenytoin. Amiodarone, an antiarrhythmic drug, caused two- to three-fold increases of phenytoin plasma levels in three patients. Inhibition of phenytoin metabolism was suspected (50).

Diazoxide

Phenytoin. Diazoxide was found to reduce phenytoin binding; the free fraction increased, whereas the total decreased somewhat. The clinical consequences are likely to vary (51).

Verapamil

Carbamazepine. In six epileptic patients, administration of 120 mg of verapamil three times daily nearly doubled carbamazepine concentrations and slightly reduced the epoxide. Subjective complaints emerged by the fourth day of co-medication (52).

Food

Food intake has been found to have variable modest, usually enhancing, effects on phenytoin absorption (36). The mechanisms by which food could affect phenytoin absorption include saturation of the first-pass mechanisms, increased phenytoin dissolution in the stomach, and increase of the splanchnic flow (53). Lipid meals were found to increase phenytoin bioavailability somewhat (54). Protein-rich diet had the same effect on phenytoin acid but not on the sodium salt (55). It has been recommended to maintain a steady relationship in time between food intake and ingestion of phenytoin (36,53,55).

Psychotropic Drugs

Phenothiazines

Phenytoin. Chlorpromazine, prochlorperazine (2), and thioridazine (56) have caused phenytoin accumulation and intoxication in some patients. In other studies a lowering effect by phenothiazines was observed (57). In general, phenothiazine drugs do not cause significant alterations of plasma phenytoin levels in the majority of patients (58).

Phenobarbital. Thioridazine caused elevations of phenobarbital levels in three of five subjects (59). In another study, therapy with phenothiazines including chlorpromazine, thioridazine, or prochlorperazine had a lowering effect on phenobarbital levels in psychiatric patients (57).

Valproate. Chlorpromazine reduced valproate levels and increased its clearance in 11 subjects who received a 400-mg test-dose of valproate (60).

Methylphenidate

Phenytoin. Methylphenidate effect on plasma phenytoin level has varied among patients. A rise has been observed in a few patients (2,61), but no change occurred in others (62), probably the majority.

Primidone. In one child receiving primidone, methylphenidate was found to increase both the primidone and phenobarbital levels but has had no such effect in others (61).

Tricyclic Antidepressants

Phenytoin. Imipramine has caused elevations of phenytoin levels in one study (63); in other studies no significant alteration of phenytoin kinetics has been found. It appears that the tricyclic antidepressants rarely necessitate phenytoin dosage adjustments.

Valproate. Amitriptyline slightly increased the elimination half-life and volume of distribution of a 400-mg test-dose of valproate in depressed patients, possibly due to changes in binding (64).

Trazodone

Phenytoin. An elevation of phenytoin level from 17 to 46 μg/ml occurred in a patient within a few weeks after the onset of trazodone administration. Clinical intoxication was present, and phenytoin dose was reduced (65).

Lithium

Carbamazepine. In some patients stabilized on lithium, ataxia, drowsiness, and tremors have been observed soon after the addition of carbamazepine in average doses. The carbamazepine levels were not particularly high, and lithium levels did not change markedly. At this time it is unclear whether this is a pharmacokinetic or pharmacodynamic interaction or both (14,66).

Vitamins

Folic Acid

Phenytoin. Several studies indicate lowering of phenytoin level by folic acid. The mechanism of this interaction is complex but is apparently related to biotransformation. A recent study in folate-deficient subjects is of interest in this respect. Administration of 1 mg folate daily caused up to a 45% drop of phenytoin levels, which were greatest in subjects with lowest K_m for phenytoin (67). Dosage adjustments may be needed.

Nicotinamide

Carbamazepine. Nicotinamide given in high doses increased carbamazepine blood levels in two patients. Nicotinamide has a modest antiepileptic activity on its own, and this combination was found to be beneficial in some hard-to-control patients. The elevation of carbamazepine blood level was thought to be due to inhibition of its metabolism by nicotinamide (68).

Primidone. Primidone biotransformation was reduced by nicotinamide in animals and in patients. This resulted in higher primidone concentration and reduced production of phenobarbital, which were thought to be beneficial in regard to seizure control, since an increase in the primidone/phenobarbital ratio produced a better therapeutic index against maximal electroshock stimulation in animals (68).

Miscellaneous Agents

Disulfiram

Phenytoin. Accumulation of phenytoin and clinical phenytoin intoxication in the majority of patients taking disulfiram together with phenytoin have been reported (69). When disulfiram was discontinued, the plasma phenytoin levels declined slowly (65), probably due to slow elimination of disulfiram. In a study with normal volunteers, disulfiram reduced phenytoin clearance from approximately 50 ml/min to 34 ml/min (70). Dosage adjustments of phenytoin are necessary if these two drugs are administered together.

Ethanol

Phenytoin. Chronic alcoholism has been reported to reduce the plasma phenytoin level (71), attributable to induction. Ongoing moderate or heavy intake of ethanol, on the other hand, elevated phenytoin levels (2). It appears that a dual action is likely; chronic intake may have an inducing effect and acute intake an inhibiting effect. The need for dosage adjustments based on this interaction is variable.

Tolbutamide

Phenytoin. Tolbutamide displaced phenytoin from the binding sites and reduced plasma phenytoin levels in patients (7). A dose of 1,000 mg tolbutamide daily in patients stabilized on phenytoin caused a 10% decline of the total plasma phenytoin level in the majority of the 17 study patients. The unbound phenytoin concentration increased at first and then declined, but the percent free remained elevated. The clinical effects of this interaction in the majority of patients are likely to be minor.

Activated Charcoal

Phenytoin, phenobarbital, carbamazepine. Delayed and reduced absorption of test-doses of these drugs was demonstrated in volunteers (5,72). Activated charcoal is being used in the treatment of drug overdoses; early application followed by intensive effective purge is important for highest benefits from charcoal.

Danazol

Carbamazepine. Danazol increased carbamazepine concentrations by 50–100% in six subjects and reduced the epoxide, transdiol, and the ring-hydroxy metabolites of carbamazepine, indicating inhibition of several pathways (73).

CLINICAL INTERACTIONS IN WHICH THE KINETICS OF OTHER DRUGS ARE ALTERED BY ANTIEPILEPTIC DRUGS

Analgesics-Antipyretics

Antipyrine

Phenobarbital. Reduction of antipyrine half-life by phenobarbital is a classic indicator of enzyme induction (3). Phenytoin has the same effect.

Acetaminophen

Phenytoin. Acetaminophen elimination is facilitated to some extent by phenytoin, perhaps through acceleration of its biotransformation (1). Antipyrine undergoes a similar fate.

Phenobarbital. It is thought that phenobarbital induces acetaminophen metabolism and increases the production of a toxic product. The epileptic patient might stand at higher risk in case of acetaminophen overdose (74).

Meperidine

Phenytoin. Meperidine half-life decreased from 6.4 to 4.3 h, and the AUC of the primary metabolite of meperidine increased after phenytoin was started. The clinical implication of this phenomenon is that patients receiving phenytoin may need higher doses of meperidine (75).

Phenobarbital. Acceleration of meperidine demethylation by phenobarbital resulting in decrease of meperidine concentrations and increase of normeperidine concentration, possibly increasing toxicity, has been suggested (76).

Methadone

Phenytoin. The AUC of methadone blood level diminished by 50% in five methadone maintenance patients after phenytoin had been given for 3 weeks. Several patients started to suffer from withdrawal signs and symptoms on the previously adequate methadone maintenance dose. Induction of methadone metabolism by phenytoin is likely to have occurred (77).

Phenobarbital. Addition of phenobarbital reduced trough and peak methadone levels in a subject and allowed withdrawal signs and symptoms to occur with the previously adequate methadone maintenance dose (78).

Antiasthma Agents

Theophylline

Phenytoin. In ten volunteers, doses of 300–400 mg of phenytoin per day, producing blood levels of 10–20 μg/ml, reduced intravenously given theophylline half-life by 40% and increased its clearance. In other patients, 20–50% increases of theophylline clearance have been observed. It is suggested that patients receiving phenytoin may need higher and/or more frequent doses of theophylline (79,80).

Phenobarbital. A 17–33% increase of plasma clearance with decrease of elimination half-life of theophylline was seen in subjects who had received 90 mg of phenobarbital for 2–4 weeks (79).

Carbamazepine. Addition of carbamazepine caused up to a 47% decline of theophylline half-life in two epileptic patients (79).

Antimicrobial Agents

Chloramphenicol

Phenytoin. Reduction of chloramphenicol levels by phenytoin was observed in epileptic patients. Higher doses of chloramphenicol may be needed during co-medication (81).

Phenobarbital. Phenobarbital has been found to induce the metabolism of chloramphenicol (82).

Doxycycline

Phenytoin, phenobarbital and carbamazepine. An increase in the elimination rate of doxycycline was observed in patients receiving the above agents (83).

Griseofulvin

Phenobarbital. Decreased levels of griseofulvin have been noted in patients taking phenobarbital. It is thought that this manifestation is caused by interference with griseofulvin absorption and/or acceleration of its metabolism or both (84).

Anticoagulants

Bishyrdoxycoumarin

Phenytoin, phenobarbital, carbamazepine. Reduction of the anticoagulant effect of bishydroxycoumarin after the onset of administration of inducing antiepileptic drugs has been reported (85). Appropriate dosage adjustments of anticoagulant guided by prothrombine time determinations are then made. If the antiepileptic drugs are discontinued, the anticoagulant dose is readjusted and this potentially dangerous interaction seldom leads to grave consequences.

Warfarin

Carbamazepine. The metabolism of warfarin was found to be increased and the anticoagulation effect decreased by carbamazepine, necessitating dosage regulation guided by prothrombin times (86).

Phenytoin. The effect of phenytoin on warfarin has been variable. It is of interest, though, that Nappi in 1979 (87) reported two patients in whom phenytoin increased the prothrombin time, suggesting inhibition of warfarin metabolism in these patients.

Antiulcer Agents

Cimetidine

Phenobarbital. Phenobarbital was found to reduce cimetidine levels and increase its clearance. Elimination of urinary cimetidine products, however, was reduced, which was interpreted as an indication of acceleration of metabolism as well as reduction of absorption (88).

Diuretics

Furosemide

Phenytoin. Furosemide efficacy is reduced by phenytoin to some degree. There is evidence that phenytoin reduces furosemide absorption, but an interference with furosemide action in the kidney may take place as well (89,90).

Cardiac Drugs

Quinidine

Phenytoin. Phenytoin was found to reduce quinidine half-life up to 50% and necessitate use of high doses of quinidine in order to maintain effective quinidine plasma levels (1). After discontinuation of phenytoin, the quinidine dose needs to be readjusted. Induction of quinidine metabolism is the likely mechanism in this interaction.

Digitoxin

Phenytoin. Digitoxin levels in some patients receiving phenytoin were found to be reduced to a modest extent (91).

Disopyramide

Phenytoin. Phenytoin was found to accelerate the rate of dealkylation of disopyramide. Since the metabolite is also pharmacologically active, a loss of effectiveness may not occur (92).

Immunosuppressants

Cyclosporine

Phenytoin. Reduced maximal concentration, AUC, and the half-life of cyclosporine were caused by phenytoin along with increased clearance; the clinical efficacy was reduced (93).

Phenobarbital. Addition of phenobarbital markedly reduced the levels and the desired clinical effects of cyclosporine in a 4-year-old child (94). Conversely, experimental cyclosporine nephrotoxicity was reduced in animals treated with phenobarbital (95). The mechanism in these interactions was thought to be induction of cyclosporine metabolism.

Psychotropic Agents

Chlorpromazine

Phenobarbital. The effect of phenobarbital on chlorpromazine levels was studied in six schizophrenic patients receiving 300 mg of chlorpromazine daily for 2 weeks. The mean blood levels of chlorpromazine ranged from 25 to 35 ng/ml. Then phenobarbital (150 mg daily) was given for 3 weeks. Soon after the onset of phenobarbital administration, chlorpromazine levels declined to near 20 ng/ml. The clinical effectiveness of chlorpromazine evaluated by psychiatric rating scores was considered not to be adversely influenced by phenobarbital in these patients (96).

Thioridazine

Phenobarbital. Addition of phenobarbital to the medication schedule altered the thioridazine levels little, if at all, but reduced considerably the levels of the metabolite, i.e., mesoridazine (97).

Haloperidol

Phenobarbital. Haloperidol levels decreased considerably after the addition of phenobarbital (97).

Carbamazepine. Since the increased use of carbamazepine in psychiatric practice, decreases of haloperidol concentration have been noticed (98–100). Up to 50% reduction occurred in all 11 patients after administration of 1,000–1,200 mg carbamazepine daily, while psychiatric rating scale changed little, if any (99). In another study clinical worsening was seen in two of five patients whose haloperidol level declined to near zero (100). Thus clinical consequences of this interaction have varied.

Tricyclic Antidepressants

Phenobarbital. Phenobarbital has reduced desipramine levels in occasional patients. In a study of epileptic patients whose medication included phenobarbital or primidone, the steady-state nortriptyline levels were lower than in nonepileptic subjects (101). It appears that induction by phenobarbital can lower the plasma levels of tricyclic antidepressant drugs, and a need to adjust dosages may occur.

Steroids

Oral Contraceptives

Phenobarbital, phenytoin, possibly carbamazepine. Contraceptive failures among epileptic women taking oral steroid contraceptives have occasionally occurred (1). In one study, breakthrough bleeding occurred in over 50% of 52 subjects taking phenobarbital and was positively correlated with the phenobarbital dose; in the control population, the incidence of breakthrough bleeding was only 4% (102). Laboratory studies usually show reduced free hormone concentrations and an increase of sex hormone binding protein (SHBP). It is generally recommended that patients taking inducing antiepileptic drugs use medium- or high-dose steroid preparations (103,104).

Dexamethasone

Phenytoin. The metabolism of dexamethasone is induced considerably by phenytoin. The elimination half-life of 3.5 h was reduced to 1.8 h after addition of phenytoin (105). In six patients dexamethasone levels dropped by 50% with phenytoin co-medication (106). Failure of low-dose dexamethasone test in patients receiving phenytoin has been reported. Dosage adjustments may be needed. Similarly, failure of the metyrapone test has occurred by the same mechanism (107). Reduced effectiveness of prednisone and prednisolone has been noted in patients receiving inducing drugs (1).

Vitamins

Vitamin D

Antiepileptic drugs. Bone disease induced by antiepileptic drugs has occurred in some epileptic patients. Usually low plasma levels of 25-hydroxycholecalciferol, the active metabolite of vitamin D, are seen in these patients. The mechanism producing this manifestation appears to be complex and incompletely understood. Induction of microsomal enzymes seems to be involved since studies of the rate of clearance of radioactive cholecalciferol indicated that the clearance was faster in induced (epileptic) patients than in normal subjects. Since the rate of synthesis of 25-hydroxycalciferol was the same in both groups, it was concluded that some of the calciferol was metabolized by a different route in the induced patients, perhaps producing inactive metabolites (108). The same conclusions have been reached on the basis of animal experiments. Environmental factors such as the amount of sunlight and the content of vitamin D in the diet seem to be the factors determining which patients develop clinical osteomalacia. Treatment of symptomatic patients is usually 4,000 units of vitamin D daily; the active hydroxy metabolites also have been used. In a recent study vitamin D2 was found primarily to increase the bone mass, whereas vitamin D3 increased calcium excretion in patients treated with 4,000 units daily (109). Prophylactic treatment with vitamin D of patients taking antiepileptic drugs is generally not recommended.

Folic Acid

Phenytoin. Plasma folate levels have been found to be reduced in patients taking phenytoin, sometimes leading to macrocytic anemia. The mechanism of this manifestation is complex: altered absorption, utilization, and biotransformation all seem to play a role. Manifest drug-induced folate deficiency is treated with 1–5 mg folic acid daily (1).

Miscellaneous

Misonidazole

Phenytoin. Phenytoin reduces the half-life of misonidazole and accelerates its demethylation. This may reduce the toxicity of misonidazole while not reducing its effectiveness as an enhancer in radiotherapy (110).

Psoralen

Phenytoin. Psoralen blood levels were reduced in patients taking phenytoin. This was accompanied by a reduction of effectiveness of psoralen as an intensifier of ultraviolet therapy in the treatment of psoriasis (111).

Fatty Acids

Valproate. Competing for binding sites, valproate may cause rapid increases of free fatty acid concentrations. This is particularly noticeable with high valproate concentrations (near 100 mg/L). Conversely, fatty acids may modify the free fraction of valproate (112).

CONCLUSIONS

Numerous pharmacokinetic interactions occur between antiepileptic drugs and other drugs. Due to induction or inhibition of biotransformation and/or competition in plasma protein binding, some changes of half-life, clearance, and/or volume of distribution can be demonstrated. These changes may often be inconsequential in clinical management. However, if these changes cause considerable accumulation or depletion, intoxication or loss of effectiveness becomes evident. The same drug combination may have different outcomes depending on the genetic and environmental constellations in individual patients. This makes assigning significance to drug combinations somewhat tenuous.

Among agents that have the potential for relatively frequent clinically significant interactions are antibiotics and antiulcer agents. Elevation of phenytoin level by chloramphenicol occurs with some regularity. Isoniazid has caused accumulation of phenytoin, primidone, and carbamazepine; erythromycin causes carbamazepine accumulation. In antiulcer therapy, antacids may reduce bioavailability of phenytoin and can be avoided by staggering the administration times. Cimetidine has caused phenytoin accumulation.

Other interactions of importance are phenytoin accumulation caused by disulfiram (nowadays often taken by AIDS patients) and sulthiame. Carbamazepine accumulation caused by verapamil may necessitate dosage adjustment. Finally, inducing antiepileptic drugs often make it necessary to adjust anticoagulant dosages, which is carried out under guidance of prothrombin times.

Prophylactic change of dosages when adding a potentially interacting drug is generally not practical. Monitoring the drug concentrations and adjusting the dosages as the need arises is prudent.

REFERENCES

1. Perucca E. Pharmacokinetic interactions with antiepileptic drugs. *Clin Pharmacokinet* 1982;7:57–84.
2. Kutt H. Interactions between anticonvulsants and other commonly prescribed drugs. *Epilepsia* 1984;25 (suppl 2):S118–S131.
3. Vesell ES, Page JG. Genetic control of the phenobarbital-induced shortening of plasma antipyrine half-lives in man. *J Clin Invest* 1969;48:2202–9.
4. Bochner F, Hooper WD, Tyrer JH, Eadie MJ. Factors involved in an outbreak of phenytoin intoxication. *J Neurol Sci* 1972;16:481–7.
5. Welling PG. Interactions affecting drug absorption. *Clin Pharmacokinet* 1984;9:404–34.
6. Marano AR, Caride VJ, Prokop EK, Tronacale FJ, McCallum RW. Effect of sucralfate and an aluminum hydroxide gel on gastric emptying of solids and liquids. *Clin Pharmacol Ther* 1985;37:629–32.
7. Wesseling H, Molsthurkow I. Interaction of diphenylhydantoin (DPH) and tolbutamide in man. *Eur J Clin Pharmacol* 1975;8:75–8.
8. Fraser DG, Ludden TM, Evens RP, Sutherland EW. Displacement of phenytoin from plasma binding sites by salicylate. *Clin Pharmacol Ther* 1980;27:165–9.
9. Paxton JW. Effects of aspirin on serum phenytoin kinetics in healthy subjects. *Clin Pharmacol Ther* 1980;27:170–8.
10. Abbott FS, Kassam J, Orr JM, Farrell K. The effect of aspirin on valproic acid metabolism. *Clin Pharmacol Ther* 1986;40:94–100.
11. Dam M, Christensen JM, Brandt J, Hansen BS, Hvidberg EF, Angelo H, Lous P. Antiepileptic drugs: interaction with dextropropoxyphene. In: Johannessen SI, Morselli PL, Pippenger CE, Richens A, Schmidt D, Meinardi H, eds. *Antiepileptic Therapy: Advances in Drug Monitoring.* New York: Raven Press, 1980:299–304.
12. Kutt H, Verebely K. Metabolism of diphenylhydantoin by rat liver microsomes. I. Characteristics of the reaction. *Biochem Pharmacol* 1970;19:675–86.
13. Dam M, Kristensen B, Hansen SB, Christensen JM. Interactions between carbamazepine and dextropropoxyphene in man. *Acta Neurol Scand* 1977;56:603–7.
14. Baciewicz AM. Carbamazepine drug interactions. *Ther Drug Monit* 1986;8:305–17.
15. Townsend RJ, Fraser DG, Scavone JM, Ox SR. The effects of ibuprofen on phenytoin pharmacokinetics. *Drug Intell Clin Pharm* 1985;19:477–8.
16. Hansen JM, Kristensen M, Skovsted DL, Christensen LK. Dicoumarol-induced diphenylhydantoin intoxication. *Lancet* 1966;2:265–6.
17. Christensen LK, Skovsted L. Inhibition of drug metabolism by chloramphenicol. *Lancet* 1969;2:1397–9.
18. Koup JR. Interaction of chloramphenicol with phenytoin and phenobarbital. A case report. *Clin Pharmacol Ther* 1978;24:571–5.
19. Wong YY, Ludden TM, Bell Rd. Effect of erythromycin on carbamazepine kinetics. *Clin Pharmacol Ther* 1983;33:460–4.
20. Fincham RW, Schottelius DD. Decreased phenytoin levels in antineoplastic therapy. *Ther Drug Monit* 1979;1:277–83.

21. Witmer DR, Ritschel WA. Phenytoin-isoniazid interaction: a kinetic approach to management. *Drug Intell Clin Pharm* 1984;18:483–6.

22. Brennan RW, Deheija H, Kutt H, Verebely K, McDowell F. Diphenylhydantoin intoxication attendant to slow inactivation of isoniazid. *Neurology* 1970;20:687–93.

23. de Wolff F, Vermeij P, Ferrari MD, Buruma OJS, Breimer DD. Impairment of phenytoin parahydroxylation as a cause of severe intoxication. *Ther Drug Monit* 1983: 5:213–5.

24. van Wieringen A, Vrijlandt CM. Ethosuximide intoxication caused by interaction with isoniazid. *Neurology* 1983;33:1227–8.

25. Ochs HR, Greenblatt DJ, Roberts GM, Dengler HJ. Diazepam interaction with antituberculosis drugs. *Clin Pharmacol Ther* 1981;29:671–8.

26. Kay L, Kampmann JP, Svendsen TL, Vergman B, Molholm-Hansen JE, Skovsted L, Kristensen M. Influence of rifampin and isoniazid on the kinetics of phenytoin. *Br J Clin Pharmacol* 1985;20:323–6.

27. Molholm Hansen J, Kampmann JP, Siersbaek-Nielsen K, Lumholtz IB, Arroe M, Abilgaard U, Skovsted L. The effect of different sulfonamides on phenytoin metabolism in man. *Acta Med Scand* 1979;624(suppl):106–10.

28. Jensen JC, Gugler R. Interaction between metronidazole and drugs eliminated by oxidative metabolism. *Clin Pharmacol Ther* 1985;37:407–10.

29. Rolan PE, Somogyi AA, Drew MR, Cobain WG, South D, Bochner F. Phenytoin intoxication during treatment with parenteral miconazole. *Br Med J* 1983;287:1760.

30. Bollini P, Riva R, Albani F, Nicola I, Cacciari L, Bollini C, Baruzzi A. Decreased phenytoin level during antineoplastic therapy: a case report. *Epilepsia* 1983;24:75–8.

31. Sylvester RK, Lewis FB, Caldwell KC, Lobell M, Perri R, Sawchuk RA. Impaired phenytoin bioavailability secondary to cisplatinum, vinblastin and bleomycin. *Ther Drug Monit* 1984;6:302–5.

32. Carter BL, Garnett WR, Pellock JM, Stratton MA, Howell JR. Effect of antacids on phenytoin bioavailability. *Ther Drug Monit* 1981;3:333–40.

33. D'Arcy PF, McElnay JC. Drug-antacid interactions of clinical importance. *Drug Intell Clin Pharm* 1987;21:607–17.

34. O'Brien LS. Failure of antacids to alter pharmacokinetics of phenytoin. *Br J Pharmacol* 1978;6:176–7.

35. Kulshrestha VK, Thomas M, Wadsworth J, Richens A. Interaction between phenytoin and antacids. *Br J Clin Pharmacol* 1978;6:177–9.

36. Cacek AJ. Review of alterations in oral phenytoin bioavailability associated with formulation, antacids and food. *Ther Drug Monit* 1986;8:166–71.

37. Garnett WR, Small RE, Pellock JM. Effects of three antacids on the bioavailability of valproic acid. *Clin Pharm* 1982;1:244–7.

38. Bartle WR, Walker SE, Shapero T. Dose-dependent effect of cimetidine on phenytoin kinetics. *Clin Pharmacol Ther* 1983;33:649–55.

39. Salem RB, Breland BD, Mishra SK, Jordan GE. Effect of cimetidine on phenytoin serum level. *Epilepsia* 1983;24:284–8.

40. Levine M, Jones MW, Sheppard I. Differential effect of cimetidine on serum concentrations of carbamazepine and phenytoin. *Neurology* 1985;35:562–5.

41. Telerman-Toppet N, Duret ME, Coers C. Cimetidine interaction with carbamazepine. *Ann Intern Med* 1981;94:544.
42. Dalton MJ, Powell JR, Messenheimer JA. Cimetidine and carbamazepine: a complex pharmacokinetic interaction. *Drug Intell Clin Pharm* 1985;19:456.
43. Webster LK, Mihaly GW, Jones DB, Smallwood RA, Phillips JA, Vajda FJ. Effect of cimetidine and ranitidine on carbamazepine and sodium valproate pharmacokinetics. *Eur J Clin Pharmacol* 1984;27:341–3.
44. Watt RW, Hetzel DJ, Hallpike JF, Hann CS, Shearman DJC. Lack of interaction between ranitidine and phenytoin. *Br J Clin Pharmacol* 1983;15:499–500.
45. Mitchard M, Harris A, Mullinger BM. Ramitidine drug interaction. A literature review. *Pharmacol Ther* 1987;32:293–325.
46. Solomon H, Shrogie JJ. The effect of phenyramidol on the metabolism of diphenylhydantoin. *Clin Pharmacol Ther* 1967;8:554–6.
47. Pugh RNH, Geddes AM, Yeoman WB. Interaction of phenytoin and chlorpheniramine. *Br J Clin Pharmacol* 1975; 2:173–4.
48. Vajda FJE, Prineas RJ, Lowell RRH. Interaction between phenytoin and the benzodiazepines. *Br Med J* 1971;1:346.
49. Richens A. Interactions with antiepileptic drugs. *Drugs* 1977;13:266–75.
50. McGovern B, Geer VR, Laraia PJ, Garan H, Ruskin JN. Possible interaction between amiodarone and phenytoin. *Ann Intern Med* 1984;101:650–51.
51. Roe TF, Podosin RL, Blaskovics ME. Drug interaction: diazoxide and diphenylhydantoin. *J Pediatr* 1975;87:480–4.
52. MacPhee GJ, Thompson GG, McInnes GT, Brodie MJ. Verapamil potentiates carbamazepine neurotoxicity: a clinically important inhibitory interaction. *Lancet* 1986;1:700–3.
53. Melander A, Brante G, Johansson O, Lindberg T, Wallin-Boll E. Influence of food on the absorption of phenytoin in man. *Eur J Clin Pharmacol* 1979;15:269–74.
54. Sekikawa H, Nakano M, Takada M, Arita T. Influence of dietary components on the bioavailability of phenytoin. *Chem Pharm Bull (Tokyo)* 1980;22:2443–9.
55. Kennedy MC, Wade DN. The effect of food on the absorption of phenytoin. *Aust NZ J Med* 1982;12:258–61.
56. Vincent FM. Phenothiazine-induced phenytoin intoxication. *Ann Intern Med* 1980;93:56–7.
57. Haydukewyck D, Rodin EA. Effects of phenothiazines on serum antiepileptic drug concentrations in psychiatric patients with seizure disorders. *Ther Drug Monit* 1985;7:401–5.
58. Sands CD, Robinson JD, Salem RB, Stewart RB, Muniz C. Effect of thioridazine on phenytoin serum concentration. A retrospective study. *Drug Intell Clin Pharm* 1987;21:267–72.
59. Gay PE, Madsen JA. Interaction between phenobarbital and thioridazine. *Neurology* 1983;33:1631–2.
60. Ishizaki T, Chiba K, Saito M, Kobavashi K, Izuka R. The effect of neuroleptics (haloperidol and chlorpromazine) on the pharmacokinetics of valproic acid in schizophoric patients. *J Clin Psychopharmacol* 1984;4:254–61.
61. Garrettson LK, Perel JM, Dayton PG. Methylphenidate interactions with both anticonvulsant and biscoumacetate. *JAMA* 1969;207:2053–6.

62. Kupferberg HJ, Jeffrey W, Hunninghake DB. Effect of methylphenidate on plasma anticonvulsant level. *Clin Pharmacol Ther* 1972;13:201–4.
63. Perucca E, Richens A. Interaction between phenytoin and imipramine. *Br J Clin Pharmacol* 1977;4:485–6.
64. Pisani F, Primerano G, D'Agostino AA, Spina E, Facio A. Valproic acid-amitriptyline interaction in man. *Ther Drug Monit* 1986;8:382–3.
65. Dorn JM. A case of phenytoin toxicity possibly precipitated by trazodone. *J Clin Psychiatry* 1986;47:89–90.
66. Shukla S, Goodwin CD, Long LEB, Miller MG. Lithium-carbamazepine neurotoxicity and risk factors. *Am J Psychiatry* 1984;141:1604–6.
67. Berg MJ, Fischer LJ, Rivey MP, Vern BA, Schottelius DD. Phenytoin and folic acid interaction: a preliminary report. *Ther Drug Monit* 1983;5:389–94.
68. Bourgois BFD, Dodson WE, Ferrendelli JA. Interaction between primidone, carbamazepine and nicotinamide. *Neurology* 1982;32:1122–6.
69. Olesen OV. The influence of disulfiram and calcium carbimide on the serum diphenylhydantoin. *Arch Neurol* 1967;16:642–4.
70. Svendsen TL, Kristensen M, Hansen JM, Skovsted L. The influence of disulfiram on the half-life and metabolic clearance rate of diphenylhydantoin and tolbutamide in man. *Eur J Clin Pharmacol* 1976;9:439–41.
71. Kater RMH, Roggin G, Tobon F, Zieve P, Iber FL. Increased rate of clearance of drugs from circulation of alcoholics. *Am J Med Sci* 1969;258:35–9.
72. Neuvonen PJ, Elonen E. Effect of activated charcoal on absorption and elimination of phenobarbitone, carbamazepine and phenylbutazone in man. *Eur J Clin Pharmacol* 1980;17:51–7.
73. Kramer G, Theisohn M, von Unruh GE, Eichelbaum M. Carbamazepine-danazol interaction: its mechanism examined by a stable isotope technique. *Ther Drug Monit* 1986;8:387–92.
74. Prescott LF, Critchley JAJH, Balali-Mood M, Pentland B. Effects of microsomal enzyme induction on paracetamol metabolism in man. *Br J Clin Pharmacol* 1981;12:149–54.
75. Pond SM, Kretschzmar KM. Effect on phenytoin on meperidine clearance and nor-meperidine formation. *Clin Pharmacol Ther* 1981;30:680–6.
76. Stambaugh JE, Hemphili DM, Wainer IW, Schwartz I. A potentially toxic drug interaction between pethidine (meperidine) and phenobarbital. *Lancet* 1977;1:398–9.
77. Tong TG, Pond SM, Kreek MJ, Jaffry NF, Benowitz NL. Phenytoin-induced methadone withdrawal. *Ann Intern Med* 1981;94:349–51.
78. Liu SJ, Wang RIH. Case report of barbiturate-induced enhancement of methadone metabolism and withdrawal syndrome. *Am J Psychiatry* 1984;141:1287–8.
79. Jonkman JHG, Upton RA. Pharmacokinetic drug interactions with theophylline. *Clin Pharmacokinet* 1984;9:309–34.
80. Sklar SJ, Wagner JC. Enhanced theophylline clearance secondary to phenytoin therapy. *Drug Intell Clin Pharm* 1985;19:34–6.
81. Bloxham RA, Durbin GM, Johnson T, Winterborn MH. Chloramphenicol and phenobarbitone—a drug interaction. *Arch Dis Child* 1979;54:70.
82. Krasinski K, Kusmiesz M, Nelson JD. Pharmacologic interactions among chloramphenicol, phenytoin and phenobarbital. *Pediatr Infect Dis* 1982;1:232–5.

83. Neuvonen PJ, Penttila O, Lehtovaara R, Aho K. Effects of antiepileptic drugs on the elimination of various tetracycline derivatives. *Eur J Clin Pharmacol* 1975;9:147–54.

84. Beurey J, Weber M, Vignaud JM. Treatment of tinea capitis: metabolic interference of griseofulvin with phenobarbital. *Ann Dermatol Venereol* 1982;109:567–70.

85. Hansen JM, Siersbaek-Nielsen K, Kristensen M, Skovsted L, Christensen LK. Effect of diphenylhydantoin on the metabolism of dicoumarol in man. *Acta Med Scand* 1971;189:15–9.

86. Hansen JM, Siersbaek-Nielsen K, Skovsted L. Carbamazepine-induced acceleration of diphenylhydantoin and warfarin metabolism in man. *Clin Pharmacol Ther* 1971;12:539–43.

87. Nappi J. Warfarin and phenytoin interaction. *Ann Intern Med* 1979;90:852.

88. Somogyi A, Gugler R. Drug interaction with cimetidine. *Clin Pharmacokinet* 1982;7:23–41.

89. Ahmad S. Renal insensitivity to furosemide caused by chronic anticonvulsant therapy. *Br Med J* 1974;3:657–9.

90. Williamson HE. Interaction of furosemide and phenytoin in the rat. *Proc Soc Exp Biol Med* 1986;182:322–4.

91. Solomon HM, Reich S, Spirt N, Abrams WB. Interaction between digitoxin and other drugs in vitro and in vivo. *Ann NY Acad Sci* 1971;79:362–9.

92. Aitio ML, Mansbury L, Tala E, Haataja M, Aitio A. The effect of enzyme induction on the metabolism of disopyramide in man. *Br J Clin Pharmacol* 1981;11:279–86.

93. Freeman DJ, Laupacis A, Keown A, Stiller CR, Carruthers SG. Evaluation of cyclosporin-phenytoin interaction with observations on cyclosporin metabolites. *Br J Clin Pharmacol* 1984;18:887–93.

94. Cartstensen H, Jacobsen N, Dieperink H. Interactions between cyclosporin and phenobarbitone. *Br J Clin Pharmacol* 1986;21:550–1.

95. Schwass DE, Saaki AW, Houghton DC, Benner KE, Bennett WM. Effects of phenobarbital and cimetidine on experimental cyclosporine nephrotoxicity: preliminary observations. *Clin Nephrol* 1986;25(suppl 1):117–20.

96. Loga S, Curry S, Lader M. Interactions of orphenadrine and phenobarbitone with chlorpromazine: plasma concentrations and effects in man. *Br J Clin Pharmacol* 1975;2:197–208.

97. Linnoila M, Viukari M, Vaisanen K, Auvinen J. Effects of anticonvulsants on plasma haloperidol and thioridazine levels. *Am J Psychiatry* 1980;137:819–21.

98. Fast DK, Jones BD, Kusalic M, Erickson M. Effect of carbamazepine on neuroleptic plasma levels and efficacy. *Am J Psychiatry* 1986;143:117–8.

99. Kidron R, Auerbuch I, Klein E, Belmaker RH. Carbamazepine-induced reduction of blood levels of haloperidol in chronic schizophrenia. *Biol Psychiatry* 1985;20:219–22.

100. Arana GW, Goff DC, Friedman H, Ornsteen M, Greenblatt DJ, Black B, Shader RI. Does carbamazepine-induced reduction of plasma haloperidol level worsen psychotic symptoms? *Am J Psychiatry* 1986;143:650–1.

101. Braithwaite RA, Flanagan RA, Richens A. Steady state plasma nortriptyline concentrations in epileptic patients. *Br J Clin Pharmacol* 1975;2:469–71.

102. Hempel E, Klinger W. Drug stimulated biotransformation of hormonal steroid contraceptives: clinical implications. *Drugs* 1976;12:442–8.
103. Orme MLE. Clinical pharmacology of oral contraceptive steroids. *Br J Clin Pharmacol* 1982;14:31–42.
104. Mattson RH, Cramer JA. Epilepsy, sex hormones and antiepileptic drugs. *Epilepsia* 1985;26(suppl) 1:S40–S55.
105. Chalk JB, Ridgeway K, Brophy T, Yelland JDN, Eadie MJ. Phenytoin impairs the bioavailability of dexamethasone in neurological and neurosurgical patients. *J Neurol Neurosurg Psychiatry* 1984;47:1087–90.
106. Wong DD, Longenecker RG, Liepman M, Baker S, La Vergne M. Phenytoin-dexamethasone: a possible drug-drug interaction. *JAMA* 1985;254(15):2062–3.
107. Meikle AW, Jubiz W, Matsakura S, West CD, Tyler FH. Effect of diphenylhydantoin on the metabolism of metyrapone and release of ACTH in man. *J Clin Endocrinol Metab* 1969;29:1553–8.
108. Hunter J. Effects of enzyme induction on vitamin D3 metabolism in man. In Richens A, Woodford FP, eds. *Anticonvulsant Drugs and Enzyme Induction.* Amsterdam: Elsevier Excerpta Medica North Holland, 1976;77–84.
109. Tjellesen L, Gotfredsen A, Christiansen C. Different actions of vitamin D2 and D3 on bone metabolism in patients treated with phenobarbitone/phenytoin. *Calcif Tissue Int* 1985;37:218–22.
110. Williams K, Begg E, Wade D, O'Shea K. Effects of phenytoin, phenobarbital and ascorbic acid on misonidazole elimination. *Clin Pharmacol Ther* 1983;33:314–21.
111. Starberg B, Hueg B. Interaction between 8-methoxypsoralen and phenytoin. Consequences for PUVA therapy. *Acta Derm Venereol (Stockh)* 1985;65:553–5.
112. Patel JH, Levy RH. Valproic acid binding to human serum albumin and determination of free fraction in the presence of anticonvulsants and free fatty acids. *Epilepsia* 1979;20:85–90.

4

Clinically Relevant Antiepileptic Drug Interactions

B. J. Wilder and Rogelio J. Rangel

Veterans Administration Medical Center and University of Florida College of Medicine, Gainesville, Florida, U.S.A.

Drug interactions occur when two or more drugs are dosed in combination and produce effects that do not occur when either drug is used alone. Two types of drug interaction occur: pharmacodynamic and pharmacokinetic. Pharmacodynamic drug interactions occur at the neuronal membrane or synaptic site of action in the case of the antiepileptic drugs. Most of the interactions occur as a result of changes in drug pharmacokinetics (absorption, protein binding, metabolism, or elimination). Pharmacokinetic drug interactions occur commonly in patients receiving two or more antiepileptic drugs. They most often are caused by drug-induced alterations in protein binding or metabolism.

PROTEIN BINDING

Many drugs, hormones, and other substances are bound to plasma proteins and in this state are biologically inactive. Only the unbound fraction of drug, hormone, etc., can cross membranes and exert biologic activity. Alterations in protein binding of a drug may result in highly significant changes in drug action. For example, if a drug is 90% bound to plasma proteins, an interaction that decreases binding to 80% would result in a 100% increase in drug available for biologic action. In such a situation total drug levels, as measured by most clinical laboratories, would not reflect any change in unbound drug concentration. If a protein-binding drug interaction is suspected, the clinician should request protein-free or unbound drug levels.

Many of the commonly used antiepileptic drugs are highly bound to plasma proteins, mainly albumin. Table 4-1 gives the range of binding of the major drugs.

Table 4-1. Protein Binding

Drug	Protein binding (%)
Phenytoin	85–93
Carbamazepine	73–88
Valproate	70–95[a]
Phenobarbital	45–55
Primidone	0–30
Ethosuximide	0–10

[a] Binding is concentration dependent.

When phenytoin (PHT), carbamazepine (CBZ), valproate (VA), diazepam (DZ), and phenobarbital (PB) are used in combinations of two or more, protein-binding interactions may occur. The clinically relevant interactions most often involve the use of VA in combination with one of these drugs. Polypharmacy with VA frequently results in clinically significant protein-binding interactions.

VA protein binding is concentration-dependent, and as total concentrations increase the ratio of free to bound drug also increases. At a total VA concentration of 50 μg/ml, 95% may be bound (1). However, at total levels of 100 μg/ml, only 70% is bound (2). VA has a greater affinity for protein-binding sites on serum albumin than do other drugs (3,4). Therefore, when VA is dosed in combination with PHT and CBZ, increasing plasma levels of VA displace PHT and/or CBZ from binding sites and may result in a significant increase in biologically available unbound CBZ or PHT. Such an increase in bioactive drug can produce clinical toxicity without altering the measured total drug level (5,6). Therefore, it is important to measure the free serum levels of the drugs involved and correlate these with clinical signs and symptoms when this situation is suspected. This interaction is more likely to occur when the Na$^+$ salt and acid formulations of the drug are used. Sodium VA in the liquid formulation and valproic acid in the soft gelatin capsule are rapidly absorbed and after dosing reach peak plasma concentrations within 30–60 min. The absorption of enteric coated divalproex (sodium, hydrogen dimer of VA) is slower and is delayed for several hours. Clinical signs and symptoms resulting from the displaced drug occur when concentrations of VA reach their peak after dosing.

One of our patients, a 9-year-old boy who was chronically receiving PHT, had a particularly significant acute PHT toxicity interaction when VA was added to his treatment regimen. Within 45 min after taking VA he would become severely ataxic and experience vertigo. Laboratory drug monitoring on one occasion revealed that before receiving a dose of VA, total PHT and free unbound PHT serum levels were 10.1 and 1.0 μg/ml, respectively. Forty-five min after receiving 250 mg of VA the total PHT level remained unchanged; however, free unbound PHT rose to 3.1 μg/ml and coincided with central nervous system PHT toxicity (unpublished data).

We have had many patients maintained on CBZ in the high therapeutic range of 9–12 μg/ml who experienced transient CBZ central nervous system toxicity (blurring of vision and diplopia, sometimes headache and mental confusion) after each dose of concurrently administered VA. Such problems usually respond to altering dosing schedules (changing b.i.d. or t.i.d. VA dosing to q.i.d. or dosing VA with meals, which slows absorption).

Somnolence, stupor, or coma have been reported when VA is added to patients chronically receiving PB (7–9). However, this interaction probably represents an as yet undefined pharmacodynamic interaction rather than a pharmacokinetic protein-binding interaction. A metabolic interaction resulting in changes in NH_3^+ metabolism has been reported when VA is added to patients receiving other antiepileptic drugs (10–12). VA also inhibits the metabolism of PB (13).

METABOLIC INTERACTIONS

The most common and clinically significant drug interactions occur as a result of induction or inhibition of drug or metabolite metabolism of one drug by another when drugs are used concurrently. Drug metabolism occurs in the liver by the microsomal P450 system. Most of the antiepileptic drug metabolic reactions involve oxidation, reduction, or hydroxylation followed by conjugation with glucuronic acid. Inactivation of the antiepileptic drugs or their metabolites usually occurs by hydroxylation. Oxidative metabolism results in the formation of active metabolites [PB from primidone (PR); CBZ, 10, 11-epoxide from CBZ; 2-en, 3-en, and 4-en valproate from VA].

Many of the antiepileptic drugs act as inducers or inhibitors of the metabolism of other drugs. Thus, they either stimulate or depress the metabolism of other antiepileptic drugs or nonepileptic drugs. Some act as inducers of some drugs and inhibitors of others. Inhibition or induction may be concentration-dependent. Only ethosuximide (ETH) has little or no effect on the metabolism of the other antiepileptic drugs. Table 4-2 lists inducers and inhibitors (13,14).

PHT, PB, and ETH are hydroxylated into single inactive metabolites that are conjugated in the liver with glucoronic acid and excreted in the urine. Only very small amounts of PHT and ETH are excreted in the urine unchanged. Approximately 50% of PB, depending on urinary pH,

Table 4-2. Inducers and Inhibitors

Inducers	Inhibitors
Phenytoin[a]	Valproate (13,14)
Carbamazepine[b]	
Phenobarbital[a]	
Primidone	

[a]Phenobarbital and phenytoin may reciprocally inhibit each other if plasma levels are in the higher ranges (PHT > 15, PB > 30).
[b]Carbamazepine inhibits phenytoin metabolism with a resulting decrease in phenytoin clearance of 20–40%.

is excreted unchanged in the urine. Alkalinization of the urine increases and acidification decreases PB excretion (15).

PR is metabolized into two active metabolites, PB and phenylethylmalonamide, and some is hydroxylated to an inactive metabolite. Small amounts are excreted unchanged in the urine.

Valproic acid is metabolized into an inactive metabolite and a number of active metabolites, and some is excreted unchanged in the urine.

The major metabolic pathway of CBZ is to an active epoxide metabolite, CBZ-10, 11-epoxide. This metabolite is then metabolized by epoxide hydroxylase into an inactive compound, conjugated, and excreted (16). The metabolites of PR, CBZ, and VA may play an important role in toxic reactions when these compounds are used in polypharmacy in the treatment of epilepsy.

Enzyme induction and inhibition commonly occur with polypharmacy. Enzyme induction occurs when drugs such as PHT, CBZ, PR, and PB are dosed with VA. This results in a significant decrease in the half-life of VA and corresponding increase in dosage requirements of VA. Often the dose of VA required to achieve therapeutic plasma levels is increased by 100–200% after co-medication with these drugs (17–19). Table 4-3 shows the

Table 4-3. Metabolism: VA Polypharmacy and Monotherapy

Treatment	Daily dose (mg/kg)	Serum levels (μg/ml)
Valproate + PHT or CBZ	32–54 (38)	38–71 (51)
Valproate monotherapy	18–29 (23)	65–114 (78)

Sixteen patients switched from VA polypharmacy to VA monotherapy.

Table 4-4. Metabolism: Primidone Polypharmacy to Monotherapy

Treatment	PRM dose (mg/kg)	PRM (μg/ml)	PB (μg/ml)
Primidone + PHT or CBZ	9.25[a]	7–14 (9)	27–58 (37)
Primidone monotherapy	9.25	13–30 (18)	7–28 (19)

Ten patients switched from primidone two- or three-drug polypharmacy to primidone monotherapy.

[a] Individual daily doses ranged from 7 to 13 mg/kg/day and remained unchanged when patients went on monotherapy.

relationship between VA dosing and plasma levels after PHT or CBZ is withdrawn to achieve VA monotherapy.

A similar induction of PR metabolism occurs when co-medicated with PHT or CBZ. Table 4-4 gives the changes that occur in PR and PB levels when either CBZ or PHT is withdrawn from concomitant dosing with PR. When PR is used in monotherapy, the PB/PR ratio at steady state ranges between <1 and 1.5. However, when PR is dosed with PHT or CBZ, the ratio increases to 3:6. In such a situation PHT and CBZ induce PR metabolism, leading to its conversion to PB, and resulting in PB adverse reactions (15). PHT is a potent inducer of CBZ metabolism.

When phenytoin is withdrawn from a regimen of CBZ and PHT, CBZ serum levels increase and the dosage requirement drops, as seen in Table 4-5.

Although CBZ is a potent inducer of VA and PR metabolism, it acts as an inhibitor of PHT metabolism (20–22). Table 4-6 shows how PHT levels decrease after CBZ is withdrawn from patients receiving both drugs.

Our data show that PB and PHT may act as reciprocal inhibitors or inducers when plasma levels of one or the other are either high or low. If PHT levels are in the high therapeutic or low toxic range, concurrently administered PB usually inhibits the rate of PHT metabolism and vice versa (15). These relationships are subject to great interpatient variation.

VA administered concurrently with CBZ interacts with CBZ and its

Table 4-5. Metabolism: CBZ Induction by PHT

Treatment	Daily dose (mg/kg)	Trough serum level μg/ml
CBZ + PHT	17–25 (20.5)	4–11 (7.3)
CBZ monotherapy	7–14 (12.5)	7–12 (8.6)

Ten patients on two-drug therapy with phenytoin and carbamazepine were converted to CBZ monotherapy.

Table 4-6. Metabolism: CBZ Inhibition of PHT
Metabolism

Treatment	Trough serum levels
Phenytoin + CBZ	15–24 μg/ml (19)
Phenytoin monotherapy	9–16 μg/ml (13)

Six patients who were receiving PHT and CBZ had CBZ
withdrawn. PHT dose remained constant.

epoxide metabolite. CBZ levels may decrease because of increased free
levels of CBZ, which is then more readily metabolized. CBZ-10, 11-epox-
ide levels increase because of VA inhibition of epoxide hydroxylase activity. The resulting clinical picture may be similar to that of CBZ toxicity
with normal or subnormal CBZ levels and high CBZ 10-11 epoxide levels
(23,24). Unfortunately most clinical laboratories do not measure CBZ
epoxide levels.

We recently encountered such a situation. A 6-year-old child was receiving CBZ and VA for generalized and partial seizures. The child became ataxic, complained of headaches, and had a poor appetite. The serum
VA level wsa 64 μg/ml and CBZ was 5.6 μg/ml. The treating physician
requested an epoxide level of 4.2 μg/ml. The patient's adverse reaction
was attributed to epoxide toxicity secondary to VA/CBZ interaction.

Metabolite induction or inhibition occurs when drugs that are metabolized to active compounds are dosed with other drugs that are inducers
or inhibitors. Table 4-7 list the situations in which this may occur. Inducers are shown on top of the reaction and inhibitor on the bottom.

The use of VA in polypharmacy significantly increases the risk of serious idiosyncratic reactions. In children less than 2 years old placed on
polypharmacy with VA, the incidence of liver failure and death has been
found to be 1/500, whereas on monotherapy this incidence drops to 1/

Table 4-7. Metabolite Induction and Inhibition

Primidone	$\xrightarrow{\text{PHT, CBZ}}$	Phenobarbital
Carbamazepine	$\xrightarrow{\text{PHT, PB}}$	CBZ-10,11-epoxide
Valproate	$\xrightarrow{\text{PHT, CBZ, PB}}$	2-en, 3-en, 4-en Valproate
CBZ-10,11-epoxide	$\xrightarrow[\text{VA}]{}$	Epoxide hydroxide

An increased rate of metabolite formation occurs as a result of induction of the
above reactions by CBZ, PHT, and PB.
VA decreases or slows the rate of CBZ-10,11-epoxide hydroxylation.

10,000 (25). The mechanism of this interaction is unknown. The induction of the toxic 4-en metabolite has been proposed as a possible mechanism (26).

When VA and PB are dosed together, a significant pharmacodynamic interaction may occur. Rangel (7) and others (8,9) have reported mental confusion, somnolence, and stupor and associated EEG changes without apparent changes in NH_3 metabolism.

DZ and PB may interact as the synaptic site in a pharmacodynamic interaction to produce respiratory depression or arrest. PB prolongs postsynaptic inhibition, and DZ enhances postsynaptic inhibition; when both are parenterally administered concurrently, respiratory arrest may occur.

A number of interactions occur when antiepileptic drugs are co-administered with non-antiepileptic drugs. The clinician should anticipate such interactions. The most clinically relevant interactions involve changes in drug metabolism, inhibition, or induction. Tables 4-8 and 4-9 (27–40) list some of the more commonly encountered interactions that may occur when non-antiepileptic drugs are co-medicated with antiepileptic drugs.

The purpose of this chapter is to discuss clinically relevant antiepileptic drug interactions. The authors have stressed those interactions that commonly occur in epileptic patients when polypharmacy is practiced. The common denominators of such interactions are toxicity and reduced drug efficacy. Toxicity most commonly results from protein-binding interactions and inhibition of drug metabolism or induction of active metabolites. Decreased drug efficacy results from induction of metabolism and the resulting difficulty of achieving or maintaining therapeutic plasma levels of the induced drug. Reduced efficacy and poor seizure control often

Table 4-8. Metabolism: Enzyme Inhibition

Drug causing enzyme inhibition of antiepileptic drug metabolism	Reference (no.)
Disulfiram	27
Isoniazid	28, 29
Propoxyphene	30
Erythromycin	31, 32
Calcium channel blockers	33, 34
Chloramphenicol	35
Sulfonamides	36
Cimetidine	37
Ethanol	38

Antiepileptic drug metabolism may be significantly inhibited with resulting toxicity by the above nonepileptic drugs.

Table 4-9. Metabolism: Enzyme Induction

Enzyme induction of nonepileptic drugs by antiepileptic drugs (PHT, CBZ, PB, PR)	Reference (no.)
Oral contraceptives	39
Coumadin	
Theophylline	
Steroids	
Vitamin K	
Quinidine	
Digitoxin	40

The efficacy of the above drugs are reduced by co-medication with some of the antiepileptic drugs.

accompany polypharmacy (41,42). Toxicity and adverse drug reactions increase in proportion with the number of drugs used.

REFERENCES

1. Bruni J, Wilder BJ. Valproic acid: review of a new antiepileptic drug. *Arch Neurol* 1979;36:393–8.
2. Patel IH, Levy RH, Cutler RE. Phenobarbital-valproic acid interaction. *Clin Pharmacol Ther* 1980;27:515–21.
3. Fleitman JS, Bruni J, Perrin JH, Wilder BJ. Albumin-binding interaction of sodium valproate. *J Clin Pharmacol* 1980;20;514–7.
4. Patel IH, Levy RH. Valproic acid binding to human serum albumin and determination of free fraction in the presence of anticonvulsants and free fatty acids. *Epilepsia* 1979;20:85–90.
5. Rodin EA, Garcia De Sousa, Haidukewych D, Lodhi R, Berchov RC. Dissociation between free and bound phenytoin levels in presence of valproate sodium. *Arch Neurol* 1981;38:240–2.
6. Perucca E, Hebdige S, Frigo GM, Gatti G, Lecchini S, Crema A. Interaction between phenytoin and valproic acid: plasma protein binding and metabolic effects. *Clin Pharmacol Ther* 1980;28:779–789.
7. Rangel RJ, Warner JJ, Wilder BJ. Valproic acid encephalopathy. *J Epilepsy* 1988;1:197–202.
8. Sackellares JC, Lee SI, Dreifuss FE. Stupor following administration of valproic acid to patients receiving other antiepileptic drugs. *Epilepsia* 1979;20:697–703.
9. Marescaux C, Warter JM, Micheletti G, Rumback L, Coquillat G, Kurtz D. Stuporous episodes during treatment with sodium valproate: report of seven cases. *Epilepsia* 1982;23:297–305.
10. Zaccara G, Paganini M, Campostrini R, et al. Effect of associated antiepileptic

treatment on valproate-induced hyperammonemia. *Ther Drug Monit* 1985;7(2):185–90.

11. Zaret BS, Beckner RR, Marini AM, Wagle W, Passarelli C. Sodium valproate induced hyperammonemia without clinical hepatic dysfunction. *Neurology* 1982;32:206–8.
12. Coulter DL, Allen RJ. Secondary hyperammonemia: a possible mechanism for valproate encephalopathy. *Lancet* 1980;1:1310–1.
13. Bruni J, Wilder BJ, Perchalski RJ, Hammond EJ, Villarreal HJ. Valproic acid and plasma levels of phenobarbital. *Neurology* 1980;30:94–7.
14. Bruni J, Gallo JM, Lee CS, Perchalski RJ, Wilder BJ. Interactions of valproic acid with phenytoin. *Neurology* 1980;30;1233–6.
15. Kutt H. Interactions between anticonvulsants and other commonly prescribed drugs. *Epilepsia* 1984;25(suppl 2):S118–S131.
16. Bertilsson L, Tomson T. Clinical pharmacokinetics and pharmacological affects of carbamazepine and carbamazepine-10, 11 epoxide. An update. *Clin Pharmacokinet* 1986;11(3):177–98.
17. May T, Rambeck B. Serum concentrations of valproic acid: influence of dose and comedication. *Ther Drug Monit* 1985;7:387–90.
18. Sackellares JC, Sato S, Dreifus FE, Penry JK. Reduction of steady-state valproate levels by other antiepileptic drugs. *Epilepsia* 1981;22:437–41.
19. Henriksen O, Johannessen SJ. Clinical and pharmacokinetic observations on sodium valproate. A 5 year follow up study in 100 children with epilepsy. *Acta Neurol Scand* 1982;65:504–23.
20. Zielinski JJ, Haidukewych D, Leheta BJ. Carbamazepine-phenytoin interaction: elevation of plasma phenytoin concentrations due to carbamazepine comedication. *Ther Drug Monit* 1985;7(1):51–3.
21. Zielinski JJ, Haidukewych D. Dual effects of carbamazepine-phenytoin interaction. *Ther Drug Monit* 1987;9(1):21–3.
22. Browne TR, Szabo GK, Evans JE, Evans BA, Greenblatt DJ, Mikati MA. Carbamazepine increases phenytoin serum concentration and reduces phenytoin clearance. *Neurology* 1988;38:1146–50.
23. Brodie MJ, Forrest G, Rapeport WG. Carbamazepine 10, 11 epoxide concentrations in epileptics on carbamazepine alone and in combination with other anticonvulsants. *Br J Clin Pharmacol* 1983;16(6):747–9.
24. McKauge L, Tyrer JH, Eadie MJ. Factors influencing simultaneous concentrations of carbamazepine and its epoxide in plasma. *Ther Drug Monit* 1981;3(1):63–70.
25. Dreifuss EE, Santilli N, Langer DH, Sweeney KP, Moline KA, Menander KB. Valproic acid hepatic fatalities: a retrospective review. *Neurology* 1987;37:379–85.
26. Rettie AE, Rettenmeier AW, Howald WN, Baillie TA. Cytochrome P-450-catalized formation of 4-VPA, a toxic metabolite of valproic acid. *Science* 1987;235:890–3.
27. Svendsen TL, Kristensen M, Hansen JM, Skovsted L. The influence of disulfiram on the half-life and metabolic clearance rate of diphenylhydantoin and tolbutamide in man. *Eur J Clin Pharmacol* 1976;9:439–41.
28. Brennan RW, Dehejia H, Kutt H, Verebely K, McDowell F. Diphenylhydantoin intoxication attendant to slow activation of isoniazid. *Neurology* 1970;20:687–93.

29. Miller RR, Porter J, Greenblatt DJ. Clinical importance of the interaction of phenytoin and isoniazid. *Chest* 1979;75:356–8.
30. Yu YL, Huang CY, Chin D, Woo E, Chang CM. Interaction between carbamazepine and dextropropoxyphene. *Postgrad Med J* 1986;62(725):231–3.
31. Jaster PJ, Abbas D. Erythromycin-carbamazepine interaction. *Neurology* 1986;36(4):594–5.
32. Goulden KJ, Camfield P, Dooley JM, Fraser A, Meek DC, Ranton KW, Tibbles JA. Severe carbamazepine intoxication after coadministration of erythromycin. *J Pediatr* 1986;109(1):135–8.
33. Macphee GJ, McInnes GT, Thompson GG, Brodie MJ. Verapamil potentiates carbamazepine neurotoxicity: a clinically important inhibitory interaction. *Lancet* 1986;1:700–3.
34. Brodie MJ, MacPhee GJ. Carbamazepine neurotoxicity precipitated by diltrazem. *Br Med J* 1986;292(6529):1170–1.
35. Christensen LK, Skovsted L. Inhibition of drug metabolism by chloramphenicol. *Lancet* 1969;2:1397–9.
36. Molholm Hansen J, Kampmann JP, Siersbaek-Nielsen K, Lumholtz IB, Arre M, Abilgaard U, Skovsted L. The effect of different sulfonamides on phenytoin metabolism in man. *Acta Med Scand* 1979;624(suppl):106–10.
37. Dalton MJ, Powell JR, Messenheimer JA Jr, and Clark J. Cimetidine and carbamazepine: a complex drug interaction. *Epilepsia* 1986;27(5):553–8.
38. Sandor P, Sellers EM, Drumbrell M, Khouw V. Effects of short and long-term alcohol use on phenytoin kinetics in chronic alcoholics. *Clin Pharmacol Ther* 1981;30:390–7.
39. Diamond MP, Green JW, Thompson JM, Vanhooydonk JE, Wentz AC. Interaction of anticonvulsants and oral contraceptives in epileptic adolescents. *Contraception* 1985;31(6):623–32.
40. Rameis H. On the interaction between phenytoin and digotin. *Eur J Clin Pharmacol* 1985;29(1):49–53.
41. Schmidt D. Reduction of two drug therapy in intractable epilepsy. *Epilepsia* 1983;24:368–76.
42. Shorvon SD, Reynolds EH. Reduction in polypharmacy for epilepsy. *Br Med J* 1979;2:1023–5.

5

Antiepileptic Drug Interactions in Clinical Use: Summary

Richard H. Mattson and Joyce A. Cramer

*Department of Neurology, Yale University School of Medicine,
New Haven, Connecticut, and Epilepsy Center, Veterans Administration
Medical Center, West Haven, Connecticut, U.S.A.*

Antiepileptic drug interactions are changes in pharmacodynamics or pharmacokinetics of one drug that occur when co-administered with one or more other drugs or exogenous substances. Interactions may also occur with circulating endogenous substances. The significance of such interactions depends in part on their frequency and severity. A reproducible, consistent, and statistically significant change in drug clearance of 5% rarely would be of any clinical importance. In general, important interactions lead to changes in control or side-effects unless dosage modifications are made in one of the drugs. Changes resulting from interactions may occur not only with addition, but also with discontinuation of one or more in a combination of substances. The timing, frequency, and seriousness of the interactions are important issues.

The available antiepileptic drugs often possess insufficient efficacy to provide complete seizure control or require dosages resulting in unacceptable side-effects, particularly for patients with partial (symptomatic) epilepsy (1). This incomplete control with single drug treatments has led to use of combinations of two or more compounds in order to obtain additive, if not synergistic, effects. The search also continues for new, more effective, less toxic compounds. Although it is hoped that a single agent can be found that effectively controls all seizures, such a possibility seems unlikely. The existence of multiple seizure types and epilepsy syndromes makes it probable that many pathophysiologic epileptic mechanisms exist. No one drug or "silver bullet" can be expected to come from the laboratory that will control all seizures found in all epilepsy syndromes. Improved seizure control will depend not only on optimal utilization of single drugs (the 11th commandment for those providing antiepileptic drug treatment), but also on employment of the most advantageous combinations of drugs to achieve overall improvement in control. Unfortunately, antiepileptic drug combinations frequently result in interactions that are disadvantageous. In the development of new drugs, both favorable and unfavorable interactions must be anticipated.

Early drug trials evaluate new compounds by adding them to existing antiepileptic drug regimens. Interactions resulting from use of a new drug may also occur with a wide variety of adjunct drugs, as well as with endogenous substances. For these reasons, a review of our current clinical experience and understanding of drug interactions is of considerable importance. The likelihood and severity of wanted or unwanted effects can be understood, or perhaps anticipated, by our current knowledge of clinical drug interactions (Chapter 3), particularly those involved with antiepileptic drugs (Chapter 4). This understanding also requires reliable methods of testing (Chapter 1) and an awareness of mechanisms (Chapter 2).

DEFINITIONS

Drug interactions may be defined as changes in the pharmacologic properties of one or more co-administered drugs, causing the ultimate effects on target tissue or other tissues to be different than when one or more of these drugs is administered alone. In addition to recognized therapeutic agents, other exogenous substances such as insecticides, environmental toxins, or ethanol may cause important antiepileptic drug interactions. Endogenous circulating substances such as hormones, proteins, and fatty acids also must be considered.

Interactions occur through changes in pharmacokinetics or pharmacodynamics of drug action. Pharmacokinetic changes may increase or decrease concentration of one or more of the drugs distributed to the target tissue or other organ systems. These changes include alterations of absorption, distribution, protein binding, biotransformation, and elimination. Metabolism may be altered to produce different types or quantities of intermediates that may be active and effective, toxic, or inert (Chapters 2–4). Pharmacodynamic effects of drug combinations are those having effects on the patient and causing clinical efficacy or toxicity. These pharmacodynamic effects in combinations of drugs may be *additive* or *supra-additive* (potentiating, synergistic) as well as *infra-additive* or *antagonistic* (Chapter 14). Both desired efficacy and toxicity can be affected by such interactions, and these can be independent of one another. Consequently, two drugs given in combination may be desirable if efficacy is additive and toxicity is infra-additive, or if they are supra-additive and the toxicity is no more than additive (2). Although combinations of drugs are most often given to enhance pharmacodynamic efficacy directly at the receptor site, some act by altering pharmacokinetics, such as use of carbidopa, which allows distribution of a higher concentration of L-Dopa to the brain.

At times, drug interactions are described as being *favorable* or *unfavorable*. Such descriptions often are of limited value, because the same interaction may be helpful or harmful under different circumstances, even in the same individual. For example, the amount of carbamazepine in the body may be increased by the administration of an enzyme-inhibiting drug such as erythromycin (Chapter 3). If the carbamazepine level initially was low and seizure control was suboptimal, the effect of a higher level may be beneficial. On the other hand, if the carbamazepine concentration at the time of erythromycin administration already was close to maximal tolerance, further inhibition of metabolism and increase in concentration would be likely to elicit side-effects. Although interactions between antiepileptic drugs often are assumed to be unwanted adverse occurrences, most combinations are given in the expectation of a beneficial effect. For example, synergistic pharmacodynamic action is usually desired in combined antibiotic use. On the other hand, increased respiratory and central system depression from combinations, such as concurrent use of alcohol and sedatives, can prove life threatening (3). The negation of pharmacodynamic effects usually is undesirable but in specific circumstances can be beneficial, such as pharmacodynamic antagonism of naloxone to morphine or reversal of heparin action by protamine binding.

Aronson and Grahame-Smith (4) have used the terms *object drugs* and *precipitant drugs* to describe interactions. However, these unidirectional effects are unusual among antiepileptic drug interactions because more than one mechanism is often involved and both compounds may be affected. For example, the addition of phenobarbital to a regimen of valproate monotherapy increases clearance of valproate due to enzyme induction. Lower valproate concentrations are a result unless dosage is increased. At the same time, valproate often inhibits metabolism of phenobarbital, causing unacceptable phenobarbital side-effects after accumulation of the barbiturate. Less predictable are interactions that, at different concentrations, may cause enzyme induction or inhibition. For example, acute administration of large quantities of alcohol inhibits phenytoin clearance (5), but moderate, chronic use causes enzyme induction and more rapid clearance of compounds metabolized by the cytochrome P-450 system (6). At the same time, the alcohol has paradoxical pharmacodynamic effects on seizures. Antiepileptic properties are additive to antiepileptic drugs acutely, but they are infra-additive during withdrawal (7).

FREQUENCY

No precise incidence or prevalence figures are available to provide a clear idea of the frequency of antiepileptic drug interactions. Murad and

Table 5-1. Properties of Drugs Making
Interactions More Probable

Low therapeutic index
Metabolism by microsomal mixed function
  Oxidases
Enzyme-inducing properties
Enzyme-inhibiting properties
High protein binding
Chronic usage

Gilman (8) suggested that the incidence of all drug interactions is 3–5% in patients receiving several medications. Hatshorn (9) reported in 1987 that he found nearly 500 articles on drug interactions published in 1986 and states, "The problem is overwhelming, or is it? Although there are exceptions to this, the object drugs of clinical concern can be counted on your fingers." However, of the 10 drugs most frequently reported in interaction articles, phenytoin is the third and carbamazepine is the seventh in frequency. In other years, phenobarbital must have been among the top 10, and valproate is likely to join the group. In short, the primary antiepileptic drugs are high on the list of those expected to be associated with drug interactions. A number of characteristics of these drugs makes pharmacokinetic interactions frequent and potentially important (Table 5-1). Many antiepileptic drugs possess more than one of these characteristics. For example, drug interactions can be expected in the majority of patients given combinations of valproate, an enzyme-inhibiting and highly protein-bound drug, when co-administered with one of the enzyme-inducing antiepileptic drugs such as carbamazepine, phenobarbital, or phenytoin (10). The problem is further complicated by special characteristics such as nonlinear pharmacokinetics. Thus, administration of an enzyme-inhibiting drug, such as cimetidine, is especially likely to affect the saturable enzymes that metabolize phenytoin.

The frequency of occurrence of various interactions is affected by multiple factors. Among the most important are genetic determinants that lead to considerable interindividual variability (see Chapter 3). The dosages and blood concentrations of one or more drugs may be of considerable importance. For example, phenytoin is a potent inducer of the mixed-function oxidase system involved in metabolism of valproate. Thus, valproate is cleared more rapidly when co-administered with phenytoin than when given as monotherapy. This effect is dose-dependent. Our studies demonstrate disinduction in some patients when the phenytoin dose has decreased to 100–200 mg daily; other patients continue to show evidence of induction until phenytoin is discontinued. Another interaction between phenytoin and valproate involves protein binding. Valproate has a higher affinity for plasma albumin, causing phenytoin to be displaced from protein and resulting in a higher free fraction of the physiologically active phenytoin (11,12). This effect is greater with higher concentrations of valproate (often given in quantities of several grams each day), which saturates binding sites (13). In contrast, despite a strong affinity and high protein binding, diazepam has no significant effect on valproate binding (14). This is probably because the therapeutic blood concentration of valproate is a thousand times greater than that of diazepam.

It should be emphasized that the true frequency of interactions is difficult to state for a number of reasons. An increase in side-effects or seizures might escape notice by the physician, or the cause may erroneously be attributed to noncompliance or other factors influencing seizure frequency (stress, menses, etc.). Some interactions may go unrecognized if caused by an unsuspected environmental toxin or even cigarette smoking. Cigarette smoke contains a polycyclic aromatic hydrocarbon mixture known to induce cytochrome P-450 isozymes (15). Cessation of smoking markedly decreases the quantity of enzyme available for drug metabolism, leading to higher drug levels. The self-administered dosage of such nonpharmaceutical agents often varies, causing inexplicable changes in drug pharmacokinetics and pharmacodynamic effects. Attempts to control these factors are important in a drug trial, but little can be done in clinical practice other than to question the patient about use of all prescription and nonprescription drugs, smoking habits, and drinking habits. Other interactions occur, but, being expected, do not warrant a special report. For example, the increased clearance observed when phenobarbital or phenytoin is added to other drug regimens would be unlikely to cause particular attention in view of these well-known properties. As a consequence, the frequency of interactions or, at least those involving antiepileptic drugs, is probably considerably underestimated.

TIMING

The timing of interactions is variable and depends on the mechanism of interaction and the drugs involved. Changes in protein binding often occur relatively rapidly. For example, displacement of phenytoin or carbamazepine by valproate occurs in less than an hour and may be as rapid as a few minutes. We have analyzed total and free levels of valproate administered with phenytoin or carbamazepine, followed by valproate dosing used alone. Changes in total and free drug concentrations occurred in parallel when samples were obtained hourly (13,16–18). Interactions in the intestinal tract resulting in disturbance of absorption, chemical binding complexes such as protamine with heparin, or alteration in renal excretion associated with pH changes may exert a relatively rapid effect observed within minutes to hours. The results of enzyme inhibition can cause drug accumulation and possible clinical effects within hours or days. The results of enzyme induction are more gradual and depend on individual drug clearance rate. The consequences of interaction may not be fully apparent until steady state is reached, which may take weeks for drugs with a relatively long half-life. For example, the time required for maximal enzyme induction or disinduction to occur may be variable and prolonged when developed during chronic alcohol use, and there can be a persistent effect on phenytoin clearance for up to 4–8 weeks (19). In addition to the time for the interaction to occur, time for re-equilibration of steady-state drug concentrations is required and also can be prolonged. On the other hand, the effects of interactions on drugs with relatively rapid clearance, such as valproate and carbamazepine, may be seen within a day or two.

The time course of disinduction should be inversely related to the terminal half-life of the inducing drug, and dependent on the declining serum concentration. Assuming equivalent inducing potency, microsomal enzyme capacity should decrease more rapidly after stopping carbamazepine than phenobarbital because of the fourfold to eightfold difference in elimination rates between these drugs. As described earlier, co-administration of phenytoin and valproate is associated with enzyme induction and rapid clearance of valproate. Discontinuation of phenytoin results in disinduction and a significant rise in valproate levels as clearance slows. In clinical practice, the discontinuation of phenytoin is usually carried out in a tapering pattern, and our studies indicate that the time of disinduction is difficult to predict. In some individuals, evidence of disinduction and rising valproate levels may be seen as phenytoin dosage decreases to 2–3 mg/kg (about 100–200 m daily), but in other patients this is not seen until after total discontinuation of the drug. The levels are seen to rise approximately 4–7 days later. Clearly, the decreasing dose of phenytoin has a lesser effect on enzyme induction over time. We found that the period of disinduction during a crossover pattern may vary by as much as 4 weeks among individuals.

The timing of some interactions can be relatively short and can escape detection. For example, both phenytoin and carbamazepine are displaced from albumin binding by valproate, causing changes in concentrations of physiologically active free drug (11,12,17,20). When dosing of valproate gives peak levels in a patient whose total carbamazepine or phenytoin levels are high, the resultant displacement from protein and increase in free carbamazepine or phenytoin may well cause toxicity. When the valproate levels decline over several hours, the process will reverse and symptoms resolve. Careful studies of multiple total and free drug levels correlated with clinical findings over 8 h or more may be required to detect these transient but important interactions.

Some interactions can be temporary. Cimetidine inhibits microsomal oxidation, and carbamazepine metabolism is slowed by half when cimetidine is started. However, Dalton et al. (21) demonstrated that the inhibition was transient, lasting only 3–4 days.

The variable and unpredictable periods of time needed for completion of pharmacokinetics and pharmacodynamic effects of drug interactions pose a special problem in the design of clinical drug testing. Initiation of the test drug or placebo in addition to current treatment may yield groups in whom concentration of the primary drug or metabolites is not comparable to that of the control group for many weeks. The lower concentration of the primary drug phenytoin, after addition of the test drug vigabatrin, is such an example (22). The problem of timing of induction or disinduction is even more problematic in crossover designs. The effects of a study drug on co-administered standard antiepileptic drug, mediated through interactions, may persist for weeks after the study drug has been discontinued and cleared from the body during the "wash out." Consequently, the probability, severity, and significance of drug interactions are variable and are often not easily predicted. The time of occurrence and the consequences of these interactions are variable and are predictable only with careful considerations of the factors involved in specific combinations.

PURPOSE OF DRUG COMBINATIONS

Most, but not all, combinations of drugs are prescribed in hopes of achieving a *supra-additive, synergistic* effect. Successful examples include the use of amphotericin B combined with flucytosine in treatment of cryptococcal meningitis. The benefit is believed to be greater than with maximal use of either drug alone, and the combination allows dose-related side-effects to be minimized. Complete control of tonic–clonic seizures and absence seizures in generalized idiopathic epilepsy is much better by combining ethosuximide with phenytoin, phenobarbital, or carbamazepine, than is possible by using any of these drugs singly, even in maximally tolerated dosage. Other well-proven examples of the synergistic effects in epilepsy therapy are few. Simple additive effects may be useful if the combination improves the therapeutic index (Chapter 14). However, no studies exist to indicate any drug combination that is more than additive in controlling partial or secondarily generalized tonic–clonic seizures. For example, motor dysfunction, including diplopia and incoordination, are typical dose-limiting side-effects with carbamazepine or phenytoin. Although drug effects are additive, extra efficacy may not be possible if dosage of one drug is already limited by side-effects (23). However, the rationale for combined drug use often does not rest with expected *supra-additive, synergistic* effects, but with an improved therapeutic index.

The addition of a second drug, such as phenobarbital, to phenytoin may allow additive drug efficacy to the already maximally tolerated dose of the phenytoin drugs, because the side-effects of sedation may be different than the motor-limiting side-effects of the phenytoin. Cumulative toxicity may be tolerated and infra-additive, leading to improved therapeutic index. It must be emphasized that such a theoretical benefit of the two drugs has never been proven in controlled clinical trials. The major study by Yahr et al. (24) indicating a superior outcome for this combination was carried out before blood level determinations and double-blind design for methods were commonly used in studies. The Veterans Administration Cooperative Study indicated that drug combinations improved efficacy in difficult patients, but side-effects also increased (1). Finally, animal studies of these drugs have failed to show that combinations improved the protective (therapeutic) index (2,23).

IMPORTANCE

It is difficult to state what constitutes an important antiepileptic drug interaction. Unequivocally significant reactions are those leading to serious permanent residuals or even life-threatening effects. For example, discontinuation of administration of phenobarbital, an enzyme-inducing drug, may cause elevation of warfarin levels leading to prolonged prothrombin times and risk of potentially fatal bleeding (Chapter 3). Synergistic pharmacodynamic interactions have major potential adverse consequences. The combination of high doses of alcohol and barbiturates or benzodiazepines may produce serious depression of consciousness and respiration. At the other end of the spectrum are effects of interactions that can be detected by minimal changes in serum concentrations or with special pharmacokinetic studies, but have little or no effect on the clinical course.

Some interaction effects on normal physiology may also be important. Failure of oral contraceptives leading to unplanned pregnancy or other changes in endocrine function can occur when enzyme antiepileptic drugs are administered. Enhanced metabolism of steroids and increased concentrations of sex hormone binding globulin during use of these drugs lead to lower than expected circulating hormone levels (25).

In addition to changes in concentration of drugs used in combination, important metabolic changes may occur through production of new or significantly different quantities of active metabolites, e.g., phenobarbital from primidone (26), or carbamazepine 10-11 epoxide from carbamazepine (27). These sometimes hidden changes can alter efficacy and toxicity. Of greater concern is the production of the toxic metabolites, as has been shown following phenobarbital enzyme induction of valproate metabolism increasing the hepatotoxic 4-en valproate metabolite (Chapter 4).

Potential interactions that might lead to loss of seizure control or side-effects may be important. Even if such interactions are unpredictable in terms of frequency and severity among individuals, their potential may lead the physician to advise an additional visit or two to the laboratory or office to insure that no serious decrease in serum levels has occurred that could risk seizure breakthrough. Similarly, assessment of blood levels or clinical examination may be advisable to detect evidence of impending toxicity that might interfere with school or employment. Consequently, even in these asymptomatic patients, the addition or removal of a drug with potential for a clinically important interaction may require additional evaluations, take time away from normal life activities, and cause physical discomfort and expense. If one accepts these minimal factors as evidence of the important effects of drug interactions, it is clear that such problems are going to occur frequently with antiepileptic drug use. The issue is of major importance in day-to-day treatment as well as in clinical investigation and development of new antiepileptic drugs.

CONCLUSIONS

Drug interactions of both pharmacodynamic and pharmacokinetic type between antiepileptic drugs and other drugs or endogenous substances are frequent and important. Indeed, these interactions may be more common than in any other field of medical treatment. Although most interactions are generally thought to be undesirable, many are helpful and intentional. Indeed, future drug development should be aimed, in part, at finding interactions that will have desired synergistic pharmacodynamic or advantageous pharmacokinetic effect to increase the therapeutic index of treatment regimens.

Acknowledgment: This work was supported by NINCDS Grant 5PONS06208-22 and the Veterans Administration Medical Research Service.

REFERENCES

1. Mattson RH, Cramer JA, Collins JF, Smith DB, Esuceta AVD, Browne TR, Williamson PD, Treiman DM, et al. Comparison of carbamazepine, phenobarbital, phenytoin and primidone in partial and secondary generalized tonic-clonic seizures. *N Engl J Med* 1985;313:145–51.
2. Bourgeois BFD, Wad N. Combined administration of carbamazepine and phenobarbital: effect on anticonvulsant activity and neurotoxicity. *Epilepsia* 1988;29:482–7.
3. Curry SH, Scales AH. Interaction of phenobarbitone and ethanol studied from dose-response curves and drug concentrations in blood. *J Pharm Pharmacol* 1973;25:142.

4. Aronson JK, Grahame-Smith DG. Adverse drug interactions. *Br Med J* 1981;282:288–91.
5. Hoensch H. Ethanol as enzyme inducer and inhibitor. *Pharmacol Ther* 1987;33:121–8.
6. Sandor P, Sellers EM, Dumbrell M, Khouw V. Effect of short- and long-term alcohol use in phenytoin kinetics in chronic alcoholics. *Clin Pharmacol Ther* 1981;30:390–7.
7. Mattson RH, Cramer JA. Valproate acid. In: Browne TR, Feldman RG, eds. *Epilepsy, Diagnosis and Management.* Boston: Little, Brown, 1983:225–34.
8. Murad F, Gilman AG. Drug interactions. In: Gilman AG, Goodman LS, Rall TW, Murad F, eds. *Goodman and Gilman's: The Pharmacological Basis of Therapeutics.* 7th edition. New York: MacMillan, 1985:1734–50.
9. Hatshorn EA. *Drug Interactions Update—1986.* American Society of Hospital Pharmacists, 1987.
10. Mattson RH. Interactions with other drugs. In: Woodbury DM, Penry JK, Pippenger CE, eds. *Antiepileptic Drugs.* New York: Raven Press, 1982:579–89.
11. Mattson RH, Cramer JA, Williamson PD, Novelly R. Valproic acid in epilepsy: clinical and pharmacological effects. *Ann Neurol* 1978;3:20–5.
12. Cramer JA, Mattson RH. Valproic acid: in vitro plasma protein binding and interactions with phenytoin. *Ther Drug Monit* 1979;1:105–16.
13. Cramer JA, Mattson RH, Bennett DM, Swick CT. Variable free and total valproic acid concentrations in sole and multi-drug therapy. In: Levy RH, et al., eds. *Metabolism of Antiepileptic Drugs.* New York: Raven Press, 1984:105–14.
14. Dhillon S, Richens A. Valproate acid and diazepam interaction in vivo. *Br J Clin Pharmacol* 1982;13:553–60.
15. Loi CM, Vestall RE. Drug metabolism in the elderly. *Pharmacol Ther* 1988;36:131–49.
16. Scheyer RD, Mattson RH, Cramer JA. Unbound valproate clearance in sole and multi-drug therapy. *Neurology* 1988;38(suppl 1):346.
17. Mattson GF, Mattson RH, Cramer JA. Interaction between valproic acid and carbamazepine: an in vitro study of protein binding. *Ther Drug Monit* 1982;4:181–4.
18. Riva R, Albani F, Conten M, Perucca E, Ambrosetto G, Gobbi G, Santucci M, Procaccianti G. Time dependent interaction between phenytoin and valproate acid. *Neurology* 1985;35:510–5.
19. Iber FL, Brzechn A, Press AW, Kirby S, Creuss DF, Adir J. Comparison of steady state phenytoin metabolism in alcoholics immediately after drinking ceases and three weeks later. *Curr Alcohol* 1979;7:109–13.
20. Levy RH, Morselli PL, Bianchetti G, Guyot M, Brachet-Liermain A, Loiseau P. Interaction between valproic acid and carbamazepine in epileptic patients. In: Levy RH, et al., eds. Metabolism of Antiepileptic Drugs. New York: Raven Press, 1984:45–51.
21. MJ Dalton, Powell JR, Messenheimer JA, Clark J. Cimetidine and carbamazepine: a complex drug interaction. *Epilepsia* 1986;27:553–8.
22. Browne TR, Mattson RH, Penry JK, Smith DB, Treiman DM, Wilder BJ, Ben Menachem E, Napoliello MJ. Vigabatrin for refactory complex partial seizure. *Neurology* 1987;37:184–9.

23. Morris JC, Dodson WE, Hatlelid JM, Ferrendelli JA. Phenytoin and carbamazepine, alone and in combination: anticonvulsant and neurotoxic effects. *Neurology* 1987;37:1111–8.
24. Yahr MD, Sciarra D, Carter S. Evaluation of standard anticonvulsant therapy in 319 patients. *JAMA* 1952;150:663–7.
25. Mattson RH, Cramer JA, Darney PD, Naftolen F. Use of oral contraceptives by women with epilepsy. *JAMA* 1986;256:238–40.
26. Gallagher BB, Baumel IP, Mattson RH. Metabolic disposition of primidone and its metabolites in epileptic subjects after single and repeated administration. *Neurology* 1972;22:1186–92.
27. Tomson T, Bertilsson L. Potent therapeutic effect of carbamazepine-10,11 epoxide in trigeminal neuralgia. *Arch Neurol* 1984;41:598–601.

II. Interactions During Drug Development

6

Recommendations for Antiepileptic Drug–Drug Interaction Studies Before Controlled Clinical Trials

David M. Treiman

*Department of Neurology, University of California at Los Angeles School
of Medicine, Reed Neurological Research Center,
Los Angeles, California, U.S.A.*

Because even a single epileptic seizure may pose a substantial risk of morbidity or even mortality, published guidelines for the development of antiepileptic drugs preclude the testing of a new drug as a sole therapeutic agent until at least some evidence of antiepileptic efficacy in man has been developed (1). Thus, current practice is to carry out initial pilot and controlled clinical trials of such drugs using one or another "add-on" experimental design, in which the drug to be tested is given to a patient who is already taking one or more marketed antiepileptic drug. Because of the necessity for such add-on designs in antiepileptic drug trials, potential drug interactions must be dealt with much earlier in antiepileptic drug development than in the development of other classes of drugs that can be tested as single agents. Thus, it becomes important to consider what sort of drug–drug interaction studies should be carried out prior to the testing of antiepileptic drugs in controlled clinical trials.

Drugs may interact in many ways, some of which are discussed in other chapters in this volume. The goal of this chapter is to consider what questions are necessary to answer regarding drug–drug interactions before carrying out a controlled clinical trial of an antiepileptic drug. The objective of such pretrial drug interaction studies is to anticipate drug–drug interactions that may occur in controlled add-on trials of antiepileptic drugs so that neither patient safety nor the power of the study to evaluate the potential efficacy of the experimental drug is compromised.

Nafimidone (1-[2-naphthoylmethyl] imidazole hydrochloride) (Fig. 6-1) is an imidazole derivative synthesized in the late 1970s that has anticon-

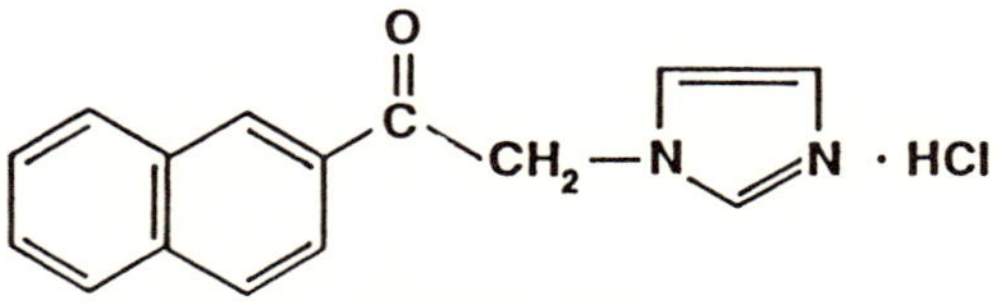

NAFIMIDONE

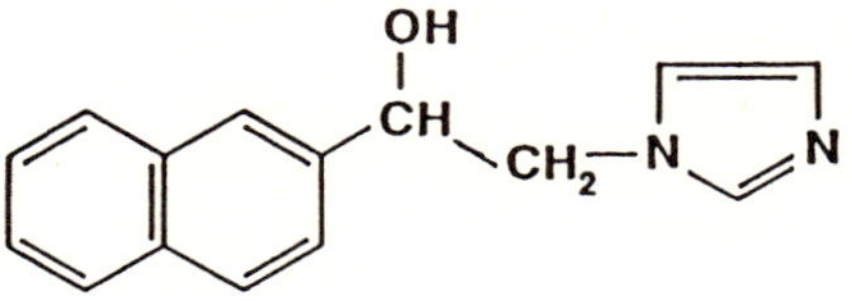

NAFIMIDONE ALCOHOL

FIG. 6-1. Structure of nafimidone and nafimidone alcohol. Note the imidazole moiety on the right-hand side of each structure.

vulsant activity in animal models of both generalized tonic–clonic seizures and partial seizures (2). Starting in 1983, we tested the drug in man for its efficacy in the treatment of intractable partial seizures (3). We were surprised to observe that nafimidone is a potent inhibitor of the metabolism of both phenytoin and carbamazepine (4). This drug interaction was not known prior to our clinical trials of nafimidone, although it might have been predicted from the chemical structure of the compound. Thus, a consideration of the development of nafimidone may be instructive in a consideration of how pretrial drug–drug interaction studies of antiepileptic drugs should be carried out.

The inhibitory effect of nafimidone on phenytoin and carbamazepine metabolism was, as indicated above, not anticipated at the time the first pilot clinical trial of the drug was initiated. In that first study nafimidone was added to a preexisting drug regimen of carbamazepine and phenytoin. The addition of nafimidone (3 mg/kg/day) produced an increase in the serum concentration of carbamazepine and phenytoin within the first 24 h, as illustrated in Fig. 6-2. By the second day of nafimidone treatment, carbamazepine concentration increased sufficiently to produce characteristic toxic symptoms. The toxic symptoms cleared when carbamazepine and phenytoin levels returned to the therapeutic range after reduction of carbamazepine and phenytoin doses, even though the nafimidone dose was simultaneously increased.

Table 6-1 and Fig. 6-3 illustrate the quantitative effect nafimidone had on the elimination of carbamazepine in each of six patients during the 14-week pilot study. For each patient, a dose/plasma concentration ratio was calculated for each clinic visit by dividing the total dose during the preceding 24 h by the trough serum concentration (9–14 h postdose). Such

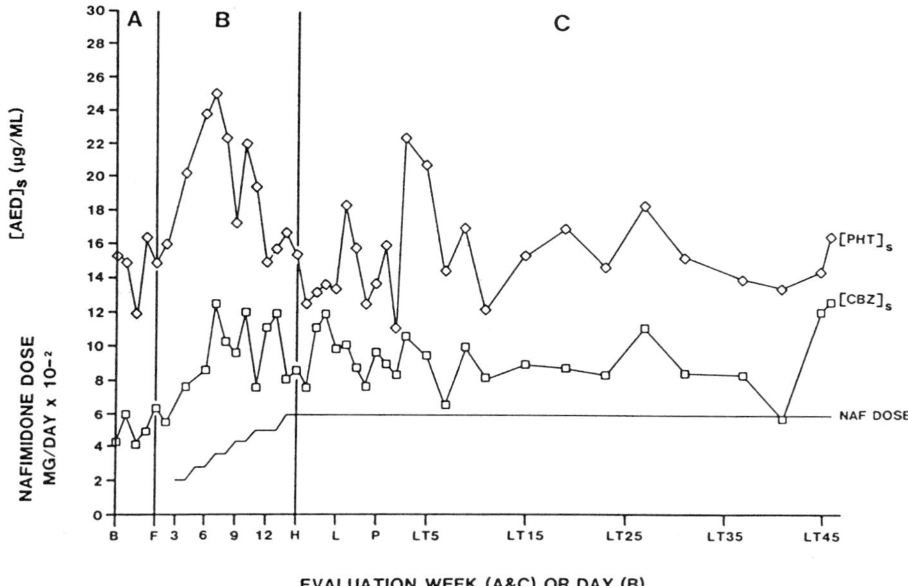

FIG. 6-2. Serum concentration of carbamazepine ([CBZ]s; squares) and phenytoin ([PHT]s; triangles) before and after the addition of nafimidone in one patient. Vertical lines divide the data into three segments: baseline (**A**), where each point represents a weekly visit; hospitalization (**B**), where each point represents a hospital day; and outpatient observation (**C**), where gradations on the x-axis represent weeks. Nafimidone was added during hospitalization; the dose is indicated by the line without symbols. CBZ and PHT levels rose rapidly after the addition of nafimidone, until their doses were lowered to compensate for the inhibition of elimination caused by nafimidone. CBZ dose was 800 mg/day during **A**. It was decreased to 300 mg/day during **B** in response to rising CBZ levels, and was then maintained at 300 mg/day throughout **C**. PHT dose was 400 mg/day during **A** and was reduced to 200 mg/day during **B**; 200 mg/day was maintained throughout **C**. [Reproduced from Treiman and Ben-Menachem (4) with permission.]

calculations were made only when the carbamazepine daily dose and serum concentration were at steady state. The mean of the dose/concentration ratios during the 4-week baseline period and during the 8-week outpatient observation period is shown in Table 6-1. There was a 78–87% decrease in the carbamazepine dose/concentration ratios compared with baseline after the addition of nafimidone, which necessitated a marked reduction of carbamazepine doses to avoid side-effects from excessively high carbamazepine levels.

Table 6-2 shows the effect nafimidone had on elimination of phenytoin in the six patients. Phenytoin elimination was estimated by calculating a

Table 6-1. Serum Concentrations and Dose/Concentration Ratios for Carbamazepine During Baseline, Outpatient Observation, and Long-term Follow-up Phases of the Study

Patient/weight	Phase of study	Mean daily dose (mg)	Mean trough [CBZ]s[a] (μg/ml)	Mean dose/ concentration ratio (l/d)	Percentage of decline in ratio from baseline
CP1/69 kg	Baseline	1,200	5.8 ± 1.0	216 ± 45	
	Observation	300	12.0 ± 3.0	27 ± 10	87
	Long-term (53 wks)	200	7.2 ± 1.6	30 ± 9	86
CP2/80 kg	Baseline	1,00	4.6 ± 0.4	221 ± 22	
	Observation	300	12.0 ± 1.1	25 ± 3	86
	Long-term (52 wks)	200	6.8 ± 1.7	31 ± 9	86
CP3/67 kg	Baseline	800	6.2 ± 1.1	135 ± 24	
	Observation	200	11.3 ± 0.6	18 ± 1	87
	Long-term (52 wks)	200	9.4 ± 1.7	22 ± 5	84
CP4/69 kg	Baseline	700	4.7 ± 2.2	170 ± 44	
	Observation	313	8.7 ± 1.5	37 ± 5	78
CP5/69 kg	Baseline	800	5.4 ± 0.9	154 ± 28	
	Observation	300	9.6 ± 1.4	32 ± 5	79
	Long-term (46 wks)	331	9.2 ± 1.7	37 ± 9	76
CP6/71 kg	Baseline	1,000	4.1 ± 0.7	253 ± 48	
	Observation	300	8.5 ± 1.8	37 ± 8	85
	Long-term (52 wks)	300	8.0 ± 1.3	39 ± 6	85

The observation phase was 8 weeks. The duration of long-term follow-up is indicated in the table for each patient.
Reproduced from Treiman and Ben-Menachem (11) with permission.
[a]Carbamazepine steady-state concentration.

24-h dose/trough concentration ratio for each hospital day or clinic visit while at steady state, as for carbamazepine. There was a 38–77% decrease in the phenytoin dose/concentration ratios after the addition of nafimidone. In the cases in which pre- and post-nafimidone/phenytoin concentrations were different, the post-nafimidone/phenytoin concentrations were, with one exception (patient CP3), always lower than the pre-nafimidone levels. Lower phenytoin concentrations would be expected to be associated with an increase in the clearance of phenytoin. Therefore, it is likely that the observed decrease in the phenytoin dose/concentration ratio was due to an inhibitory effect of nafimidone on phenytoin metabolism.

Table 6-3 displays the mean serum concentrations of carbamazepine during baseline, observation, and long-term follow-up. For nine patients receiving carbamazepine, a mean 100% increase in the serum carbamazepine levels during the 8-week observation period occurred with the introduction of nafimidone, and a mean 44% increase over baseline occurred during the long-term follow-up.

The unanticipated interaction between nafimidone and phenytoin and carbamazepine was unfortunate, because the rise in phenytoin and carbamazepine levels not only compromised patient safety but also the evaluation of the efficacy of nafimidone in the treatment of partial seizures. Gastrointestinal symptoms, dizziness, diplopia, and ataxia, which appeared in the first two patients when carbamazepine and phenytoin levels rose, disappeared when carbamazepine and phenytoin concentrations returned to therapeutic ranges. Even after carbamazepine and phenytoin doses were adjusted downward in order to prevent toxic carbamazepine and phenytoin concentrations with the addition of nafimidone, there was still a twofold increase in the mean carbamazepine serum concentrations during the 8-week observation period compared with the 4-week baseline period in this study. This doubling of the carbamazepine blood levels compromised the power of the study to determine whether the improvement in seizure control observed in these patients was due to efficacy of nafimidone or the increase in carbamazepine concentrations.

This example illustrates the need for a systematic approach to the evaluation of potential drug–drug interactions prior to the initiation of controlled clinical trials of antiepileptic drugs. There are four questions that might be asked early in the development of an antiepileptic drug in order to anticipate possible drug–drug interactions. The remainder of this chapter will address these four questions:

1. Can potential drug–drug interactions be predicted from the chemical structure of the drug?

2. What can be learned about drug–drug interactions from in vitro studies of microsomal metabolism?

3. What can be learned from in vivo pharmacokinetic studies in ani-

CP1
CBZ DOSE/CONCENTRATION RATIO (L/DAY)
350 300 250 200 150 100 50 0
B F 3 6 9 12 H L P LT5 LT15 LT25 LT35 LT45 LT52
EVALUATION DAY
CP2
CBZ DOSE/CONCENTRATION RATIO (L/DAY)
350 300 250 200 150 100 50 0
B F 3 6 9 12 H L P LT5 LT15 LT25 LT35 LT45 LT52
EVALUATION DAY
CP3
CBZ DOSE/CONCENTRATION RATIO (L/DAY)
350 300 250 200 150 100 50 0
B F 3 6 9 12 H L P LT5 LT15 LT25 LT35 LT45 LT52
EVALUATION DAY
CP4
CBZ DOSE/CONCENTRATION RATIO (L/DAY)
350 300 250 200 150 100 50 0
B F 3 6 9 12 H L P LT5 LT15 LT25 LT35 LT45 LT52
EVALUATION DAY

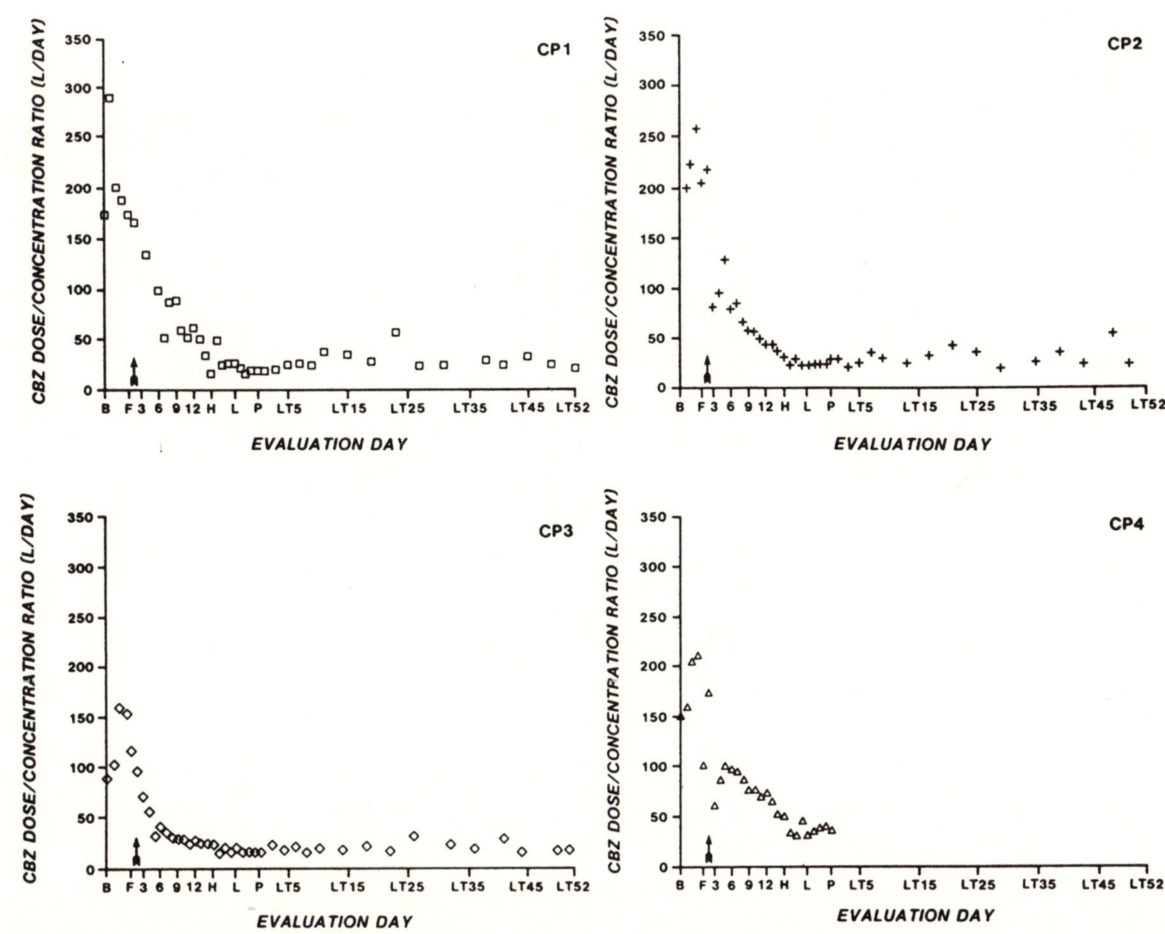

94

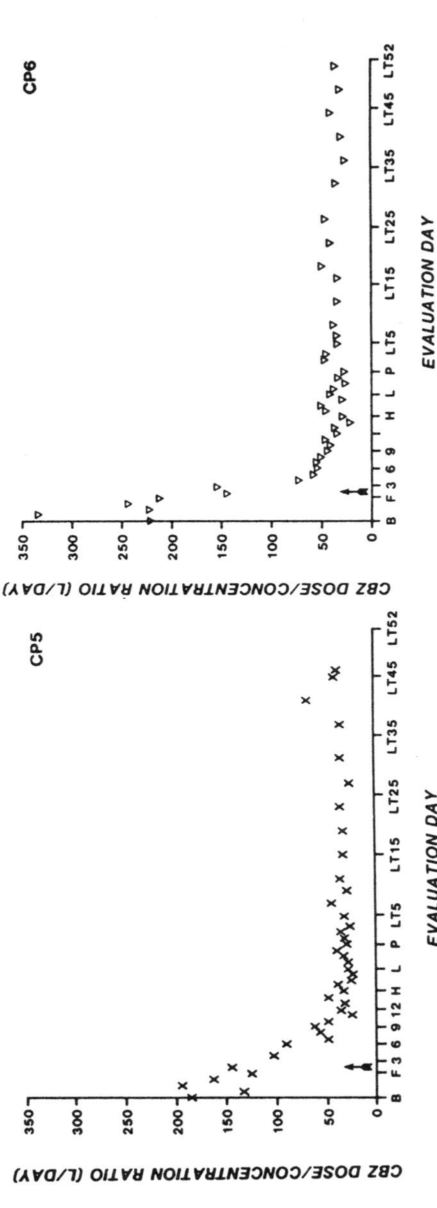

FIG. 6-3. Carbamazepine dose/concentration ratios for six patients before and after the addition of nafimidone. The F visit represented the first hospital day. Nafimidone was begun on the second hospital day, at which time the ratios began to fall as nafimidone doses were increased. Inhibition of carbamazepine elimination persisted throughout the first year of long-term follow-up. Patient CP4 did not enter long-term follow-up.

Table 6-2. Serum Concentrations and Estimated Elimination Rates of Phenytoin During Baseline, Outpatient Observation, and Long-term Follow-up Phases of the Study

Patient/weight	Phase of study	Mean daily dose (mg)	Mean trough [PHT]s[a] (μg/ml)	Mean estimated dose/concentration ratio (l/d)	Percentage of decline in ratio from baseline
CP1/69 kg	Baseline	500	26.5±1.7	19±1	
	Observation	200	19.3±1.6	10±1	45
	Long-term (53 wks)	224	12.0±3.2	21±9	−11
CP2/80 kg	Baseline	500	28.2±0.7	18±1	
	Observation	200	22.4±2.6	10±1	49
	Long-term (52 wks)	200	12.5±3.9	19±9	− 5
CP3/67 kg	Baseline	230	11.2±2.3	22±5	
	Observation	75	17.8±7.3	5±1	77
	Long-term (52 wks)	90	13.6±3.3	7±2	67
CP4/69 kg	Baseline	400	21.7±2.0	19±2	
	Observation	175	16.9±7.2	12±3	38
CP5/69 kg	Baseline	400	14.5±1.6	28±3	
	Observation	200	14.1±1.8	14±2	49
	Long-term (46 wks)	201	15.8±2.8	13±2	53
CP6/71 kg	Baseline	450	12.2±2.8	40±12	
	Observation	223	11.2±4.1	22± 7	44
	Long-term (52 wks)	270	13.1±3.9	22± 5	45

The observation phase was 8 weeks. The duration of long-term follow-up is indicated in the table for each patient.
Reproduced from Trieman and Ben-Menachem (11) with permission.
[a]Phenytoin steady-state concentration.

Table 6-3. Mean Carbamazepine Serum Concentrations

Patient	Baseline (4 weeks)	Observation (8 weeks)	Percentage of change	Long-term follow-up (19–56 weeks)	Percentage of change
CP1	5.8	12.0	108	7.2	24
CP2	4.6	12.0	162	6.8	50
CP3	6.2	11.3	82	9.4	52
CP4	4.7	8.7	85	—	—
CP5	5.4	9.6	79	9.2	72
CP6	4.1	8.5	108	9.2	96
WP2	4.9	11.9	143	—	—
WP4	8.9	10.8	21	8.2	−8
WP5	5.5	12.8	133	9.0	64

mals, normal volunteers, and epileptic patients in Late Phase I pilot studies?

4. When should studies of pharmacodynamic drug interactions be done?

STRUCTURE–ACTIVITY RELATIONSHIPS AND DRUG INTERACTIONS

Certain classes of compounds have a predictable inhibitory or inductive effect on the metabolism of other drugs. It thus should be possible to predict, on the basis of similarities of chemical structure, that compounds belonging to that same chemical class are likely to have similar effects. An important characteristic of nafimidone is that it is a substituted imidazole compound. In 1972, Wilkinson and his colleagues demonstrated that many 1- and 4(5)-substituted lipophilic imidazoles are potent inhibitors of hepatic microsomal epoxidation and hydroxylation, due to their capacity to bind both cytochrome P-450 and closely related substrate binding sites (5,6). 1-Alkylated imidazoles have also been shown to be potent inhibitors of cholesterol biosynthesis in vitro (7) and of liver microsomal drug oxidations (8). Certain 1-arylimidazoles are inhibitors of adrenal steroid hydroxylases (9). An awareness of these observations would have led to the prediction that compounds containing the imidazole moiety might be potent inhibitors of the metabolism of antiepileptic drugs. In addition to nafimidone, two other imidazole compounds that are used clinically have been shown to inhibit the metabolism of phenytoin and carbamazepine. Iyer and Kutty (10) reported an elevation of phenytoin levels when metronidazole was added to patients' therapeutic regimens. Cimetidine, an imidazole guanidine, is widely prescribed for the treatment of peptic ulcer disease because of its ability to antagonize histamine H2 receptors. This

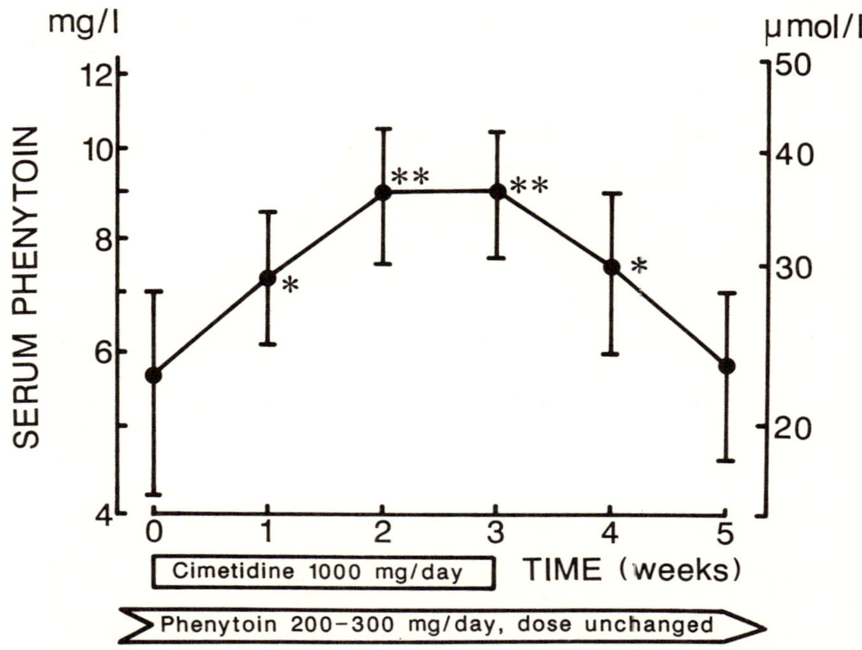

FIG. 6-4. Effect of cimetidine on serum phenytoin concentration in nine patients after 2–4 months on phenytoin (mean ± SEM). Asterisk indicates significant difference (p < 0.05 *; < 0.01 **) from values at 0 and 5 weeks. [Reproduced from Neuvonen et al. (14) with permission.]

compound has been reported to inhibit the metabolism of phenytoin and carbamazepine in a number of studies (11–18). Neuvonen et al. (11) studied the effect of cimetidine on serum phenytoin concentrations in nine patients who had been stabilized on fixed doses of phenytoin for 2–4 months. They demonstrated a significant increase in phenytoin concentrations within 2 weeks after the addition of 1,000 mg/day cimetidine (Fig. 6-4). The phenytoin concentrations returned to baseline within 2 weeks after cimetidine was discontinued. Bartle et al. (14) observed a concentration-dependent inhibition of phenytoin elimination after a 250-mg dose was given intravenously in eight normal volunteers who had been treated with 1,200 or 2,400 mg of cimetidine for 3 days (Fig. 6-5).

Similar effects have been observed on carbamazepine metabolism. Grasela and Rocci (17) studied the effect of cimetidine on carbamazepine elimination after the administration of a 25 mg/kg dose of carbamazepine given intravenously concomitantly with 50 mg/kg of cimetidine in Sprague-Dawley rats. They observed a mean reduction in the slope of the elimination curve of 45% compared with that of the control rats, which only

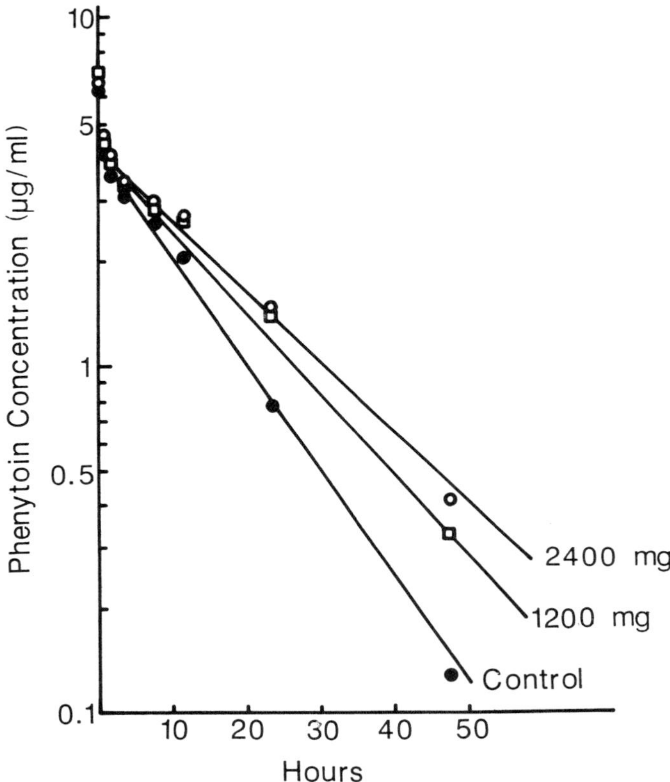

FIG. 6-5. Plasma phenytoin concentrations following a 250-mg intravenous injection before and after 3 days of 1,200-mg and 2,400-mg cimetidine. Data are from one representative subject. [Reproduced from Bartle et al. (14) with permission.]

received carbamazepine (Fig. 6-6). There was a 40% reduction in the clearance of carbamazepine and an 82% increase in the half-life of carbamazepine after the addition of cimetidine.

IN VITRO MICROSOMAL METABOLISM

If the structure of an experimental antiepileptic drug suggests that it is likely to have an inhibitory effect on the metabolism of phenytoin, carbamazepine, or any other antiepileptic drug that is anticipated as a co-medication in a clinical trial, then the possibility of such a drug–drug interaction may be tested initially in vitro using a hepatic microsomal system. Such studies should be carried out prior to in vivo studies of such pharmacokinetic interactions. Unfortunately, in vitro studies, followed by ani-

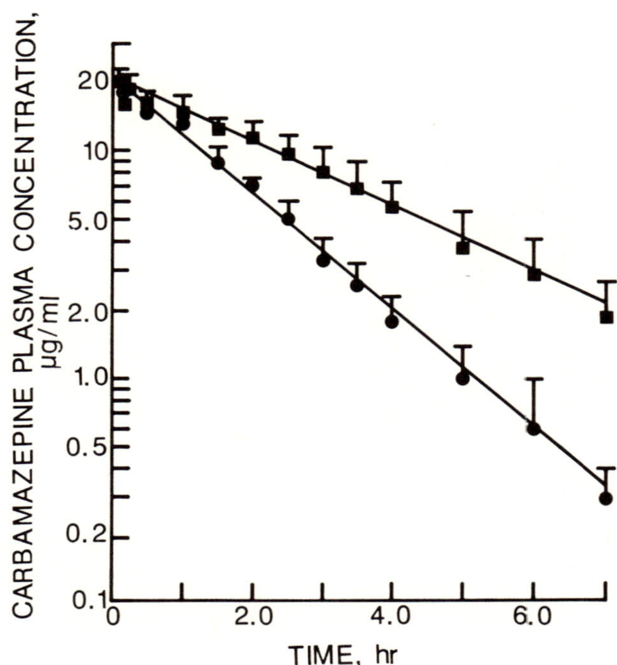

FIG. 6-6. Mean ± SD carbamazepine plasma concentrations following a 25-mg/kg intravenous dose of carbamazepine (closed circles) and in combination with a 50-mg/kg intravenous dose of cimetidine (closed boxes) in rats. There was a 45% reduction in the slope of the elimination curve from the cimetidine treated animals. [Reproduced from Graselai and Rocci (17) with permission.]

mal studies, followed by studies in normal volunteers, followed by studies in patients, is not always carried out in this order. For example, because of our observation of an inhibition of carbamazepine and phenytoin metabolism by nafimidone in our pilot study, Kapetanovic and Kupferberg (19) examined the effects of nafimidone and its metabolite (reduced nafimidone) on p-hydroxylation of phenytoin using hepatic microsomes from rats pretreated with phenytoin. Figure 6-7 graphically demonstrates the inhibition of p-hydroxylation of phenytoin to HPPH in the absence of, and in the presence of, reduced nafimidone. The inhibition of microsomal, p-hydroxylation of phenytoin by nafimidone and reduced nafimidone was concentration-dependent for the effect of both nafimidone and reduced nafimidone. Table 6-4 shows the effect of rising concentrations of nafimidone and its metabolite on microsomal p-hydroxylation. A marked inhibition of p-hydroxylation of phenytoin occurred at submicromolar concentrations of nafimidone or its metabolite. This is an important observation

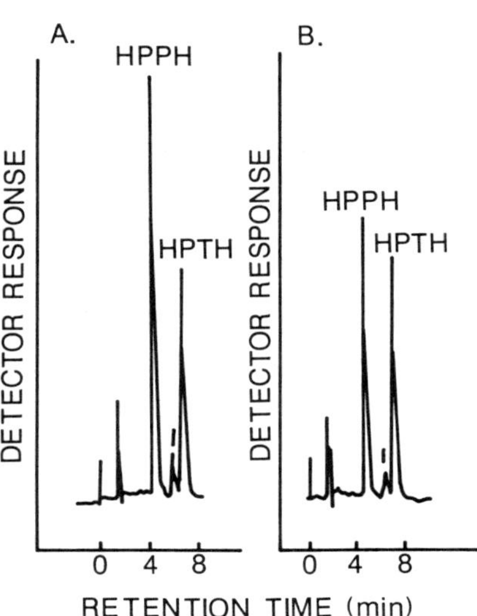

FIG. 6-7. Graphic demonstration of the inhibition of parahydroxylation of phenytoin HPPC by reduced nafimidone. Panel A demonstrates the high-performance liquid-chromatogram of extracts of microsomal p-hydroxylation of phenytoin in the absence of reduced nafimidone, whereas Panel B illustrates the high-performance liquid-chromatogram in the presence of reduced nafimidone. [Reproduced from Kapetanovic and Kupferberg (19) with permission.]

Table 6-4.   Concentration-Dependent Inhibition of Microsomal p-Hydroxylation of Phenytoin by Nafimidone and Reduced Nafimidone

Phenytoin (μM)	Inhibitor	Inhibitor (μM)	Inhibition (%)
3.17	Nafimidone	0.15	11.0
3.17	Metabolite	0.15	23.5
3.17	Nafimidone	0.29	35.6
3.17	Metabolite	0.29	47.4
3.17	Nafimidone	1.17	72.3
3.17	Metabolite	1.09	70.9
23.8	Nafimidone	0.15	27.6
23.8	Metabolite	0.15	32.2
23.8	Nafimidone	0.29	41.6
23.8	Metabolite	0.29	50.9
23.8	Nafimidone	1.17	69.2
23.8	Metabolite	1.17	77.6

Reproduced from Kapetanovic and Kupferberg (19) with permission.

because in order to extrapolate the results of in vitro microsomal metabolism studies to animals and man, the concentration at which an inhibitory effect is demonstrated should be equal to or lower than the free-drug concentration, which is likely to be seen by the hepatic microsomes in in vivo studies. Kapetanovic and Kupferberg have also used similar techniques to demonstrate inhibition of phenobarbital p-hydroxylation by valproate (20).

The studies cited above demonstrate that much can be learned about potential drug–drug interactions from microsomal metabolism studies. If add-on clinical trials of antiepileptic drugs that use specific standard concomitant antiepileptic drugs for specific seizure types are to be done, then in vitro studies of inhibition of microsomal metabolism should be routinely carried out on those drugs planned for use as concomitant drugs.

IN VIVO PHARMACOKINETIC STUDIES

Much information regarding possible drug–drug interactions between an experimental and standard antiepileptic drug can be gained by carrying out in vivo pharmacokinetic studies of the two drugs alone and when given in combination. Such studies are traditionally performed during the Phase I clinical evaluation of a new antiepileptic drug. However, there is no reason that pharmacokinetic studies, using designs similar to those planned for humans, could not be carried out initially in small animals in order to predict possible drug–drug interactions in man.

The argument is sometimes made that it is difficult to extrapolate rat data to humans, and thus rat pharmacokinetic studies are of little value. However, such problems can be overcome, and pharmacokinetic studies in rats be made quite useful, if an effort is made to anticipate the plasma concentrations of the experimental drug that are likely to be studied during human trials. In 1969 Brodie and Reid (21) addressed the problem of extrapolating animal data to humans. They pointed out, ". . . there are vast individual and species differences in the metabolism of a large number of pharmacodynamic agents, but in many instances the pharmacological responses are similar for equal plasma levels of drug. This suggests that receptors for this type of drug may be quite similar in various mammalian species." This concept, which has become known as the Brodie-Reid hypothesis, appears to be valid for antiepileptic drugs, as indicated in Table 6-5 (22). From Table 6-5 it can be seen that the effective therapeutic range when these drugs are used for the treatment of partial onset seizures in humans is similar to the therapeutic range observed for various experimental models of epilepsy in animals.

The experimental models listed in Table 6-5 are all models of chronic epilepsy. We have recently demonstrated that plasma antiepileptic drug concentrations effective in stopping generalized convulsive status epilep-

Table 6-5. Therapeutic Range of Antiepileptic Drugs in Partial-Onset Seizures and Experimental Models of Epilepsy

Experimental model	Phenytoin[a]	Phenobarbital[a]	Primidone[a]	Carbamazepine[a]	Valproate[a]
Human: partial onset and GTC seizures	10–25	15–45	6–12	4–12	50–150
Photomyoclonus					
Papio papio	10–20	15–25	8–12	effective	
Epileptic fowl	8–14	4–14	<22		105–250
Alumina cream (monkeys)	5–21	10–25	Traces–4; 10–25 (PB)	>2	50–150
Kindled seizures (baboons and cats)	10–30	20–25		10–12	50–150

Modified from Woodbury (22).
[a] Serum concentrations in μg/ml.

Table 6-6. Effect of Various Antiepileptic Drugs in the Treatment of Experimental Secondarily Generalized Convulsive Status Epilepticus in the Rat

					Response to treatment[a]		
Drug	No.	Dose/kg body weight	Mean serum concentration/ml (range)	Mean time (min) from treatment to sample (range)	No success	Partial success	Complete success
Phenytoin	7	100–150 mg	19.4 μg (8.2–29.5)	79.9 (58–153)	2/7	4/7	1/7
Phenobarbital	3	60 mg	64.3 μg (58.1–67.7)	78.0 (68–97)	0/3	1/3	2/3
Diazepam	3	2.5 mg	40 ng (38–41)	164.5 (145–184)	2/3	1/3	0/3
Diazepam	3	5.0 mg	137 ng (91–166)	101.0 (68–161)	0/3	2/3	1/3
Lorazepam	6	2.5 mg	539 ng (197–795)	64.0 (59–70)	0/6	1/6	5/6
Propylene glycol	4	0.2–1.5 ml	n/a	n/a	4/4	0/4	0/4

Reproduced from Walton and Treiman (23) with permission.

[a] No success—both behavioral and electrical seizures continued. Partial success—behavioral seizures stopped, ictal activity continued on EEG. Complete success—both behavioral and electrical seizures stopped.

ticus in the rat are approximately the same as those necessary to stop generalized convulsive status epilepticus in humans (23). These data are illustrated in Table 6-6.

The data presented in Tables 6-5 and 6-6 suggest that information gained in animal studies can be extrapolated to humans if care is taken to carry out the animal studies at plasma levels comparable to those anticipated in humans, even if this means that the animals receive markedly different doses of the drug than anticipated for man.

Recently published data suggest that the Brodie-Reid hypothesis should be extended from a consideration of the total plasma concentration of a drug to a consideration of the concentration of free or unbound drug. Macdonald and McLean (24) have demonstrated that drug suppression of sustained repetitive firing of action potentials that have been induced by intercellularly applied current pulses in spinal cord neurons correlates well with the ability of the test drug to inhibit maximal electroshock seizures. Effectiveness of an antiepileptic drug in protecting against maximal electroshock seizures is a good predictor of the effectiveness of that drug against partial onset seizures in man. Macdonald and McLean showed that drugs such as phenytoin and carbamazepine are able to inhibit sustained repetitive firing in neuron tissue cultures at concentrations that approximate free levels of these drugs in man (24). Figure 6-8 demonstrates the concentration dependence of limitation of repetitive firing of spinal cord neurons by phenytoin and carbamazepine. The effect appears maximal at 2 μg/ml for phenytoin and 1 μg/ml for carbamazepine. Both these drugs

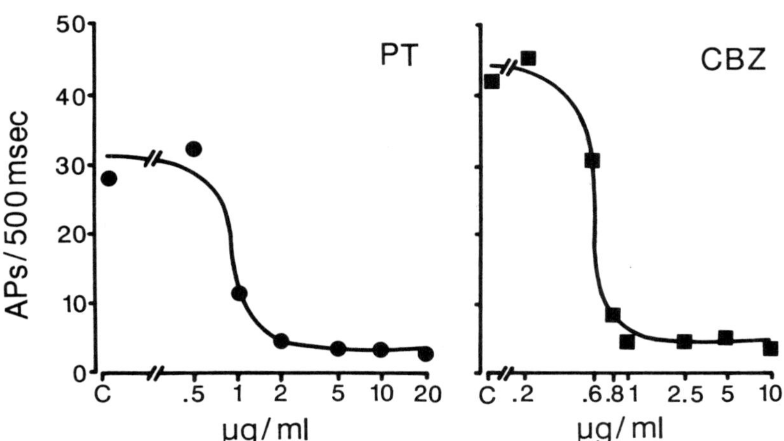

FIG. 6-8. Concentration dependence of limitation of repetitive firing of spinal cord neurons by phenytoin and carbamazepine. Reductions occurred at therapeutic CSF concentrations (1–2 μg/ml for phenytoin; 0.8 to 5 μg/ml for carbamazepine). [Reproduced from Macdonald and McLean (24) with permission.]

are approximately 90% protein-bound. Therefore, these concentrations are comparable to the free concentrations observed in man when total concentrations are 20 μg/ml for phenytoin and 10 μg/ml for carbamazepine.

A consideration of this extension of the Brodie-Reid hypothesis suggests that in order to carry out studies of antiepileptic drugs in animals that will yield the most information regarding drug behavior in humans, the animal experiments need to be designed to achieve concentrations of unbound drug comparable to those anticipated to be necessary in human studies. The same rationale can be used to predict what free level should be sought in human studies in order to achieve a desired clinical effect. Thus, study in Macdonald's system of an experimental drug that is effective against maximal electroshock seizures should allow prediction of the free-drug concentration in man necessary to be effective against partial-onset seizures.

In order to achieve comparable free concentrations of the drug under study in animals and in man, protein-binding studies will be necessary. Such studies can be carried out without difficulty in small animals and in man. Furthermore, technology is now available to measure free, as well as total, plasma concentrations of standard antiepileptic drugs (25). The same technology can be used to measure unbound concentrations of experimental drugs.

The practical impact of these concepts is that drug interaction and Phase I pilot efficacy studies should be carried out using fixed plasma concentrations (adjusted to give comparable free drug concentrations) rather than fixed doses in order to extrapolate study results across species and to reduce the effect of pharmacokinetic heterogeneity. Pharmacokinetic heterogeneity is a major problem in the design of drug trials in human subjects. For some drugs there may be large differences in pharmacokinetic parameters between two individuals. Single-dose pharmacokinetic data from a recently completed Late Phase I study of the experimental antiepileptic drug, flunarizine, are shown in Table 6-7 (26). Tenfold differences in clearance rates and volumes of distribution were observed among the 12 patients. If a rising dose design rather than a rising plasma concentration design had been used in this study, there would have been tenfold differences in plasma concentrations of the drug when the patients were given comparable doses.

ELIMINATION

Single-dose pharmacokinetic studies of a new drug provide essential information regarding absorption, distribution, and metabolism. When such studies are carried out when the experimental drug is added to a pre-existing antiepileptic drug, comparison of results from the two studies can

Table 6-7.   Single-Dose Pharmacokinetics of Flunarizine After a 30-mg Oral Dose in 12 Adult Patients

Patient	Peak (h)	$t_{1/2}-1$(h)	$t_{1/2}-2$(h)	$t_{1/2}-3$(h)	C1 (L/h)	VD (L)
J01	2.0	3.03	53.72	582.35	18.94	15,916
J02	1.5	2.24	42.26	422.56	23.72	14,463
J03	1.5	1.45	6.93	153.32	62.11	13,741
J04	3.0	2.44	44.42	287.55	25.56	10,606
J07	2.0	1.68	29.36	211.28	21.88	5,897
J08	1.5	1.96	25.48	422.56	38.28	20,920
J09	2.0				5.64	1,959
J12	3.0	3.65	25.96	455.92	32.27	15,587
J15	3.0	1.82	12.93	435.85	30.77	16,814
J17	1.5	1.47	10.07	417.47	26.39	15,615
J14	2.0	1.89	11.12	477.93	25.47	19,895
J16	1.5				61.82	5,437
Mean	2.04	2.16	26.23	386.68	31.07	13,071
SD	0.59	0.67	15.47	123.45	15.75	5,662

provide important information regarding possible drug–drug interactions. Such studies should be carried out initially without other antiepileptic drugs, in animals and normal volunteers, in order to define (a) whether the drug is eliminated following a 1-, 2-, or 3-compartment model, (b) the half-lives of the distribution and various elimination phases, (c) the clearance, and (d) the volume of distribution. Single-dose studies in both drug-free and co-medicated animals can be carried out to provide information regarding possible drug interactions. Studies in normal volunteers do not allow determination of the effect of chronic co-medication on a new drug being tested. However, normal volunteer data obtained from drug-free patients can be compared with single-dose pharmacokinetic data obtained from co-medicated epileptic patients during Late Phase I studies in order to ascertain whether there is any interaction between the experimental drug and the co-medication. In all of these studies the pharmacokinetic parameters should be determined for both the experimental drug and the concomitant drug, because it is important to know whether either drug has an effect on the pharmacokinetic behavior of the other drug.

Table 6-8 provides the serum half-life of nafimidone alcohol for six patients who were treated with 550 mg/day or 600 mg/day of nafimidone for 6–16 weeks (27). The mean half-life of nafimidone alcohol in these patients was 3.3 h, compared with about 8 h in normal volunteers (2). These data suggest that the metabolism of nafimidone alcohol was induced by the co-medications phenytoin and/or carbamazepine. An alternative ex-

Table 6-8. Nafimidone Alcohol Serum Half-life Following a 200-mg Oral Dose of Nafimidone[a]

Patient	$t_{1/2}(h)$	r
DH	3.14	0.99
GS	2.43	0.95
JS	5.26	0.99
SM	3.29	0.99
AH	3.08	0.99
WB	2.76	0.83
Mean ± SD	3.33 ± 1.00	

Reproduced from Treiman and Gunawan (27) with permission.

[a] 550–600 mg/day for 6–16 weeks.

planation is that nafimidone induced its own metabolism, because the first half-life was determined 6–16 weeks following the start of treatment with nafimidone. However, when the serum half-life of nafimidone alcohol was determined after short-term (9–10 weeks) and long-term (127–152 weeks) maintenance therapy with nafimidone at a dose of 600 mg/day, there was no difference in the mean half-lives between the two groups (Table 6-9). This suggests that, if autoinduction occurred in this group of four patients co-medicated with carbamazepine only, it must have occurred early in the nafimidone treatment period.

In addition to single-dose pharmacokinetic studies, dose interval clearance studies should be carried out at fixed plasma concentration increments. Again, such studies can be done initially in animals and later repeated in patients in late Phase I studies. Dose-interval clearances should be determined for both the experimental drug and the co-medication in order to determine whether there is an effect of one of the drugs on the metabolism of the other. By using rising increments of drug concentration, if there is an effect of the experimental drug on the metabolism of the co-medication, it can then be ascertained whether such an effect is concentration dependent.

DISTRIBUTION

Prior to the initiation of controlled clinical trials it is important to determine if there is an interaction due to competition for serum protein-binding sites between concomitant antiepileptic drugs and the experimental antiepileptic drug. Although the degree of protein binding may be different between animal models and man, in general there is a rough correspondence in the degree of binding among various species. There-

Table 6-9. Nafimidone Alcohol Half-life After Short- and Long-term Maintenance Therapy with Nafimidone[a]

Patient	$t_{1/2}(h)$	
	9–10 weeks	127–152 weeks
DA	2.01	2.89
KP	2.00	1.63
WB	2.76	2.41
WR	2.16	1.70
Mean ± SD	2.23 ± 0.36	2.16 ± 0.60

Reproduced from Treiman and Gunawan (27) with permission.
[a] 600 mg/day.

fore, if studies of protein binding and of free-drug concentrations are first done in animals, with and without the concomitant antiepileptic drugs, such studies should have the ability to predict, at least qualitatively, whether such drug interactions are likely to be observed in human patients. When such studies are done in man, they should be done at the plasma concentrations anticipated for use in the controlled clinical trial. Such studies are particularly likely to be useful in a trial that involves two drugs that are highly protein bound, especially if drugs are given in gram, as opposed to milligram, doses. Thus protein-binding studies and studies of free-drug concentrations are particularly important when designing controlled clinical trials that involve such drugs as valproic acid, which is not only highly protein bound, but is used at such high serum concentrations that it has the potential of saturating serum protein-binding sites.

PHARMACODYNAMIC STUDIES

Studies of pharmacodynamic drug–drug interactions are far more difficult to quantitate than studies of pharmacokinetic interactions. However, methods described by Bourgeois (28) and by Swinyard (29) in this volume provide an approach to the quantitative assessment of potential pharmacodynamic interactions between antiepileptic drugs. Using techniques such as described in Chapters 14 and 19, it should be possible to carry out in vivo pharmacodynamic studies in experimental animals to predict such interactions in human patients. When such studies are carried out it is important to adjust doses and routes of administration such that concentrations of unbound drug available to the receptor binding sites approximate those anticipated to be necessary in the treatment of human patients. Furthermore, there is a need for the development of techniques for the study of antiepileptic drug efficacy and particularly toxicity in experimental animals that more closely approximate human responses. The maximal electroshock and pentylenetetrazol screening tests developed by Swinyard et al., as well as the rotorod test for toxicity, have been extremely useful for screening large numbers of compounds for antiepileptic drug efficacy and toxicity (30–32). However, in order to carry out pharmacodynamic interaction studies that have better predictive value for human studies, other techniques need to be developed. This is particularly important in relation to the potential of antiepileptic drugs for cognitive and behavioral toxicity, neither of which is measured by the rotorod test.

CONCLUSIONS

Because of ethical constraints that require that new and unproven experimental antiepileptic drugs be tested in man as add-on studies, drug–drug interactions are likely to be seen in controlled clinical trials. In order to anticipate such drug interactions, so that neither patient safety nor the power of a study to detect a potentially effective antiepileptic drug is compromised, it is important to identify such potential drug–drug interactions before controlled clinical trials are begun. Many drug interactions can be predicted from the structure of a compound if other structurally similar members of the same chemical class have been observed to have inductive or inhibitory effects on the metabolism of other drugs. In vitro studies of the effect of a new drug on the microsomal metabolism of other drugs can be carried out and have the benefit of predicting inhibitory effects on epoxidation and hydroxylation metabolic pathways that are mediated by cytochrome P-450 and other hepatic enzymes. Single-dose pharmacokinetic and dose interval clearance studies of an experimental drug, with or without a concomitant antiepileptic drug, can and should be carried out in experimental animals prior to Phase I clinical studies in humans. When such studies are planned, they should be done using drug doses designed so that concentrations of unbound drug approximate those anticipated to be appropriate for the human studies. Such studies, in combination with efficacy studies in experimental animals, can be used to project appropriate target concentrations of unbound drug for the human studies. Pharmacodynamic drug interaction studies can also be done in experimental animals and should also be planned with attention to optimal concentrations of unbound drug.

Table 6-10 summarizes the stages in antiepileptic drug development at which various drug–drug interactions should be performed. The systematic incorporation of such studies into the development of antiepileptic drugs would result in a modest increase in the time required before such drugs could first be tested in humans. However, by avoiding unanticipated drug–drug interactions that may require the repetition of expen-

Table 6-10.   Recommendation for Pre-Trial Evaluation of Antiepileptic Drug Interactions

	In vitro	Animal in vivo	Early phase I (volunteers)	Late phase I (patients)
Structure/activity	X			
Microsomal metabolism	X			
Pharmacokinetic interactions				
Absorbtion			X	
Distribution		X	X	
Elimination		X		X
Pharmacodynamic interactions				
Efficacy		X		X
Toxicity		X		X

sive clinical trials, a systematic study of potential drug–drug interactions during preclinical and Phase I antiepileptic drug development may have the effect that useful new antiepileptic drugs may actually be brought to the market earlier than is possible under the current system of nonsystematic and relatively haphazard early study of potential drug–drug interactions.

Acknowledgment: Support for studies from which some of the data were cited was provided in part by Contracts NO1-NS-81-2377, T.O. #1 and #2 from the Epilepsy Branch NINCDS; by USPHSCRC Grant RROO865; and by grants from Syntex Research.

REFERENCES

1. Guidelines for clinical evaluation of anticonvulsant drugs. FDA Publication No. 77-3045, Sept., 1977.
2. Buhles WC, Wallach MB, Chaplin MD, Treiman DM. Nafimidone. In: Meldrum BS, Porter RJ, eds. *New Anticonvulsant Drugs.* London: John Libbey, 1986:203–14.
3. Treiman DM, Wilensky AJ, Ben-Menachem E, et al. Efficacy of nafimidone in the treatment of intractable partial seizures: report of a two-center pilot study. *Epilepsia* 1985;26:607–11.
4. Treiman DM, Ben-Menachem E. Inhibition of carbamazepine and phenytoin metabolism by nafimidone, a new antiepileptic drug. *Epilepsia* 1987;28:699–705.
5. Wilkinson CF, Hetnarski K. Imidazole derivatives—a new class of microsomal enzyme inhibitors. *Biochem Pharmacol* 1972;21:3187–92.
6. Wilkinson CF, Hetnarski K, Hicks LJ. Substituted imidazoles as inhibitors of

microsomal oxidation and insecticide synergists. *Pesticide Biochem Physiol* 1973;4:299–312.

7. Atkin SD, Morgan B, Baggaley KH, Green J. The isolation of 2,3-oxidosqualene from the liver of rats treated with 1-dodecylimidazole, a novel hypocholesterolaemic agent. *Biochem J* 1972;130:153–7.
8. Palmer ED, Cawthorne MA. The effects of l-alkylimidazoles on hepatic drug-metabolizing enzyme activity. *Xenobiotica* 1974;4:209–17,
9. Johnson AL, Kauer JC, Sharma DC, Dorfman RI. The synthesis of 1-arylimidazoles, a new class of steroid hydroxylation inhibitors. *J Med Chem* 1969;12:1024–8.
10. Iyer KS, Kutty AG. Influence of metronidazole and chloral hydrate on the activity of other drugs. *Indian J Physiol Pharmacol* 1974;18:49–52.
11. Neuvonen PJ, Tokola RA, Kaste M. Cimetidine-phenytoin interaction: effect on serum phenytoin concentration and antipyrine test. *Eur J Pharmacol* 1981;21:215–20.
12. Hetzel DJ, Bochner F, Hallpike JF, Shearman DJC, Hann CS. Cimetidine interaction with phenytoin. *Br Med J* 1981;282:1512.
13. Algozzine GJ, Stewart RB, Springer PK. Decreased clearance of phenytoin with cimetidine. *Ann Intern Med* 1981;95:244–5.
14. Bartle WR, Walker SE, Shapero T. Dose-dependent effect of cimetidine on phenytoin kinetics. *Clin Pharmacol Ther* 1983;33:649–55.
15. Salem RB, Breland BD, Mishra SK, Jordan JE. Effect of cimetidine on phenytoin serum levels. *Epilepsia* 1983;24:284–88.
16. Telerman-Toppet N, Duret ME, Coers C. Cimetidine interaction with carbamazepine. *Ann Intern Med* 1981;94–544.
17. Grasela DM, Rocci ML Jr. Inhibition of carbamazepine metabolism by cimetidine. *Drug Metab Dispos* 1984;12:204–8.
18. Sonne J, Luhdorf K, Larsen NE, Andreasen PB. Lack of interaction between cimetidine and carbamazepine. *Acta Neurol Scand* 1983;68:253–6.
19. Kapetanovic IM, Kupferberg HJ. Nafimidone, an imidazole anticonvulsant, and its metabolite as potent inhibitors of microsomal metabolism of phenytoin and carbamazepine. *Drug Metab Dispos* 1984;12:560–4.
20. Kapetanovic IM, Kupferberg HJ. Inhibitions of microsomal phenobarbital metabolism by valproic acid. *Biochem Pharmacol* 1981;30:1361–3.
21. Brodie BB, Reid WD. Is man a unique animal in response to drugs? *Am J Pharm* 1969X:21–7.
22. Woodbury DM. Convulsant drugs: mechanisms of action. In: Glaser GH, Penry JK, Woodbury DM, eds. *Antiepileptic Drugs: Mechanisms of Action*. New York: Raven Press, 1980:249–303. (Advances in neurology; vol 27.)
23. Walton NY, Treiman DM. Experimental secondarily generalized convulsive status epilepticus induced by D,L-homocysteine thiolactone. *Epilepsy Res* 1988:2;79–86.
24. MacDonald RL, McLean MJ. Anticonvulsant drugs: mechanisms of action. In: Delgado-Escueta AV, Ward AA, Woodbury DM, Porter RJ, eds. *Advances in Neurology: Basic Mechanisms of the Epilepsies: Molecular and Cellular Approach*. New York: Raven Press, 1986;44:713–36. (Advances in neurology; vol 44.)
25. Cramer JA. Practical considerations and techniques used to monitor free drug

levels. In: Porter RJ ed. *Advances in Epileptology, 15th Epilepsy International Symposium.* New York: Raven Press, 1984;143–8.

26. Treiman DM, DeGiorgio CM, Kapetanovic I, Kupferberg H. Single dose and steady state pharmacokinetics of flunarizine in epileptic patients. *Epilepsia* 1986;27:649.

27. Treiman DM, Gunawan S. Pharmacokinetics of nafimidone in patients with chronic intractable epilepsy. *Clin Pharmacokinet* 1987;12:433–9.

28. Bourgeois BFD, Dodson WE. Antiepileptic and neurotoxic interactions between antiepileptic drugs. In: Pitlick WH, ed. *Antiepileptic Drug Interactions.* New York: Demos Publications, 1989:209–19.

29. Swinyard EA, Woodhead JJ, Wolf HH. Use of isobolograms in predicting drug interactions. In: Pitlick WH, ed. *Antiepileptic Drug Interactions.* New York: Demos Publications, 1989:261–75.

30. Swinyard EA. Laboratory assay of clinically effective antiepileptic drugs. *Am Pharm Assoc* 1949;38:201–4.

31. Swinyard EA. Introduction. In: Woodbury DM, Penry JK, Pippenger CE, eds. *Antiepileptic Drugs.* New York: Raven Press, 1982:1–9.

32. Swinyard EA, Kupferberg HJ. Antiepileptic drugs: detection quantification and evaluation. *Fed Proc* 1985;44:2629–33.

7

Interactions Between Novel and Standard Antiepileptic Drugs in Clinical Trials: Progabide, Felbamate, and MK-801

Ilo E. Leppik

University of Minnesota,
Minneapolis, Minnesota, U.S.A.

INTRODUCTION

Phase II clinical studies are performed to determine the efficacy and safety of novel antiepileptic compounds (1). For reasons detailed elsewhere in this volume (2), the most common designs for these studies involve protocols in which the novel compound is added to existing antiepileptic drug treatment. Unfortunately, these designs permit a number of interactions in the pharmacokinetic and pharmacodynamic arenas (Table 7-1). Appropriately sophisticated clinical trials must be designed and performed to fully factor in all of the potential confounding variables.

In the pharmacokinetic arena, interactions include alteration in absorption, distribution, protein binding, and elimination. Although phase I clinical trials ideally should detect these interactions (3) and animal in vivo and in vitro models may give some information regarding potential interactions (4), phase II clinical trials must be prepared to deal with interactions that have been predicted or be able to detect interactions that might have gone unnoticed. Concentrations of the novel drug may be increased or decreased by a standard drug, and the concentration of a standard drug may in turn be increased or decreased by the novel drug. Furthermore, each standard drug may have opposite effects on the novel drug and vice versa. Thus, phenytoin (PHT) might increase the concentrations of a novel drug, whereas carbamazepine (CBZ) does just the opposite. In any study

Table 7-1. Summary of the Possible Interactions Between a Novel and a Standard
Antiepileptic Agent[a]

Effect of novel agent	Increase	Decrease	No change
Pharmacokinetic			
Absorption	X	X	X
Distribution	X	X	X
Protein binding	X	X	X
Clearance	X	X	X
Pharmacodynamic			
Receptor site for			
efficacy	X	X	X
Receptor site for			
side-effects	X	X	X

[a]The standard agent may affect the novel substance as well. Introduction of a second standard antiepileptic compound complicates the pattern even more.

of efficacy, it is important to maintain the concentrations of the concomitant medications within a narrow range of the baseline concentrations to avoid erroneous interpretation of results. The classic example is that of sulthiame being judged to be an effective substance before it was determined that it could elevate PHT concentrations (5). A more recent example is that of progabide, where a double-blind study in which PHT levels were controlled showed no significant efficacy (6), contradicting results from previous studies in which PHT concentrations were not controlled (7–9).

In this chapter, alterations of PHT and CBZ concentrations related to use of progabide (PGB) and felbamate (FBM) are discussed. In addition, some data regarding the effect of concomitant medication on MK-801 clearance is presented.

PROGABIDE

PGB is a synthetic compound with γ-aminobutyric acid (GABA)-agonist properties (10,11). A controlled study designed to evaluate the safety and efficacy of PGB was sponsored in the United States by the National Institutes of Health (NIH) (6). All patients in this study were required to have concomitant treatment with PHT and CBZ but no other antiepileptic drugs (AEDs). The 32 patients who completed the NIH protocol at the University of Minnesota were used for this analysis. There were 16 men and 16 women averaging 29 ± 6.0 years of age and 69.1 ± 11.2 kg. All patients had at least four partial complex seizures per month despite serum PHT and CBZ concentrations greater than 10 mg/L and 4 mg/L, respectively.

The study incorporated a randomized, double-blind, crossover, placebo-controlled design. After a stabilization period during which PHT and CBZ concentrations were brought into optimal ranges and patient compliance was verified, all patients entered a 2-month baseline period. PHT and CBZ dosage changes were not allowed during this baseline period. Serum PHT and CBZ concentrations were stable and were maintained within a range of 10–25 mg/L and 4–12 mg/L, respectively. Upon completion of baseline, patients were hospitalized for a 7–10-day period to receive Treatment I, which consisted of prior AED therapy plus either PGB or matching placebo. The PGB or placebo treatment was titrated upward to a total daily dosage of 25–30 mg/kg and administered in four divided doses. PGB and matching placebo were supplied as white, film-coated tablets by Lorex Pharmaceuticals, Inc. (Skokie, IL, U.S.A.). After 12 weeks in Treatment I, the patients were crossed over to Treatment II for another 12 weeks. During each hospitalization, blood samples were drawn prior to the morning AED doses. A protocol supplement permitted obtaining additional blood samples for CBZ and CBZ-epoxide (CBZ-E) concentrations at 1, 2, 4, 6, and 8 h after the morning dose. No medications were given during the sampling.

Patients used their own supply of PHT and CBZ during the baseline period. During the treatments, all medications were prepackaged in an ambulatory unit dose system. Each unit dose container was labeled with a patient's name, drug dosages, and dosing times to optimize medication compliance. Patients were seen in the clinic every 2 weeks throughout the entire study for evaluation of seizure control, drug side-effects, and determination of serum AED concentrations. Blood for drug assays was obtained at all clinic visits. The time between dose and blood collection was held constant for each patient throughout the study and ranged from 1 to 4 h among all patients. PHT and CBZ were measured by a standard gas–liquid chromatographic assay in a clinical toxicology laboratory that participates in a quality control program.

Throughout the study, serum PHT and CBZ concentrations were maintained within the range established at baseline for each patient, altering doses when necessary. Progabide doses were not altered. Target values were determined by the serum PHT and CBZ concentrations observed on visit 4, which was 6 weeks into the baseline period. The range was established as ± 25% of the target concentration. Previous reports have demonstrated that compliant patients have fluctuations in serum concentrations of less than 20% for PHT (12) and less than 25% for CBZ when sampling times are controlled (13). Medication counts and patient reports indicated that all subjects approached 100% compliance with their drug regimens. The serum PHT and CBZ concentrations obtained at each clinic visit were compared with the ranges established during baseline. Dosage changes for PHT or CBZ were initiated by the unblinded pharmacist if one or more of the following conditions were met: (a) if two consecutive serum concentrations were outside the established range, (b) if one serum concentration was above the upper boundary and the patient had symptoms of clinical toxicity, or (c) if the patient experienced side-effects that were verifiable by objective examination or sufficiently severe to be distressing to the patient.

Dosage adjustments were determined by an unblinded pharmacist. CBZ dosages were adjusted assuming linear pharmacokinetics. Since PHT follows nonlinear, capacity-linked pharmacokinetics, dosage changes were determined using a Bayesian forecasting technique (14). When a PHT dosage adjustment was indicated, the most recent serum concentration was used to determine a new dosage.

Data Analysis

The effect of PGB on the disposition of PHT and CBZ was analyzed in four ways: (a) the mean serum PHT and CBZ concentrations at the end of baseline were compared with those at the end of PGB and placebo treatments; (b) the number of patients requiring PHT and CBZ dosage adjustments during PGB treatment was compared with that during placebo treatment; (c) Serum PHT and CBZ concentrations/dose (C/D) ratios obtained during baseline were compared with C/D ratios during PGB and placebo treatments; and (d) Serum CBZ and CBZ-E concentrations from the area-under-the-concentration time curve (AUC) from Treatment I and Treatment II hospitalizations were compared.

A X^2 test was used to compare the frequency of dosage adjustments. A one-way analysis of variance (ANOVA) was used to test for differences in baseline, PGB, and placebo serum concentrations and C/D ratios. Student's t test was used to compare differences between groups of two. Significance was set at a $p < 0.05$. Nonlinear regression analysis was used to examine the relationship between increases in PHT concentration and variables such as patient age, weight, baseline PHT concentration, and PGB pharmacokinetics.

AUC was calculated for CBZ and CBZ-E using the trapezoidal rule (15). AUC data was available: (a) while receiving placebo, (b) after the first dose of PGB, and (c) at the end of the 10-week PGB treatment phase (steady state) for each patient. In addition to this intensive monitoring of serum concentrations, the serum concentrations obtained during clinic visits were evaluated. The mean of the four serum concentrations from the final 8 weeks of treatment phases was calculated, thus providing a mean CBZ concentration for each patient during active and placebo treatments. CBZ-E concentrations were not measured on the outpatient samples.

Sixty-nine percent (22 of 32) of the patients had PHT dosage changes during PGB treatment ($p < 0.001$) (16). All of these adjustments were dos-

Table 7-2.   Number of Patients Requiring Dosage Decreases by Treatment During Progabide Study

	Phenytoin[a]		Carbamazepine[b]	
	Progabide	Placebo	Progabide	Placebo
Decrease	22 (69%)	4 (12%)	5 (16%)	2 (6%)
No decrease	10 (31%)	28 (88%)	27 (84%)	30 (94%)

Data modified from Brundage et al. (16).
[a]$p < 0.001$.
[b]$p > 0.75$.

age decreases (Table 7-2). Twelve percent (4 of 32) of the patients had a PHT dosage decrease during placebo treatment. In 12 of the 22 patients who experienced a PHT dosage decrease during PGB treatment, the dosage was reduced due to two consecutive serum concentrations that exceeded the upper boundary. These patients may or may not have had signs or symptoms of toxicity. Six patients had increased serum PHT concentrations that remained within range, but the dose was reduced because PHT toxicity was suspected. More than 50% of the patients requiring a dosage change had their dosage reduced within 4 weeks of exposure to PGB. All patients requiring a dosage adjustment had their dosage reduced by week 10. These data indicate that the time course for this interaction to become apparent is variable but tends to occur within 4–6 weeks after PGB is started. The mean PHT dosage at the end of PGB treatment (384.7 mg/day) was less than that observed at the end of the baseline (404.7 mg/day) or placebo (395.1 mg/day) period, but the difference was not statistically significant.

The mean serum PHT concentrations at the end of baseline, placebo, and PGB treatments were statistically different ($p < 0.05$), but because of dose adjustments in both the placebo and PGB treatment periods, PHT values remained within 25% of baseline concentrations (Table 7-3). The

Table 7-3.   Maintenance of Target Serum Antiepileptic Drug Concentrations

	Baseline	Progabide	Placebo
Phenytoin (mean)	17.5 μg/ml	20.4 μg/ml[a]	16.8 μg/ml
SD	4.2	6.0	4.8
Carbamazepine (mean)	6.2 μg/ml	5.5 μg/ml	6.8 μg/ml
SD	1.9	1.9	2.2

Data modified from Brundage et al. (16).
[a]$p < 0.05$.

PHT C/D ratio during PGB treatment (0.055 ± 0.020) was significantly larger (p<0.05) than the baseline (0.044 ± 0.013) or placebo (0.044 ± 0.016) treatments.

All CBZ dosage adjustments were decreases. Adjustment was infrequent, 16% (5 of 32 patients) and 6% (2 of 32 patients), respectively (Table 7-2). Two patients had CBZ dosages decreased after two consecutive serum concentrations were above the upper boundary. Both of these patients were in placebo treatment at the time. The remaining five patients had reductions in CBZ dosage after reporting toxicity.

Of the 21 patients on whom AUC data were available, 16 had lower mean serum CBZ concentrations during the active treatment period as compared to placebo. This difference was statistically different (p=0.03, Wilcoxon Signed Rank). The mean downward deviation was 1.3 mg/L (26%) in 16 patients versus a 0.6 mg/L (9%) increase in four patients. One patient's average concentrations were identical during placebo and active treatment periods (17).

The Cpss values calculated from the inpatient AUC data confirmed this decrease in CBZ concentrations (Table 7-4). In comparison to placebo treatment, mean CBZ Cpss values were 10% lower after one dose of PGB and remained at this level for 3 months of active treatment. Individual CBZ Cpss concentrations decreased after one dose of PGB in 15 of 21 patients and at steady state in 12 of 21 patients. Mean CBZ-E Cpss values were 13% higher after one dose of PGB and rose further to 24% after 3 months of active treatment. Eighteen of 21 patients had an increase in CBZ-E Cpss after one dose of PGB, and 17 of these remained elevated at the end of the treatment period. Significant (p<0.0025) increases from placebo in the epoxide-to-parent ratio were observed after one dose of PGB and at the end of treatment. Eighty-one percent (17 of 21) of the patients had an increase of their epoxide-to-parent ratio after the first dose of PGB and 95% (20/21) at the end of the treatment period.

Table 7-4. Alterations in Carbamazepine and Carbamazepine 10,11-Epoxide Concentrations During Treatment with Progabide

	Carbamazepine (mg/day)	Carbamazepine concentration (μg/ml)			Carbamazepine-epoxide concentration (μg/ml)		
		Placebo	First dose	Steady state	Placebo	First dose	Steady state
Mean	1,119.0	5.2	4.7[a]	4.7	1.5	1.8[a]	1.9[a]
SD	312.4	1.2	0.9	1.2	0.4	0.5	0.5

Data modified from ref. 17.
[a]p<0.05 as compared to placebo.

FELBAMATE

FBM (2-phenyl-1,3-propanediol dicarbamate) is a novel AED currently undergoing clinical trials in the United States. Previous pharmacologic and toxicologic studies in laboratory animals suggest that FBM has antiepileptic potential with a significant margin of safety (18). Clinical studies to determine pharmacokinetics and/or tolerability reported increases in PHT serum concentrations, whereas CBZ serum concentrations declined or remained the same (19).

A double-blind crossover study sponsored by the epilepsy branch of the National Institute of Neurological and Communicative Disorders and Stroke (NINCDS) was carried out at the University of Minnesota and the University of Virginia, using the protocol described above for PGB with only minor modifications. The effect of FBM on PHT and CBZ serum concentrations on the 32 patients who completed the study in Minnesota is presented.

The study population consisted of 12 female and 20 male patients ranging in age from 18 to 55. Weights ranged from 51.8 kg to 110 kg with a mean of 68.6 kg.

At the beginning of each treatment period, the patients were hospitalized for 7 days while FBM or placebo was initiated and increased to its maximum dose, given t.i.d. Initially the maximum dose was 3000 mg. However, due to patient complaints of subjective toxicity, the maximum dose was reduced to 2600 mg/day after the first four patients. Previous studies detected a significant increase in PHT serum concentrations when FBM was added. Therefore, PHT doses for those patients on active drug regimen were automatically decreased 20% (20). During the second hospitalization, the drug used during Treatment I was tapered whereas Treatment II was added incrementally. PHT doses were either increased back to the baseline dose if Treatment I was active or decreased 20% if Treatment I was placebo.

PHT and CBZ were measured by a standard high-performance liquid chromatography (HPLC) assay. The coefficients of variations for PHT and CBZ over the range of concentrations observed in the study were < 8% and < 6%, respectively. FBM was determined by HPLC. The range of concentrations was 0.5–100 μg/ml. The slopes of the regression line did not vary by more than 8% on a day-to-day basis.

Throughout the study, serum PHT and CBZ concentrations were maintained within a patient-specific target range. The range for each patient was determined after completion of baseline. The serum drug concentrations on visits 2, 4, and 6 weeks of the baseline period were summed and the mean taken. The patient-specific range was determined as the baseline mean, 20% for PHT and 25% for CBZ. During the treatment phases, PHT and CBZ concentrations were determined during the biweekly clinic visit. Blood sample collection occurred at approximately the same time after a dose at all clinic visits. The AED concentrations were compared with the PHT and CBZ boundaries for the patient-specific range. If a patient was not complaining of toxicity and the concentrations were within the range, no dose changes occurred. Dose changes for PHT, CBZ, FBM, or placebo were made by the unblinded pharmacist using the same criteria as in the PGB.

Throughout the study, patients were supplied with FBM and/or matching placebo, PHT and/or matching placebo, and CBZ. All drugs were prepacked for the individual patient in daily unit dose containers to ensure compliance. The number of capsules a patient received remained constant throughout the study.

PHT dosage was changed using a Bayesian forecasting technique developed by Vozeh et al. (14). CBZ dosage was changed using linear pharmacokinetics.

The effect of FBM on the disposition of PHT and CBZ was analyzed in the following ways: (a) The average PHT and CBZ doses and serum concentrations during baseline were compared by a paired Student's t test with those during FBM or placebo treatment; and (b) PHT and CBZ apparent clearance (ml/h/kg) was calculated as: daily dose (mg/kg/day)/serum concentration (mg/L). Comparisons were made between baseline, FBM, and placebo periods by a paired Student's t test.

Despite a 20% mean reduction in PHT dose (range, 10–30%) during FBM treatment, there was no difference in PHT serum concentration when comparing FBM treatment to baseline or placebo periods (Table 7-5).

All patients receiving FBM required PHT dosage adjustments (Table 7-6). The protocol mandated a 20% decrease in PHT dose upon initiation of active FBM. Subsequently, dose changes for PHT could be made if the PHT concentrations did not stay within the patient-specific range or symptoms attributed to PHT toxicity were seen. Seventeen of 32 patients required additional PHT dosage changes. Seven patients had PHT dosage adjustments during placebo treatment because of low PHT concentrations.

CBZ concentrations decreased significantly in patients receiving active FBM. Although small (mean 1.3 /μmg/ml), a decrease occurred in 30 of 32 patients. Only three patients had CBZ dose changes. These three patients had their doses increased during the active treatment period.

MK-801

MK-801 is a (t)-10,11-dihydro-5-methyl-5H-dibeuzo [a,d] cycloheptene 5,10 imine (21). It appears to block the effect of excitatory amino acids. We performed an open dose titration study of efficacy and toxicity of MK-801 (22).

Table 7-5. Felbamate, Phenytoin, and Carbamazepine Dose, Concentration, and Clearance Data

	Felbamate	
	Mean	Range
Dose (mg)	2,400	1,400–2,600
Dose (mg/kg/day)	35.5	18.6–50.2
Serum concentration (μg/ml)	32.4	21.5–44.8
Clearance (ml/h/kg)	48.0	26.0–88.0

	Phenytoin		
	Baseline	Felbamate	Placebo
Dose (mg)	390 (80)	310 (80)[a]	390 (80)
Dose (mg/kg/day)	5.8 (1)	4.6 (1)[a]	5.8 (1)
Serum concentration (μg/ml)	16.6 (3.5)	16.1 (3.4)[a]	15.7 (3.4)
Clearance (ml/h/kg)	15.0 (3.2)	12.7 (3.4)[a]	15.0 (3.4)

	Carbamazepine		
	Baseline	Felbamate	Placebo
Dose (mg)	1,200 (300)	1,200 (300)	1,200 (300)
Dose (mg/kg/day)	17.7 (5.7)	17.8 (5.7)	17.8 (5.7)
Serum concentration (μg/ml)	6.3 (1.3)	5.0 (1.1)[a]	6.4 (1.4)
Clearance (ml/h/kg)	120 (40)	154 (68)[a]	116 (36)

[a]$p < 0.05$ as compared with baseline and placebo and after-dose adjustments.

A total of 14 patients were entered into the study. These included 4 females and 10 males ranging from 19 to 54 years of age (mean, 30.3 years). All patients were hospitalized at the University of Minnesota Epilepsy Treatment Unit. During this hospitalization, concomitant antiepilep-

Table 7-6. Number of Patients Requiring Dosage Adjustments During the Felbamate Study

	Felbamate	Placebo
Phenytoin	32/32 (100%)[a]	7/32 (22%)
	17/31 (53%)[b]	
Carbamazepine	3/32 (9%)	1/32 (3%)

[a]Mandated by protocol.
[b]Necessary even after mandated change.

Table 7-7. Effect of Concomitant Antiepileptic Drug Treatment on MK-801 Clearance

Patient number	Concomitant AED(S)	MK-801 maximum dose (mg/day)	MK-801 maximum level (pg/ml)	MK-801 total body clearance (ml/mn/kg)
1	PHT, VPA	7.0	958	0.09571
2	PHT	7.0	500	0.15399
3	PHT, CBZ	20.0	1,478	0.21242
9	PHT, VPA, CZP	30.0	2,143	0.14350
10	VPA	6.0	2,826	0.03351
12	PHT, VPA	4.0	772	0.10017
13	PHT	12.0	634	0.26862
14	PHT, VPA	8.0	677	0.25681

tic medications were withdrawn gradually in order to promote the occurrence of seizures, which were then recorded for diagnostic purposes.

Initially, MK-801 was started at 0.2 mg t.i.d., and MK-801 was added to whatever standard antiepileptic drug therapy was being used at the end of the diagnostic phase. Seizure frequency was reviewed on a daily basis. If a significant change in seizure frequency was not observed, the dose of MK-801 was increased. The initial maximum dose was 0.2 mg per day. However, it became obvious after the first few patients that this dose had no toxicity, and seizure control was not attained. The protocol was subsequently modified several times to allow for doses to be increased until definite clinical toxicity or complete seizure control was observed. Because of lack of toxicity with lower doses, some patients had the MK-801 dose pushed to 20–30 mg per day, tenfold greater than initially permitted. Results of outcomes are presented in Table 7-7. Eight patients had received sufficient MK-801 to achieve blood levels greater than 160 pg/ml and were in the study long enough to have reliable dose and level data.

The most interesting result from this study was the great variability in MK-801 clearance (Table 7-7). Clearances were markedly influenced by concomitant medication. One patient on valproate monotherapy had clearance and dose requirements similar to that seen in human volunteers. However, persons receiving PHT and/or CBZ as co-medication had clearances tenfold greater than observed with valproate monotherapy.

DISCUSSION

Results reviewed in this chapter indicate that all of the novel agents studied interacted with or were subject to interaction with standard AEDs

Table 7-8. Summary of Effects of Progabide and Felbamate on Phenytoin and Carbamazepine Concentrations

	Progabide	Felbamate
Phenytoin	Moderate increase	Marked increase
Carbamazepine	No change or slight decrease	Moderate decrease
Carbamazepine-epoxide	Slight decrease	

(Table 7-8). PGB had not been considered to affect the metabolism of PHT prior to the NIH-sponsored study (6), yet a significant increase in PHT concentrations was observed when concentrations were monitored frequently. Because of the nonlinear kinetics of PHT, this effect would have caused PHT concentrations to rise to much higher levels, and it possibly could have affected the efficacy or toxicity results of the clinical trial if not corrected by timely dose reductions. The mean time to observe this effect was 4 weeks after institution of PGB, indicating that a small but persistent change in clearance had occurred. Because the half-life of PHT is concentration dependent, it is not unexpected that at higher concentrations, where the half-life may be measured in days, some weeks would be required to observe this effect.

Although not observed in evaluating outpatient levels (16), a small but statistically significant decrease in CBZ levels with a concomitant increase in the 10,11-epoxide concentrations was observed using the data from an 8-h time–concentration determination. This finding points to the need for using more extensive pharmacokinetic evaluation in larger numbers of patients on chronic medication than is sometimes possible with short-term pilot studies. However, because the 10,11-epoxide possesses some antiepileptic properties, the shift from parent to active metabolite in this situation may not influence the efficacy evaluation. The time course of this interaction is unusual, it is present after the first dose, and it is not changed after the complete treatment period of almost 3 months. This would suggest that the effect of PGB may be influenced by the volume of distribution of CBZ.

Some previous clinical studies found PGB to be quite effective (7–9), but these studies did not control for fluctuations in concomitant antiepileptic medications. In the study in which concentrations of PHT and CBZ were maintained within a narrow range, PGB, although helpful for a few individual patients, did not demonstrate statistically significant effectiveness for the whole study population (6) and more closely reflected the outcome of other studies (23,24).

In the case of FBM, data from the pilot and the phase I study indicated an inhibition of PHT clearance, and appropriate adjustments were made. This type of study requires the presence of an unblinded pharmacist to maintain the blind in an appropriate fashion. In spite of the predetermined 20% adjustment, more than half of the subjects still required additional adjustment of the PHT dose, either up or down. Thus, the presence of interindividual variability requires the study design to allow for dose adjustment, even when data from preliminary studies does not clearly demonstrate a pharmacokinetic interaction.

The MK-801 data explore the standard–novel drug interaction from another perspective and indicate that the metabolism of a novel drug, especially a potent compound, can be markedly affected by standard drug therapy. Only the subject on valproate monotherapy had a dose level relationship similar to that seen in volunteers. Thus, in designing efficacy and safety trials, one would need, in this circumstance, to permit dose adjustments to the novel drug.

The ideal design for safety and efficacy trials would permit for both novel and standard drugs to undergo a dose adjustment in order to maintain steady levels throughout the testing period. While it would be ideal to have drugs with no interactions, it is more likely that the novel agents will mirror the experience with standard drugs: every drug interacts with every other. Only the degree and mechanisms of interaction appear to differ. Thus, if pilot studies show interactions, the novel drug should not be deemed unworthy of further development. Rather, appropriate efficacy and toxicity studies fully utilizing the best pharmacokinetic models and implemented by researchers capable of performing these studies should be designed and implemented. Once a novel agent is proven effective, its usefulness should not be impeded in practice by the presence of interactions. Valproate use has not been significantly hampered by its interactions with phenobarbital or PHT. The role of an unblinded researcher capable of using sophisticated pharmacokinetic models to adjust the doses is essential in clinical trials of novel antiepileptic medications.

Acknowledgment: The data presented were gathered and analyzed by a number of persons working with the Comprehensive Epilepsy Program of the University of Minnesota. The major contributors were: James C. Cloyd, Nina M. Graves, Robin H. Fuerst, Richard C. Brundage, Timothy E. Welty, Gregory B. Holmes, Cynthia A. Rask, Terry Bowman-Cloyd, Karen Marienau, Margaret P. Jacobs, and William E. Rosenfeld. Major support from the Epilepsy Branch of the NINCDS was instrumental in carrying out this study under contracts P50 NS 16308 and NO1-NS-1-2371. Merck, Sharp, and Dohme provided support for the MK-801 study and Lorex Pharmaceuticals for the supplemental protocol of the Progabide study.

REFERENCES

1. Cereghino JJ, Penry K. Testing of antiepileptic drugs in humans. In: Woodbury DM, Penry JK, Pippenger CE, eds. *Antiepileptic Drugs*, 2nd ed. New York: Raven Press, 1982.
2. Pledger GW. Drug interactions in clinical trials: statistical considerations. In: Pitlick WH, ed. *Antiepileptic Drug Interactions*. New York: Demos Publications, 1989:143–56.
3. Trieman DM. Recommendations for antiepileptic drug–drug interaction studies before controlled clinical trials. In: Pitlick WH, ed. *Antiepileptic Drug Interactions*. New York: Demos Publications, 1989:89–113.
4. Remmel RP, Graves NM. Animal model systems for the study of antiepileptic drug interactions and their clinical implications. In: Pitlick WH, ed. *Antiepileptic Drug Interactions*. New York: Demos Publications, 1989:181–96.
5. Green JR, Troupin AS, Halpern LM, Friel P, Kanarek P. Sulthiame: evaluation as an anticonvulsant. *Epilepsia* 1974;15:329–49.
6. Leppik IE, Dreifuss FE, Porter R, et al. A controlled study of progabide in partial seizures: methodology and results. *Neurology* 1987;37:963–8.
7. Loiseau P, Bossi L, Guyot M, Orofiamma B, Morselli PL. Double-blind cross-over trial of progabide versus placebo in severe epilepsies. *Epilepsia* 1983;24:713–5.
8. Martinez-Lage JM, Bossi L, Morales G, Martinez Vila E, Orogiamma B, Viteri C. Progabide treatment in severe epilepsy: a double-blind crossover trial versus placebo. *Epilepsia* 1984;25:586.
9. Weber M, Vespignani B, Remy MC, Regnier F, Bossi LA. Controlled trial of progabide versus placebo in therapy-resistant epilepsies. In: Bartholini G, et al., eds. *Epilepsy and GABA Receptor Agonists: Basic and Therapeutic Research*. New York: Raven Press, 1985:353–62.
10. Worms P, Depoortere H, Durand A, Morselli PL, Lloyd KG, Bartholini G. Gamma-aminobutyric acid (GABA) receptor stimulation. I. Europharmacological profiles of progabide (SL 76002) and (SL 75102), with emphasis on their anticonvulsant spectra. *J Pharmacol Exp Ther* 1982;220:660–71.
11. Lloyd KG, Arbilla S, Beaumont K, et al. Gamma-aminobutyric acid (GABA) receptor stimulation. II. Specificity of progabide (SL 76002) and (SL 75102) for the GABA receptor. *J Pharmacol Exp Ther* 1982;220:672–77.
12. Leppik IE, Cloyd JC, Sawchuch RJ, Pepin SM. Compliance and variability of plasma phenytoin levels in epileptic patients. *Ther Drug Monit* 1979;1:475–83.
13. Graves NM, Holmes GB, Leppik IE. Compliant populations: variability in serum concentrations. *Epilepsy Res* 1988; Suppl 1:91–100.
14. Vozeh S, Murr KT, Sheiner LB, et al. Predicting individual phenytoin dosage. *J Pharmacokinet Biopharm* 1981;9:131–46.
15. Gibaldi M, Perrier D. *Pharmacokinetics*, 2nd ed. New York: Marcel Dekker, 1982.
16. Brundage RC, Cloyd JC, Leppik IE, Graves NM, Welty TE. Effect of progabide on serum phenytoin and carbamazepine concentrations. *Clin Neuropharmacol* 1987;10(6):545–54.
17. Graves NM, Fuerst RH, Cloyd JC, Brundage RC, Welty TE, Leppik IE. Pro-

gabide induced changes in carbamazepine metabolism. *Epilepsia* 1988;29:775–80.

18. Swinyard EA, Sofia RD, Kupferberg HJ. Comparative anticonvulsant activity and neurotoxicity of felbamate and four prototype antiepileptic drugs in mice and rats. *Epilepsia* 1986;27:27–34.

19. Wilensky AJ, Friel PN, Ojemann LM, Kupferberg HS, Levy RH. Pharmacokinetics of W-544 (ADD 03055) in epileptic patients. *Epilepsia* 1985;26:602–6.

20. Sheridan PH, Ashworth M, Milne K, et al. Open pilot study of felbamate (ADD 03055) in partial seizures. *Epilepsia* 1986;27:649.

21. Clineschmidt BV, Martin GE, Bunting PR. Anticonvulsant activity of (+)5-methyl-10,11-dihydro-5Hdibenzo(a,d)cyclohepten-5,10-imine (MK-801), a substance with potent anticonvulsant, central sympathomimetic, and apparent anxiolytic properties. *Drug Dev Res 2* 1982a;123–34.

22. Leppik IE, Marienau K, Graves N, Rask C. MK-801 for epilepsy: a pilot study. *Neurology* 38(1):405.

23. Dam M, Gram L, Philbert A, et al. Progabide: a controlled trial in partial epilepsy. *Epilepsia* 1983;24:127–34.

24. Schmidt D, Utech K. Progabide for refractory partial epilepsy: a controlled add-on trial. *Neurology* 1986;36:217–21.

8

Two Facets of Antiepileptic Drug Interactions as Illustrated by Stiripentol

[1]Pierre Loiseau, [2]René Levy, and [3]Jack Tor

[1]*Department of Neurology, University Hospital, Bordeaux, France;* [2]*Department of Pharmaceutics, School of Pharmacy, University of Washington, Seattle, Washington, U.S.A.; and* [3]*Laboratoires Biocodex, Montrouge, France.*

At present, untreated epileptic patients are generally prescribed only one drug (1). However, polypharmacy still exists in at least two situations: (a) in chronic, difficult-to-treat patients; and (b) during the clinical evaluation of a new drug. In those situations, drug interactions are prevalent. They are schematically of two types; some drugs induce and others inhibit the metabolism of co-prescribed drugs. A decrease in the plasma level of an induced drug may result in a lesser efficacy. An increase in the plasma level of an inhibited drug increases toxic risks. This is, in fact, an oversimplification of very complex situations. A drug is not necessarily an inducer or inhibitor of all the other drugs. For instance, valproic acid (VPA) raises the plasma level of phenobarbital (PB) but not of carbamazepine (CBZ) (2). Felbamate lowers CBZ concentration while increasing phenytoin (PHT) concentration (3). Large interindividual variations exist for a given interaction (4).

Drug interactions constitute a problem for the clinician. Plasma levels of all the drugs must be checked repeatedly. It may be impossible to achieve a satisfactory level of an induced drug. For instance, uncontrolled patients receiving VPA in polytherapy were better off when VPA remained the sole medication (5). The blind nature of clinical trials can be confounded by the dosage changes and the blood-level monitoring required in the treatment block involving the drug under investigation. Interactions involve not only parent drugs, but also metabolites, which may have their own toxicity. For instance, both valproate and valpromide increase carbamazepine-10,11-epoxide (CBZE) concentration. But valpromide is even more potent than valproate in increasing CBZE levels, and this risk is of potential clinical significance (6).

On the other hand, an inhibitory drug may be beneficial when it raises the concentration of the co-prescribed parent drug without raising its metabolites.

Stiripentol (STP) interactions exemplify the above considerations.

METHODS

STP

STP [4,4-dimethyl-1-[(3,4 methylene dioxy) phenyl]-1-penten-3-ol] is a new antiepileptic drug selected from a chemical series that contains no nitrogen (7). It has been effective with a low degree of toxicity in rodent screening models (8). Its anticonvulsant activity was documented in the alumina-cream monkey model (9,10). Its kinetics are nonlinear of the Michaelis-Menten type (11–14). In open clinical trials, STP was considered a promising new drug (15–18). It reduces the elimination clearance of concomitant antiepileptic drugs (14).

Data Collection

Available published and unpublished data were included. All of them demonstrate the importance of STP interactions. However, many blood-level determinations were difficult to use. Dosage reductions were made at various times after STP introduction because patients developed toxic signs or, later on, there was a conscious effort to avoid toxicity. Thus, inhibited drugs may not have been at steady state. The main source of data was a pharmacokinetic study done in six epileptic patients receiving other antiepileptic drugs (14). These drugs were maintained at constant dosage for at least one month before the study. The patients were compliant. STP was administered in progressively increasing dosages from day 1 to day 12. A dosage of 2,400 mg/day was maintained constant from day 13 to day 30. Other drugs were reduced when required after the addition of STP.

Plasma samples collected over 8-h dosing intervals were used to calculate area under the curve (AUC), steady-state serum concentration (C_{ss}), and apparent clearance. Clearance rather than concentration data were used to examine the interaction of STP with PHT, CBZ, and PB when subjects were not at steady states. Other figures come from various clinical trials when stable dosage or plasma levels were maintained long enough.

RESULTS

STP Metabolism Is Induced by Other Antiepileptic Drugs

The mean ($\pm$ S.D.) clearance of STP at 1,200 mg/day was 0.28 ± 0.08 L/kg/h in normal subjects (13). It was 0.85 L/kg/h in epileptic patients receiving PB, PHT, or CBZ and the same dose of STP (14), a 300% increase. The apparent in vivo Michaelis-Menten parameters K_m and V_m were determined in co-medicated epileptic patients (14) and in normal subjects (13). V_m was larger (49.3 ± 13.1 and 39.9 ± 8.5 mg/kg/day, respectively) and K_m smaller (1.35 ± 1.08 mg/kg/h and 2.20 ± 1.28 mg/h, respectively) in the co-medicated patients. A large intersubject variability in STP clearance was also noted.

STP Inhibits the Metabolism of Other Antiepileptic Drugs

PHT. In the pharmacokinetic study by Levy et al. (14), phenytoin clearance decreased in all five subjects who received this drug, from a mean ($\pm$ S.D.) control of 29.5 ± 13.4 to 6.48 ± 2.59 L/day after 30 days of STP exposure. Large intersubject variability was noted among the five patients, on day 0 as well as on day 30 (Table 8-1). Decrease in PHT clearance was associated with large rises in plasma concentration. PHT kinetics varied from patient to patient. In one, the PHT level rose slowly and then declined, with a clear lag time between the dosage change and the concentration decrease (Fig. 8-1). In another patient receiving a constant dose of PHT, the PHT level rose on day 15, continued to rise after a dosage reduction, and decreased 9 days after return to the initial dosage (Fig. 8-2). In a third patient, PHT levels peaked on day 17 and then declined without any dosage change.

When a constant dosage of PHT was maintained in patients undergoing clinical trials, STP raised the C_{ss} of PHT 50–317% (mean, 202%) (Ta-

Table 8-1. Effect of STP on PHT Clearance (L/Day)

Patient	J_0	J_{30}	Percent change
1	29.0	3.68	−87
2	27.3	7.35	−73
3	52.1	5.41	−90
4	18.1	10.50	−42
5	20.8	5.47	−74
$\overline{X}$	29.5	6.48	−78

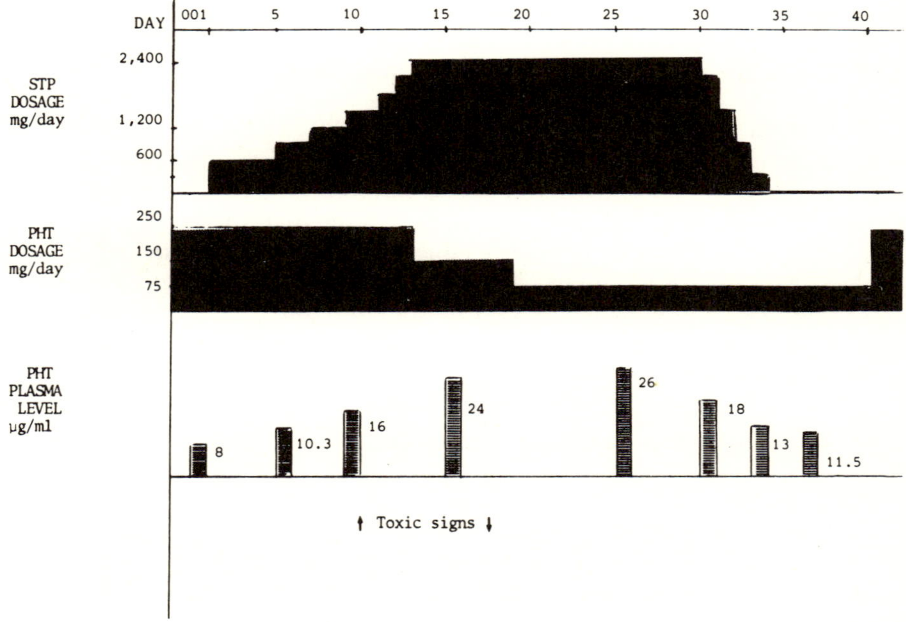

FIG. 8-1. Patient C.S.: influence of STP on the phenytoin (PHT) plasma level. A daily dosage of 250 mg of PHT was well tolerated. After the addition of STP, the PHT level rose slowly. Toxic signs appeared on day 9 with a level of 16 μg/ml. PHT dosage was reduced 3 days later. PHT levels continued to rise with a peak on day 25. PHT dosage was 75 mg/day for 7 days. PHT slowly declined during approximately 7 days.

ble 8-2). Toxic signs were noted when PHT levels increased, but they disappeared in some patients despite high PHT concentrations (Fig. 8-1). A 25–66% (mean, 49%) PHT dosage reduction was necessary to keep PHT plasma concentration constant (Table 8-2).

CBZ. In the pharmacokinetic study by Levy et al. (14), CBZ clearance decreased in the two CBZ-treated patients. In one subject (Patient D), CBZ clearance fell from 209 L/day on day 1 to 60.8 L/day on day 30. CBZ C_{ss} rose from 3.83 μg/ml on day 1 to 6.26 μg/ml on day 9 with a regular 800-mg/day CBZ dosage. Although CBZ was reduced to 600 mg/day on day 11, the plasma level continued to rise, reaching 9.86 μg/ml on day 30. In the other patient, CBZ C_{ss} rose from 4 μg/ml on day 1 to 10 μg/ml on day 30.

CBZ clearance was also measured in eight patients before and after 10 weeks of STP treatment (2,400–3,000 mg/day). Mean ($\pm$S.D.) CBZ clearance decreased from 6.1 ($\pm$1.1) to 2.0 ($\pm$0.7) L/h (19).

In clinical trials, STP addition to a constant dosage of CBZ raised the

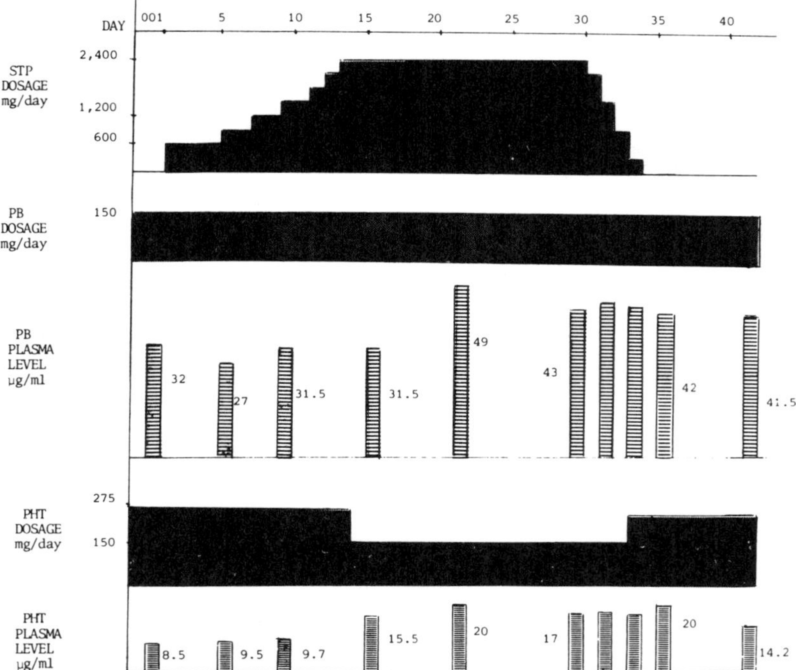

FIG. 8-2. Patient A.D.: influence of STP on the phenobarbital (PB) plasma level. PB level rose between day 16 and day 20 after the addition of STP to a regimen of PB and PHT. Despite a constant dosage of PB, the PB level decreased slightly. PHT level rose earlier, before day 15. Despite a reduction in dosage on day 13, PHT level continued to rise. It rose again with an increased dosage, but decreased on day 40, probably before a new steady state was achieved.

C_{ss} of the drug 15–182% (mean, 89%) (Table 8-3). The rise in CBZ level was generally not as great as in the case of PHT, and it was more variable. It is worthwhile to note that no toxic effect appeared with levels as high as 20 μg/ml. To maintain constant plasma levels, a 12.5–78% (mean, 47.8%) dosage reduction was necessary (Table 8-3).

STP increases CBZ concentrations probably by inhibiting the formation of CBZE. In monkeys, the CBZE/CBZ ratio dropped from 0.26 to 0.06 when STP was added and returned to 0.26 when STP administration ceased (20). In man, a CBZE/CBZ ratio (mean ± S.D., 0.06 ± 0.016) was found (19).

Two studies were designed to determine whether STP affects CBZE formation, elimination, or both (21). In Study 1, STP was administered (1,000–3,000 mg/day) to four epileptic patients on CBZ monotherapy. Both the CBZ dose/plasma concentration and the CBZE/CBZ plasma ratio re-

Table 8-2. Effect of STP on PHT

| | Constant dosage of PHT | | | | About constant level of PHT | | | | | |
| | | Level (μg/ml) | | | | Level (μg/ml) | | Dosage (mg/day) | | |
Patient	Dosage (mg/day)	Control	+STP	% change	Patient	Control	+STP	Baseline	+STP	% change
C.T.	80	3.0	4.5	+ 50	M.J.M.	4.6	6.5	200	150	−25
A.D.	300	20.0	45.0	+125	J.B.	15.5	15.5	325	200	−38
J.M.	300	13.0	30.0	+131	S.V.	10.8	8.0	210	120	−43
B.C.	100	5.5	13.0	+137	R.G.	3.2	3.2	400	200	−50
C.F.	400	12.5	31.0	+148	M.D.	25.0	20.0	300	150	−50
X.G.	400	10.2	28.0	+176	A.B.	21.2	20.0	350	150	−57
L.M.	300	7.5	17.2	+229						
M.J.R.	200	11.5	45.9	+317						

Table 8-3. Effect of STP on CBZ

| | Constant dosage of CBZ | | | | About constant level of CBZ | | | | | |
| | | Level (μg/ml) | | | | Level (μg/ml) | | Dosage (mg/day) | | |
Patient	Dosage (mg/day)	Control	+STP	% change	Patient	Control	+STP	Control	+STP	% change
V.Q.	400	8.5	10.0	+ 15	H.M.	7.0	6.7	800	700	−12.5
A.R.	1,200	9.4	13.0	+ 38	X.A.	10.3	10.7	1,200	800	−33
C.S.	400	11.8	16.5	+ 40	A.R.	7.2	7.7	1,200	600	−50
J.B.	1,000	8.2	12.9	+ 57	D.V.	9.5	10.0	800	400	−50
M.D.	1,200	6.0	10.0	+ 67	E.I.	12.0	12.4	1,200	600	−50
R.G.	400	4.9	8.2	+ 67	T.M.	7.5	7.1	800	400	−50
G.F.	1,000	6.0	11.5	+ 92	Y.L.	9.0	9.0	800	400	−50
B.B.	800	9.2	19.4	+110	P.S.	13.8	12.3	1,800	800	−56
J.S.	1,600	5.6	14.3	+155	J.B.	14.4	13.0	1,400	500	−64
J.R.	1,200	7.5	20.2	+169	L.M.	8.0	7.6	1,200	400	−66
P.R.	600	2.3	6.5	+182	R.M.	11.0	11.0	1,200	400	−64
					M.A.	10.2	12.8	1,800	600	−66
					D.M.	12.3	12.3	1,400	300	−78

quired an equilibrium time of 7–10 days following initiation of STP. After 2 weeks of STP treatment, mean ($\pm$S.D. CBZ) clearance was reduced from 120 ± 28 L/day to 55.8 ± 7.3 L/day, and the CBZE/CBZ ratio in plasma decreased from 0.137 ± 0.025 to 0.072 ± 0.012. The percent change in CBZ clearance was 27–67% and the percent change in CBZE/CBZ AUC ratio was 32–60. These results indicate that STP reduces CBZE formation and/or increases CBZE elimination. The latter hypothesis was tested in Study 2. Six normal adult volunteers each received two single oral doses of CBZE, one time with and one time without STP treatment. STP did not have a significant effect on CBZE half-life (5.89 ± 0.55 h without STP, 5.65 ± 0.54 h with STP) or plasma clearance (1.78 ± 0.24 ml/min/kg without STP, 1.98 ± 0.24 ml/min/kg with STP).

These data lead to the following conclusions: (a) STP inhibition of CBZ clearance is probably due to cytochrome P-450 inhibition; (b) STP does not inhibit epoxide hydrolase; and (C) reduction in CBZE/CBZ ratio is due to inhibition of CBZE formation.

PB. STP decreases the clearance of PB. In the study by Levy et al. (14) it dropped from 3.84 L/day on day 1 to 2.25 L/day on day 30 in one patient and from 5.06 L/day on day 1 to 3.42 L/day on day 30 in another patient. The data on plasma levels were inconclusive because the period of observation in this study was shorter than that required for PB levels to rise from one steady state to another. Nevertheless, an increase in plasma level was noted in the three patients treated by PB. It is exemplified in Fig. 8-2. In this patient, the rise was very progressive, noticeable on days 14–20. A trend toward a relative decrease was noted in this patient, whose daily dosage of PB was maintained at a constant.

In clinical trials, STP addition to a constant dosage of PB raised the C_{ss} of the drug 8–80% (mean, 44%) (Table 8-4). To maintain approximately constant plasma levels, the daily dosage was reduced 10–50% (mean, 29%) (Table 8-4).

Primidone (PRM). This interaction is exemplified in Fig. 8-3. Patient C.C. belonged to the study by Levy et al. (14). PRM dosage was maintained constant (750 mg/day) during 30 days of STP administration. A twofold rise in the PRM level was noted by day 22. It began slowly, noticeable after day 8. The PRM level was lower on days 30 and 33, without a change in PRM dosage. PB levels remained practically unchanged. In another patient, M.M., receiving 750 mg/day of PRM, baseline levels of PRM and PB were 7.5 μg/ml and 32 μg/ml, respectively. Two weeks after STP was added to her regimen, PRM level had risen to 16.5 μg/ml and reached 18.5 μg/ml 2 weeks later. Marked toxic signs were present. The patient decided on her own to stop STP. PB plasma levels were 21 μg/ml on week 2 and 17 μg/ml on week 4.

STP was added to the existing drug regimen of two adult in-patients with an intractable epilepsy. The regimen was, for patient P.R., 750 mg/

Table 8-4. Effect of STP on PB

| | | Constant dosage of PB | | | | About constant level of PB | | | | |
| | | Level (μg/ml) | | | | Level (μg/ml) | | Dosage (mg/day) | | |
Patient	Dosage (mg/day)	Control	+STP	% change	Patient	Control	+STP	Control	+STP	% change
V.L.	150	32.0	34.5	+ 8	S.V.	42.0	43.0	160	145	−10
M.B.	150	26.0	31.0	+19	M.T.M.	17.5	19.0	100	80	−20
F.M.	100	13.0	18.0	+38	M.M.	27.0	26.0	200	150	−25
A.D.	150	32.0	45.0	+41	J.B.	41.0	39.0	200	150	−25
P.L.	150	16.0	25.0	+56	M.D.	35.5	31.0	175	125	−28
B.B.	150	32.0	52.0	+62	J.M.M.	30.5	23.0	150	100	−30
P.C.	100	29.0	48.0	+66	F.E.	37.5	38.6	250	150	−40
N.Z.	100	20.0	36.0	+80	C.G.	17.5	21.0	105	60	−43
E.I.	100	18.0	36.0	+97						

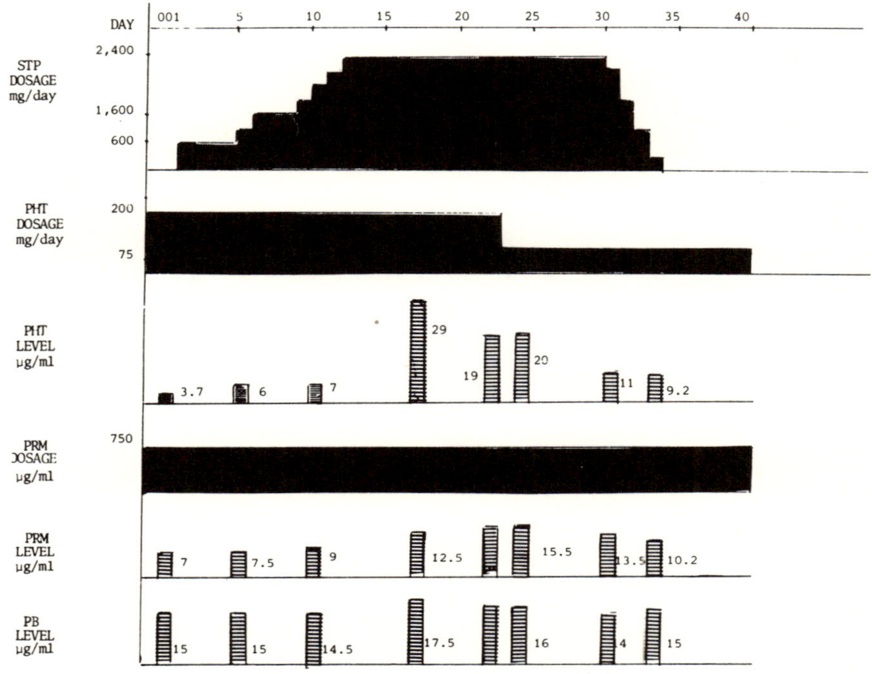

FIG. 8-3. Patient C.C.: influence of STP on primidone (PRM), PB, and PHT plasma levels. A twofold increase of the PRM level slowly appeared. A decrease occurred without a change in PRM dosage. The PB level remained practically unchanged. The PHT level increased dramatically, then decreased prior to a dosage reduction on day 23.

day of PRM, 600 mg/day of CBZ, and 2 mg/day of clonazepam and, for patient N.B., 500 mg/day of PRM, 1,000 mg/day of VPA, and 2 mg/day of clonazepam. Five PRM and PB plasma-level determinations were made the day prior to STP addition and after 2 weeks of STP exposure (1,800 mg/day and 2,400 mg/day, respectively). An increase of 53% and 64% in PRM concentration was noted. Toxic signs were present. PB levels demonstrated a slight decrease (Table 8-5). These findings suggest that STP decreases the clearance of PRM and reduces the formation of PB.

VPA. A significant rise in VPA plasma level was never observed during clinical trials. However, such large intraindividual fluctuations in VPA plasma concentrations take place during the day that there is little value in single-level determinations.

In order to elucidate the influence of STP on VPA metabolism, eight healthy volunteers received VPA (1,000 mg/day for 11 days) without, then with STP (1,200 mg/day) (22). The mean (± S.D.) VPA level at steady

Table 8-5. Effect of STP on PRM Plasma Levels (μg/ml)

| | Patient P.R. | | | | Patient N.B. | | | |
| | Control | | +STP | | Control | | +STP | |
Sampling time	PRM	PB	PRM	PB	PRM	PB	PRM	PB
8:00	5.7	27.0	10.9	24.5	4.2	20.0	8.7	19.6
11:00	10.6	30.5	14.9	27.0	7.9	24.5	11.8	17.5
14:00	9.1	30.0	14.6	29.5	6.8	22.0	10.0	17.5
16:00	11.8	34.5	16.0	27.0	5.8	20.0	8.8	20.0
19:00	8.2	32.0	13.3	27.0	4.3	21.0	7.5	19.5
$\overline{X}$	9.1	30.8	13.9	27.0	5.8	21.5	9.5	18.8

state increased from 62.6 ± 10 μg/ml to 68.5 ± 12 μg/ml. C_{max} and C_{min} increased by 14% and 13%, respectively. Such a small effect was completely explained by the lack of influence on the major metabolic pathways of VPA (glucuronidation and beta oxydation). However, a pronounced inhibition of the cytochrome P-450 mediated pathway was found. The formation clearance of the hepatotoxic metabolite, delta-4-VPA, was reduced by 32%.

DISCUSSION

STP interactions with the major anticonvulsant drugs are significant and complex. They are fairly well characterized. However, whereas a probable interaction is known before prescription, the extent of the interaction may differ from one patient to the next. When STP is added to an existing drug regimen, there may be major problems, but also repercussions beneficial for the patient.

In terms of its own anticonvulsant properties, a concentration-dependent efficacy of STP was documented in the monkey model of epilepsy (10). However, since STP metabolism is induced by CBZ, PHT, and PB, it may be very difficult to achieve plasma levels higher than 8 μg/ml in co-medicated patients. These concentrations are probably insufficient.

The metabolic inhibition by STP of other antiepileptic drugs makes the interpretation of an add-on therapy difficult. In terms of efficacy it would be logical to ascribe the reported benefit of STP in the control of seizures to the fact that it raised the plasma levels of associated drug(s). In order to evaluate the efficacy of STP, it is mandatory to maintain a constant baseline concentration of the drug(s). Some agents, such as CBZ and PRM, have active metabolites. In these cases, matching of concentrations should include both parent drug and metabolite concentrations. In terms of toxicity, the dose of background anticonvulsant(s) has to be changed according to the rise of their plasma level to avoid side-effects. Thus, the level of concomitant anticonvulsants must be monitored when STP is added to or removed from dosing regimens. Repeated sampling is necessary, because the inhibitory effect of STP on other drugs appears slowly and may persist throughout the course of long-term follow-up in many patients, but is probably more or less transitory in a few patients.

On the other hand, the inhibitory properties of STP have positive aspects. In add-on therapy with an other antiepileptic drug, nafimidone, CBZ and PHT rose within 24 h after nafimidone was added (23). The toxic risk is less important with STP, which very slowly lowers the elimination of PHT, CBZ, or PB. Some of the neurotoxic effects of CBZ are dose-related. An association of STP–CBZ alleviates the neurotoxicity of CBZ: in clinical trials, several patients tolerated CBZ concentrations well in the usually toxic range. Contradictory results on the effectiveness of PRM in humans have been reported (24). The rate of enzymatic conversion of PRM to PB is modified by STP. It will be now possible to push PRM level up to the maximum tolerated concentration without increasing PB concentration.

Metabolic interactions may be relevant for teratogenesis and hepatotoxicity. Many drugs are hydroxylated in the arene oxide pathway, in which epoxides are intermediate metabolites. Epoxides can have toxic effects through covalent binding to macromolecules like proteins and DNA (25,26). CBZE is a stable epoxide that can be determined in blood. Elevation of plasma CBZE levels by co-medication with valproate (27) and to a greater extent with valpromide (6) has been reported. High CBZE levels in pregnant women have been suggested to be teratogenic (28,29). Other epoxides of CBZ (30) and of PHT (31) are suspected. Since STP is a broad-spectrum inhibitor of cytochrome P-450 and reduces the CBZE/CBZ ratio in humans, it will reduce the formation of arene oxides. STP may therefore offer some advantages in women of childbearing age.

A large body of data indicates that delta-4-VPA is a potent hepatotoxin. This property is shared also by delta-2, 4-VPA, a further metabolite of delta-4-VPA. Recently, Rettie et al. (32) have demonstrated that the formation of delta-4-VPA from VPA is catalyzed by cytochrome P-450. The hypothesis that STP would reduce the formation of delta-4-VPA was tested and validated in humans (33). The behavior of STP is opposite to that of classical antiepileptic drugs (such as CBZ and PHT), which were found to increase the formation of delta-4-VPA in epileptic patients (33). The effects of CBZ and PHT on delta-4-VPA are consistent with the 10- to 20-fold increase in incidence of hepatotoxicity associated with polytherapy (34). Thus, one could predict that addition of STP would reduce the incidence of fatal hepatotoxicity associated with VPA.

Acknowledgment: We thank Jim Sneed and Marie-Françoise Aury for technical assistance.

REFERENCES

1. Reynolds EH, Shorvon SD. Monotherapy or polytherapy for epilepsy? *Epilepsia* 1981; 22:1–10.
2. Johanessen ST. Preliminary observations on valproic acid kinetics in patients with epilepsy. *Arzneimittelforsch* 1977; 27:1083–5.
3. Holmes GB, Graves NM, Leppik IE, Fuerst RH. Felbamate: bidirectional effects on phenytoin and carbamazepine serum concentrations. *Epilepsia* 1987; 28:578–636.
4. Wilder BJ, Willmore LJ, Bruni S, Villareal HS. Valproic acid interaction with other anticonvulsant drugs. *Neurology* 1978; 28:892–6.
5. Henriksen O, Johannessen SI. Clinical and pharmacokinetic observations on sodium valproate. *Acta Neurol Scand* 1982; 65:504–23.
6. Pisani F, Fazio A, Oteri G, Ruello C, Gitto C, Russo F, Perucca E. Sodium valproate and valpromide: differential interactions with carbamazepine in epileptic patients. *Epilepsia* 1986; 27:548–52.
7. Astoin J, Marivain A, Riveron A, Crucifix M, Lapotre M, Torrens Y. Action de nouveaux alcools alpha-ethyléniques sur le système nerveux central. *Eur J Med Chem Chim Ther* 1978; 13:41–7.
8. Poisson M, Huguet F, Savatier A, Bakri-Logeais F, Narcisse G. A new type of anticonvulsant, stiripentol. *Arzneimittelforsch* 1984; 34:199–204.
9. Lockard JS, Levy RH, Maris DO, Rhodes PH. Stiripentol in alumina-gel monkeys: 4-dexoxypyridoxine hydrochloride paradigm. *Epilepsia* 1983; 24:252.
10. Lockard JS, Levy RH, Rhodes PH, Moore DF. Stiripentol in acute/chronic efficacy test in monkey model. *Epilepsia* 1985; 26:704–12.
11. Lin HS, Levy RH. Pharmacokinetic profile of a new anticonvulsant, stiripentol, in the rhesus monkey. *Epilepsia* 1983; 24:692–702.
12. Levy RH, Lin HS, Blehaut H, Tor JA. Pharmacokinetics of stiripentol in normal man: evidence of nonlinearity. *J Clin Pharmacol* 1983; 23:523–33.
13. Levy RH, Loiseau P, Guyot M, Blehaut H, Tor J, Moreland TA. Michaelis-Menten kinetics of stiripentol in normal humans. *Epilepsia* 1984a; 25:486–91.
14. Levy RH, Loiseau P, Guyot M, Blehaut H, Tor J, Moreland TA. Stiripentol kinetics in epilepsy: nonlinearity and interactions. *Clin Pharmacol Ther* 1984b; 36:661–9.
15. Martinez-Lage M, Loiseau P, Levy RH, Gonzalez I, Strube E, Tor J, Blehaut H. Clinical antiepileptic efficacy of stiripentol in resistant partial epilepsies. *Epilepsia* 1984; 25:673.
16. Martinez-Lage M, Levy RH, Gonzalez I, Viteri C, Tor J, Blehaut H. Stiripentol in therapy-resistant and severe epileptic patients: a long-term open trial in bitherapy. In: Wolf P, Dam M, Janz D, Dreifuss FE, eds. *Advances in Epileptology, vol 16.* New York: Raven Press, 1987; 541–6.
17. Loiseau P, Tor J. Stiripentol in absence seizures. *Epilepsia* 1987; 28:579.
18. Loiseau P, Strube E, Tor J, Levy RH, Dodrill C. Evaluation neuropsycholo-

gique et thérapeutique du stiripentol dans l'épilepsie. *Rev Neurol (Paris)* 1988;144:165–72.

19. Levy RH, Martinez-Lage M, Tor J, Blehaut H, Gonzalez I, Bainbridge G. Stiripentol level-dose relationship and interactions with carbamazepine in epileptic patients. *Epilepsia* 1986; 26:544.

20. Lockard JS, Levy RH. EEG effects of stiripentol in add-on with carbamazepine in monkey model. *Epilepsia* 1986; 27:648.

21. Levy RH, Martinez-Lage M, Kern BM, Viteri C. Effect of stiripentol on the formation and elimination of carbamazepine-epoxide. *Abstracts, 17th Epilepsy International Congress.* Jerusalem, Israel: 1987:71.

22. Levy RH, Loiseau P, Guyot M, Acheampong A, Tor J, Rettenmeier AW. Effects of stiripentol on valproate plasma level and metabolsim. *Epilepsia* 1987; 28:605.

23. Buhles WC, Wallach MB, Chaplin MD, Treiman DM. Nafimidone. In: Meldrum BS, Porter RJ, eds. *Current Problems in Epilepsy. New Anticonvulsant Drugs.* London: John Libbey, 1986:203–14.

24. Fincham RW, Schottelius DD. Primidone. Relation of plasma concentration to seizure control. In: Woodbury DM, Penry JK, Pippenger CE, eds. *Antiepileptic Drugs.* New York: Raven Press, 1982:429–40.

25. Jerina DM, Daly JW. Arene oxides: a new aspect of drug metabolism. *Science* 1974; 185:573–82.

26. Clapper ML, Klein NW. Identification of a teratogenic drug-protein complex in sera of phenytoin-treated monkeys. *Epilepsia* 1986; 27:685–96.

27. McKauge L, Tyrer JH, Eadie MJ. Factors influencing simultaneous concentrations of carbamazepine and its epoxide in plasma. *Ther Drug Monit* 1981; 3:63–70.

28. Lindhout D, Höppener RJEA, Meinardi H. Teratogenicity of antiepileptic drug combinations with special emphasis on epoxidation (of carbamazepine). *Epilepsia* 1984; 25:77–83.

29. Meijer JWA, Binnie CD, Debets RMC, Van Parys JAP, De Beer-Pawlinkowski NKB. Possible hazard of valpromide-carbamazepine combination therapy in epilepsy. *Lancet* 1984(i): 802.

30. Letratanangkoon K, Morning MG. Metabolism of carbamazepine. *Drug Metab Dispos* 1982; 10:1–10.

31. Martz F, Failinger C, Blake DA. Phenytoin teratogenesis: concentration between embryopathic effect and covalent binding of putative arene oxide metabolite in gestational tissue. *J Pharmacol Exp Ther* 1977; 203:231–9.

32. Rettie AE, Rettenmeier AW, Howald WN, Baillie TA. Cytochrome P-450-catalyzed formation of delta-4-VPA, a toxic metabolite of valproic acid. *Science* 1987; 235:890–3.

33. Levy RH, Rettenmeier AN, Baillie TA, Howald WN, Wilensky AJ, Friel PN, Anderson G. Formation of hepatotoxic metabolites of valproate in patients on carbamazepine on phenytoin. *Epilepsia* 1987; 28:627.

34. Dreifuss FE, Santilli N, Langer DH, Sweeney KP, Moline KA, Menander KB. Valproic acid hepatic fatalities: a retrospective review. *Neurology* 1987; 37:379–85.

9

Drug Interactions in Clinical Trials: Statistical Considerations

Gordon W. Pledger

Technical Information Section, Epilepsy Branch, National Institutes of Health, Bethesda, Maryland, U.S.A.

The term *drug interaction* is suggestive of one drug altering the effects of another or of the combined use of drugs producing effects not entirely attributable to the effects of the individual drugs when given alone. This rather vague concept must be given a more precise meaning before it can become the subject of scientific investigation. The basis of a standard statistical approach to defining and studying interaction is presented below. However, it will be seen that the situation is not straightforward. For example, even when an intuitively meaningful definition of interaction is available, it may be at odds with an alternative, and equally reasonable, definition.

FACTORIAL DESIGNS

The type of experiment that allows the most direct assessment of interactions between factors (e.g., drugs) is called a *factorial experiment* (1). In a factorial experiment, the effects of the variables (or factors) of interest are investigated simultaneously. All possible combinations of the factors are included as treatments in the factorial design. Consider the simplest case, that of only two factors. Suppose one is interested in the effects of two drugs, standard (S) and test (T), given singly and in combination. For the sake of simplicity, suppose further that each drug is to be tested at a predetermined fixed dosage. Thus, there are two factors, S and T, and each can occur at two levels, predetermined fixed dose or zero. The resulting experimental design, referred to as a 2×2 factorial design, includes four treatment groups (here assumed to be of equal size). The treatments are as follows:

$$ST \qquad \text{(both drugs present)}$$
$$ST_p \qquad \text{(S present, T absent)}$$
$$S_pT \qquad \text{(S absent, T present)}$$
$$S_pT_p \qquad \text{(both drugs absent)}$$

where S_p (respectively, T_p) is a matching placebo for drug S (T).

The mean responses observed in the trial might be displayed as follows:

		Drug S	
		Absent	Present
Drug T	Absent	22.9	44.8
	Present	50.4	55.2

The results shown here are for illustrative purposes only. In an antiepileptic drug trial, they might represent seizure counts or reductions from baseline.

These data yield estimates of various treatment effects. For instance, the effect of the test drug, T, in the absence of the standard antiepileptic drug, S, is estimated by the difference

$$50.4 - 22.9 = 27.5$$

The effect of T when given concomitantly with S is estimated by the difference

$$55.2 - 44.8 = 10.4$$

However, if the two drugs are independent, i.e., if the presence of one does not alter the effects of the other, then the two differences computed above are estimates of the same parameter; the effect of drug T in the presence of drug S is the same as the effect in the absence of S. In this case, the effect of drug T would be better estimated by the average of the two previously computed estimates:

$$\tfrac{1}{2}(27.5 + 10.4) = 19.0$$

The standard error of this estimate, called the *main* effect of T, is $1/\sqrt{2}$ times the standard error of the earlier estimates, called *simple* effects in the statistical jargon.

If there is an interaction between S and T, then the simple effects of T are not equal; concomitant administration of drug S changes the effect of drug T in some way. In this case the interaction between the two drugs can be estimated by the difference between the simple effects

$$27.5 - 10.4 = 17.1$$

It should be noted that this situation is symmetric. The simple effects for drug S are 21.9 and 4.8, leading to an interaction estimate of

$$21.9 - 4.8 = 17.1$$

Using lower case letters to represent the observed means of the corresponding treatments, S or T or placebo (P), the estimated interaction can be expressed as

$$(st - t) - (s - p)$$

This is simply a difference of means, and testing whether the interaction is zero, e.g., by a t-test, is equivalent to testing whether S and T act independently. If S and T do act independently, then their effects are additive, i.e., the effect of the combination, ST, is the sum of the individual drug effects. This can be seen by setting the interaction equal to zero:

$$(ST - T) - (S - P) = 0$$

implies

$$(S - P) + (T - P) = (ST - P)$$

If the interaction is positive, then the effect of the combination treatment is greater than the sum of the effects of the two drugs when given alone. In this case, S and T are said to be synergistic. If the interaction is negative, then S and T are said to be antagonistic.

If the variable being observed is a measure of clinical efficacy, then the terms *synergism* and *antagonism* have intuitive meanings. For instance, there is evidence that caffeine has a synergistic relationship with certain analgesics. Caffeine, when given alone, exhibits no analgesic activity, but it enhances the analgesic effects of both aspirin and acetaminophen (2). One of the best-documented cases of antagonism is a type of drug combination that occurs in an uncountable number of over-the-counter products, those products containing both a decongestant and an antihistamine. For example, clinical trials have shown that the combination of triprolidine and pseudoephedrine is inferior to the decongestant component, pseudoephedrine, alone, with respect to relief of nasal congestion. Of course, this does not imply that such products are not useful and rational combinations. They are intended to relieve a symptom complex and, whereas the antihistamine may interfere with the action of the decongestant, it also contributes positive effects on other symptoms (sneezing, watery eyes, etc.).

In order to avoid giving an oversimplified view of the concept of interaction, several points need to be mentioned. First, although the additive model used throughout this presentation is the most commonly used model, it is not the only one. One alternative is the multiplicative model. Consider the following example in which the efficacy measure is the observed seizure frequency expressed as a proportion of the placebo rate.

<table>
<tr><td></td><td></td><td colspan="2" align="center">Drug S</td></tr>
<tr><td></td><td></td><td align="center">Absent</td><td align="center">Present</td></tr>
<tr><td rowspan="2">Drug T</td><td>Absent</td><td align="center">1</td><td align="center">0.5</td></tr>
<tr><td>Present</td><td align="center">0.4</td><td align="center">0.2</td></tr>
</table>

Under the multiplicative model, a zero interaction means that the effect of the combination is the product of the individual drug effects, as it is in this example. In some cases, the multiplicative model may be a reasonable choice. An example of such a situation is mentioned in the next section.

Even if the standard, additive model is used, the presence of an interaction may be dependent on the efficacy variable chosen. Examples can be constructed such that there is no interaction if the efficacy measure is mean seizure frequency reduction from baseline, but there is an interaction if efficacy is expressed in terms of mean percent reduction in seizure frequency. Both of these efficacy variables seem sensible and are often used. Thus, interactions can be artificial constructs; they can be made to appear or disappear. This phenomenon reflects the difficulty often encountered when one attempts to describe in precise mathematical terms an intuitive concept. It certainly suggests that caution is in order when interpreting interactions.

A final point deserves note here. In the foregoing discussion of the various effects that are estimable and testable in a factorial design, the test for the presence of an interaction was mentioned; some discussion of the practical utility of that test is needed. Although the test can be done, it often has such low power that the failure to detect an interaction constitutes only minimal evidence that in fact no important interaction exists. The standard error of the estimate of the interaction is twice that of the main-effect estimate and exceeds the simple-effects standard error by a factor of $\sqrt{2}$. In terms of statistical power, the impact of this increased variation can be huge. For instance, if a factorial trial is designed to have power 0.9 to detect a main effect equal to one standard deviation (assuming no interaction), then the power to test for an interaction of the same magnitude is only about 0.3. Thus, the underlying assumption of no interaction cannot be strongly supported on an empirical basis; it will need support from other sources such as the biological or other rationale, pilot studies, etc. This problem is exacerbated by the fact that clinical trials are usually conducted with sample sizes just large enough to test the primary hypothesis.

INTERACTIONS IN ANTIEPILEPTIC DRUG TRIALS

The examples of drug interactions mentioned in the preceding section were demonstrated in straightforward, factorial design clinical trials. Such trials are difficult to conduct in epilepsy, because groups of patients with uncontrolled seizures would be receiving only placebo or only an investigational drug. Of course, the interaction of two drugs, say a test drug and a standard, could be investigated against a standardized background treatment. For instance, patients being treated with carbamazepine monotherapy could be randomized to receive, in addition, placebo, phenytoin, a test drug, or the combination of the test drug and phenytoin. Clearly, the interaction information obtainable from such an add-on trial would not be equivalent to that available in a trial without the concomitant antiepileptic treatment, but this may not be a major problem. More important, the carbamazepine effect may leave insufficient room for additional improvement in seizure frequency, i.e., the presence of the background antiepileptic treatment may inhibit the design's ability to detect the effect of the test drug or its possible interaction with phenytoin.

The above remarks regarding the possible decreased sensitivity of add-on trials suggest what may be a common source of antagonistic interactions between drugs intended to treat the same symptom or condition. An observed antagonism is not necessarily an indication that one drug interferes pharmacologically with the action of the other. It may be that the effect of one drug simply decreases the room for additional beneficial effects. In the most extreme case, if one of the drugs abolishes the symptom, then the combination cannot do any better. In less extreme cases, the multiplicative model mentioned earlier may avoid this artificial type of negative interaction.

INTERACTIONS IN DOSE-RESPONSE DESIGNS

To this point, it has been assumed that the two dosage levels in a factorial design are zero and a specified, fixed dosage greater than zero. It is not necessary that zero be one of the tested doses. One or both drugs could be tested at a low dose and a high dose, or even at more than two doses. As an example, consider the situation described in the preceding section. One wishes to investigate the effectiveness of a new drug T as well as its interaction with a standard drug S, phenytoin in the preceding discussion. An alternative to the add-on design described above would be a design that superimposes the T versus placebo comparison on a dose response study of the standard drug S. Letting L represent a low dose of S and H represent a high dose, the design can be represented schematically as follows:

		Drug S	
		L	H
	Placebo	L	H
Test Drug			
	T	TL	TH

This design has the following features: (a) no patient is untreated; each receives at least the low dose of the standard drug; (b) half of the patients receive the test drug and half do not, so the design should provide a reasonably efficient test of the efficacy of T; and (c) an interaction between S and T corresponds to a change in the dose-response curve of S. The interaction term is

$$(TH - TL) - (H - L)$$

Here the interaction may be less informative than when $L = 0$; however, it will often have a meaningful interpretation if the doses L and H are well chosen. Ideally, L and H would be on the steep part of the dose response curve so that the difference in response to these doses is large. A positive interaction indicates that the difference in response between L and H is increased in the presence of the test drug T. It is intuitively reasonable to refer to this property as synergism (assuming, of course, that the response to TL is not less than that to L alone).

It should be noted that L and H could represent plasma drug concentrations rather than doses. In fact, the efficiency of the design is enhanced by using low and high plasma concentrations instead of doses if the plasma level–response relationship is more predictable, i.e., less variable, than is the dose–response relationship.

It should also be noted that even though this discussion has focused on factorial designs, nothing precludes investigating clinical interactions within the context of a crossover study. In fact, trials in which patients receive, in random order, each of the factorial design treatments have been conducted in certain drug classes. Generally, these have been studies in conditions where the required observation time on any particular treatment is relatively short, e.g., trials of combinations of antihypertensive drugs. Efficacy trials of antiepileptic drugs usually have treatment periods that are several months long. Studies that attempt to retain individual patients for the duration of four such treatment periods may encounter problems with dropouts. In addition, the analytical problems that arise in two-period crossover trials, such as dealing with treatment by period interactions, are much more formidable in a four-period design.

PHARMACOKINETIC INTERACTIONS

Interactions that are manifested in changes of pharmacokinetic parameters can often be investigated without conducting a full factorial design. To see this, consider the situation in which the variable of interest is the plasma concentration of standard drug S. A factorial design adequate for addressing the question of whether S interacts with test drug T would have the following treatments:

| | Drug S | |
	Absent	Present
Drug T — Absent	Placebo	S
Present	T	ST

However, if it is assumed that patients who do not take drug S will have zero plasma concentration of S, then the two treatments in the first column, placebo and T, are not needed. The interaction term,

$$(ST - S) - (T - placebo)$$

reduces to

$$(ST - S)$$

This brief derivation simply confirms intuition; the interaction between S and T is the amount by which the plasma S levels change in the presence of T as opposed to the levels when S is administered alone. Thus, the interaction between S and T could be estimated from a design that randomizes patients (or volunteers) to either a fixed dosage of S or fixed dosage of each of S and T. Alternatively, a randomized crossover design could be used to compare these two treatments. However, to my knowledge, neither of these designs is actually used in the early studies aimed at detecting interactions and dose tolerability.

A commonly used design is one that includes no randomization. It begins with a period during which stable plasma concentrations of drug S are established with a fixed dosage of S. Drug T is then added in escalating dosages. Even without randomized control, the design might provide usable estimates of the interaction if the plasma levels of S were only monitored. However, these levels typically are manipulated through dosage changes aimed at keeping the plasma levels constant. This greatly complicates the interpretation of study results. For a fixed dosage of S and T, the change in plasma S concentration can be written as

$$\Delta S = I + \epsilon$$

where I is the interaction and ϵ is a random error. This assumes that there are no extraneous changes occurring over time; if such changes are present, a controlled design is needed to detect them. An obvious estimate of I under this model is the mean change in observed plasma level of S.

Suppose now that changes in the dosage of S are permitted in response to observed changes in the plasma concentration. Furthermore, assume, for the sake of simplicity, that within the range of dosages being used in the study, the interaction is not dose dependent. Clearly, the interaction can no longer be estimated by the mean plasma S level change. In fact, if the adjustments in the dosage of S achieve their goal, then the mean change in plasma level will be near zero, regardless of the magnitude of the interaction. Construction of a reasonable interaction estimate is complicated because of the extent of the dependence in the model. The levels are dependent on the dosages, which, in turn, are dependent on the levels. Two "seat-of-the-pants" methods for handling this situation come to mind: (a) ignore all plasma levels after the first dosage change and estimate the interaction from the remaining levels; or (b) use the levels observed on the modified dosages to estimate the levels that would have been observed without dosage changes, and then use the estimated levels to estimate the interaction.

Neither of these approaches is entirely satisfactory. The first approach does become increasingly acceptable the longer the first dosage change can be delayed, i.e., the closer the study comes to using a fixed-dose design. The second approach requires some assumptions about the relationship between dosage and plasma level of S in the *presence* of T.

IMPACT OF INTERACTIONS ON TRIAL DESIGN: EXAMPLE

The Antiepileptic Drug Development Program of the National Institutes of Health recently sponsored a controlled clinical trial aimed at demonstrating efficacy and safety of felbamate. Using a two-period crossover design, felbamate was compared to placebo as add-on therapy. Each of the 57 patients was receiving concomitant treatment with both phenytoin and carbamazepine throughout the trial. Pilot study data indicated an interaction between felbamate and the concomitant treatment; when felbamate, at the doses to be tested in the controlled trial, was added to the background therapy of phenytoin and carbamazepine, plasma phenytoin levels rose by approximately 20%.

In order to account for this identified interaction and to maintain stable phenytoin levels during the trial, the design called for replacement of approximately 20% of the phenytoin dosage by matching placebo during the felbamate treatment period of the crossover study. The exact phenytoin dosage reduction varied from patient to patient; 20% was used as a guideline for the initial reduction, but subsequent adjustments were made in response to the monitored plasma levels.

Figures 1 and 2 show the actual mean dosage reductions and the resulting mean plasma phenytoin levels. Separate graphs are presented for each of the two study centers, the University of Minnesota and the University of Virginia, and for each of the two treatment sequences in the crossover design.

Consider a possible rationale for the phenytoin dosage reduction maneuver introduced into the design of the felbamate trial. (This was not the primary rationale used by the designers of the trial, but it is of theoretical interest.) If the mean seizure frequency is less during the felbamate treatment period than during the placebo treatment period, one would like to be able to attribute that difference to antiepileptic activity on the part of felbamate. However, if it is also observed that the mean plasma phenytoin level was 20% higher during the felbamate treatment period as opposed to the placebo treatment period, then this difference may represent a plausible explanation for the reduction in seizure frequency. Thus, the systematic phenytoin dosage modifications could have been included in the trial design in an attempt to eliminate a potential source of between-treatment differences in efficacy data. If this were the primary goal, then the dosage adjustment strategy would appear to be based on an underlying assumption that there is a direct relationship between plasma phenytoin level and degree of antiepileptic activity. This assumption may be tenable, but it is not self-evident, and it deserves careful consideration under the conditions of the present trial. A plasma phenytoin level resulting from a drug interaction is not necessarily equivalent to the same level achieved under different conditions, e.g., phenytoin monotherapy. It should be recognized that the type of systematic dosage changes made in this trial are not without potential costs. In eliminating systematic differences in plasma levels, the design gives rise to systematic differences in phenytoin dosage. The importance of one difference must be balanced

Felbamate Trial: Mean Phenytoin Levels

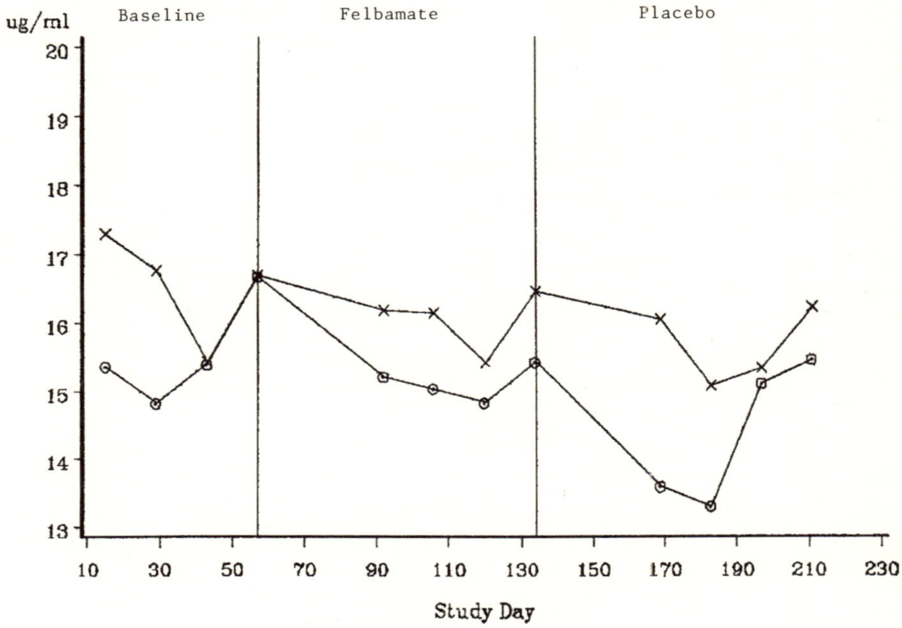

Mean Phenytoin Dosages

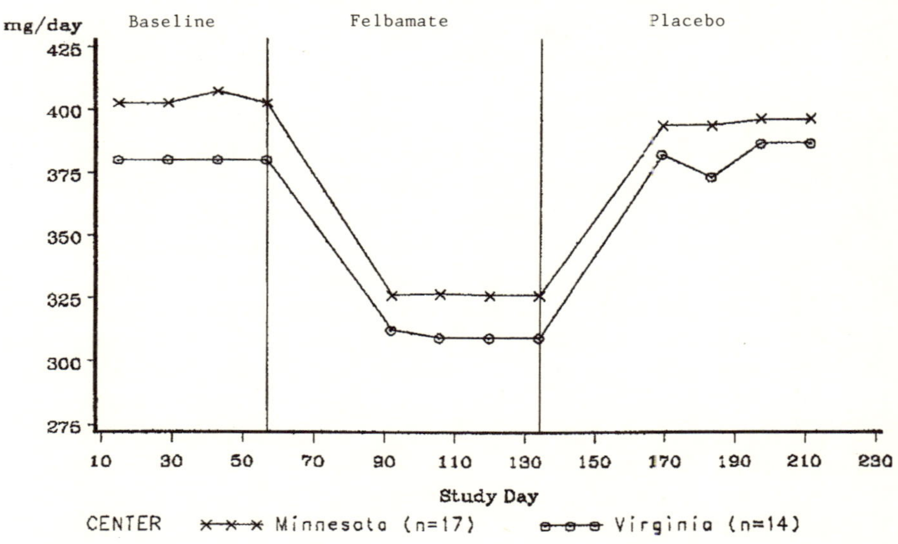

FIG. 9-1. Mean phenytoin dosages and corresponding plasma levels for patients randomized to the treatment order felbamate/placebo in the NIH-sponsored crossover trial. All patients were receiving concomitant treatment with both phenytoin and carbamazepine.

Felbamate Trial: Mean Phenytoin Levels

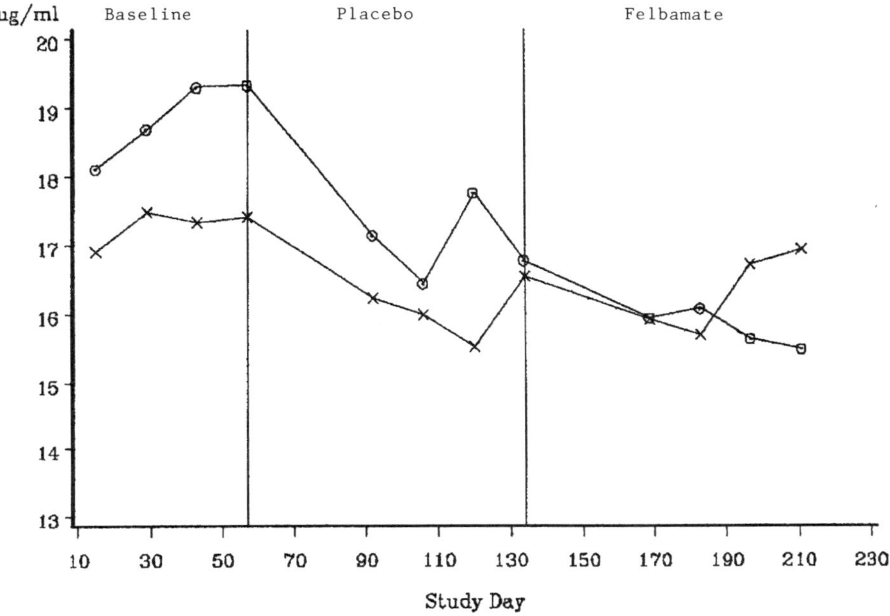

Mean Phenytoin Dosages

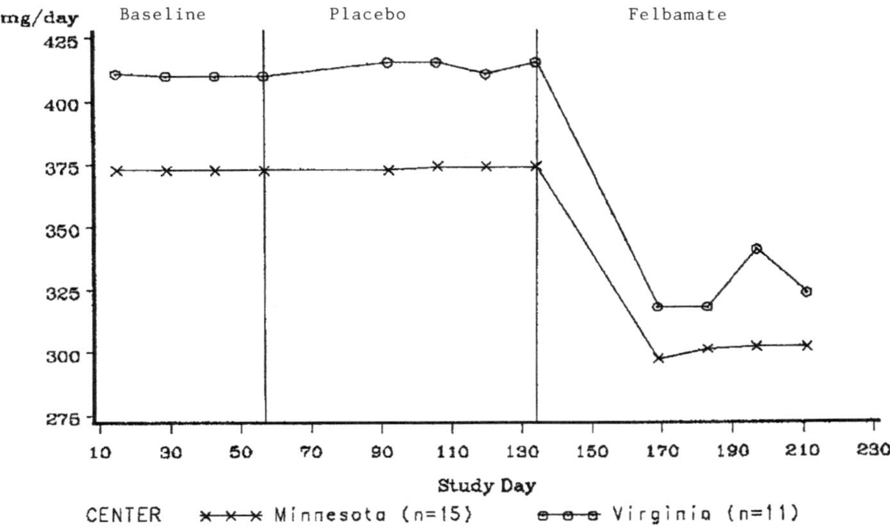

FIG. 9-2. Mean phenytoin dosages and corresponding plasma levels for patients randomized to the treatment order placebo/felbamate in the NIH-sponsored crossover trial. All patients were receiving concomitant treatment with both phenytoin and carbamazepine.

against that of the other, and the choice must be made with less than complete information.

A very different sort of rationale was actually invoked in designing the felbamate trial. Patients were not enrolled in this clinical trial unless their seizures were considered therapy resistant. Thus, one could argue that their phenytoin and carbamazepine dosages had been adjusted to achieve the maximum tolerated plasma level prior to study entry. If felbamate were added to the patient's treatment regimen, with a resulting 20% increase in plasma phenytoin level, then drug toxicity could occur and could jeopardize the blinding or even the feasibility of the study. Again, this argument assumes that drug effects, in this case adverse effects of phenytoin, are driven by the plasma level, not by the amount of phenytoin administered.

The decision whether to conduct the trial at constant phenytoin dosages or at stable plasma concentrations might have been crucial to the success of the trial. As the trial was conducted, with systematic phenytoin dosage reductions during the felbamate treatment period, the primary risk was that the design would be biased against the test drug. The treatments compared were (approximately)

$$[F + 0.80P + C] \text{ vs. } [P + C]$$

where F is felbamate, P is phenytoin, and C is carbamazepine dosage.

One would probably feel comfortable interpreting a positive study as evidence of felbamate's effectiveness, but a negative outcome in the trial would not necessarily imply that felbamate is ineffective. On the other hand, if no dosage adjustments are made, so that the comparison is $[F + P + C]$ vs. $[P + C]$, then, as discussed above, interpretation of a positive study may present problems. It needs to be recognized, however, that with either design approach, constant dose or stable plasma level, a positive study result would be meaningful. It is not a false positive simply because a rationale has been constructed that suggests that a similar result might not be achieved under different conditions, e.g., monotherapy. A positive trial will have demonstrated that administration of the drug results in a beneficial effect under the conditions of the trial. Speculations about the mechanism leading to that effect represent conjectures that require their own empirical verification.

The standard statistical formulation used in clinical trial design is hypothesis testing. This formulation is asymmetric; controlling the probability of a false positive (Type 1 error) is considered to be of paramount importance. This often leads to conservative approaches to design and analysis, i.e., the chance of a false negative (Type 2 error) may be inflated. It appears that the designers of the felbamate trial acted in accordance with this principle. A possibly inflated probability of a false negative trial was considered tolerable in order to avoid more undesirable outcomes, e.g., an increased dropout rate during the felbamate treatment period.

An additional point concerning the felbamate trial design merits discussion here. As mentioned above, the magnitude of the phenytoin dosage reduction during the felbamate treatment period was approximately, but not exactly, 20%. In addition to the planned reduction of about 20% at one point during the trial, dosage adjustments based on observed plasma phenytoin levels were allowed throughout both the felbamate and placebo treatment periods. The dosage adjustments were determined at each center by unblinded staff who monitored the plasma phenytoin concentrations. The risk of bias arising from this procedure appears to be slight, because the unblinded dose adjusters had no contact with the patients in the trial. However, there is some indication in the study data that plasma-level–driven dosage adjustments were not made by consistent criteria during the two treatment periods. Thus, this may be another illustration of the fact that it is hard to behave as if blinded if one is not blinded. It would be interesting to know how much less stable the plasma phenytoin levels would have been if only the systematic 20% dosage adjustments had been permitted.

CONCLUSIONS

Factorial designs are underutilized in clinical trials (3). These designs allow the simultaneous investigation of two (or more) drugs. In the example discussed above, one of the two drugs was a standard, but both could be experimental drugs. Thus, the efficacy of two new drugs could be studied in one trial requiring less time and fewer patients than would be needed for separate trials. At the same time, information can be gained about the interaction, although this might not be a primary objective of the clinical trial.

As pointed out above, the test for a nonzero interaction usually has low power. It may be that the perceived difficulty in detecting the interactions of primary interest has led to the situation in antiepileptic drug testing in which greater emphasis is placed on the more tractable problem of pharmacokinetic interactions. This is a useful approach if the pharmacokinetic interactions are indicative of pharmacodynamic interactions. In order to determine whether such correspondences exist, both types of interaction need to be investigated in the same trial, using a factorial design.

Acknowledgment: The author gratefully acknowledges the contributions of two true-blue Nittany Lions: Marla Dombroski, who produced the graphs in Figs. 1 and 2, and Diane Dudes, who prepared the manuscript.

REFERENCES

1. Cochran WG, Cox GM. *Experimental Designs.* 2nd ed. New York: John Wiley and Sons, Inc., 1966.
2. Laska EM, Sunshine A, Mueller F, Elvers WB, Siegel C, Ruben A. Caffeine as an analgesic adjuvant. *JAMA* 1984 251:1711–8.
3. Peto R. Clinical trial methodology. *Biomedicine* 1978; 28 (special issue):24–36.

10

Interactions of Antiepileptic Drugs During Development: Summary

Roger J. Porter

National Institute of Neurological Disorders and Stroke, National Institutes of Health, Bethesda, Maryland, U.S.A.

The development of new antiepileptic drugs is critical to the millions of patients worldwide who suffer from epilepsy. In the United States alone, there are 2,000,000 patients with seizure disorders and 200,000 who have seizures more than once a month. Most of these patients depend on drugs to control their seizures. For many patients with intractable epilepsy, hope lies in the development of more effective medications; for patients whose seizures respond to currently available medications, new drugs could potentially reduce the side-effects they must often tolerate in order to gain seizure control.

The history of the development of antiepileptic drugs is a study in both serendipity and science. Pioneer drugs—the bromides and the first barbiturate—were discovered by astute clinical observations. In 1937, however, experimental means were utilized to identify phenytoin, causing a revolution in the preclinical approach to the discovery of new drugs. Although a number of new drugs have been developed since the marketing of phenytoin (Table 10-1), progress in the last 20 years has been slow. Valproate, the last major addition to our armamentarium, was marketed in France in 1969; almost two decades have elapsed since the appearance of a major new drug for patients with epilepsy.

This volume on antiepileptic drug interactions explores a major aspect of designing studies to prove the efficiency and safety of new compounds. In drug development, however, there are other factors to be taken into account. The major considerations are listed in Table 10-2 and are discussed at length (1). Study design is addressed in detail (2).

Table 10-1. Antiepileptic Drugs Marketed in the United States

Year introduced	International nonproprietary name	U.S. trade name	Company
1912	Phenobarbital	Luminal	Winthrop
1935	Mephobarbital	Mebaral	Winthrop
1938	Phenytoin	Dilantin	Parke–Davis
1946	Trimethadione	Tridione	Abbott
1947	Mephenytoin	Mesantoin	Sandoz
1949	Paramethadione	Paradione	Abbott
1950	Phethenylate[a]	Thiantoin	Lilly
1951	Phenacemide	Phenurone	Abbott
1952	Metharbital	Gemonil	Abbott
1952	Benzchlorpropamide[b]	Hibicon	Lederle
1953	Phensuximide	Milontin	Parke–Davis
1954	Primidone	Mysoline	Ayerst
1957	Methsuximide	Celontin	Parke–Davis
1957	Ethotoin	Peganone	Abbott
1960	Aminoglutethimide[c]	Elipten	Ciba
1960	Ethosuximide	Zarontin	Parke–Davis
1968	Diazepam[d]	Valium	Roche
1974	Carbamazepine	Tegretol	Geigy
1975	Clonazepam	Clonopin	Roche
1978	Valproic acid	Depakene	Abbott
1981	Clorazepate dipotassium[d]	Tranxene	Abbott

Reproduced from Porter (1) with permission.
[a]Withdrawn in 1952.
[b]Withdrawn in 1955.
[c]Withdrawn in 1966.
[d]Approved by the FDA as an adjunct.

SPECIFIC ISSUES IN THE INTERACTIONS OF ANTIEPILEPTIC DRUGS

Drugs During Development

Drug interactions are a major concern when developing new drugs. First, one must consider interactions of currently marketed drugs that, even prior to the introduction of the test drug, may interact among themselves. At present, clinical trials in epilepsy tend to be studies with only one concomitant medication, and, therefore, the problem of established drugs interacting with each other only rarely arises. Second, one must consider the effect of the concomitant medication(s) on the new drug. Finally, one must consider the effect of the new drug on the concomitant medication.

Table 10-2. Factors to be Considered in the Development of a New
Antiepileptic Drug

Preclinical considerations
  Molecular structure and structural novelty
  Mechanism of action—usually increased inhibition or diminished excitation
  Classical empirical screening data for efficacy
  Other animal models of efficacy and toxicity

Clinical investigations
  Patient heterogeneity
  Patient exclusion criteria
  Patient seizure type
  Patient seizure frequency
  Concomitant medications (and interactions)
  The dose of the test compound
  Study design

Of these last two considerations, investigators usually focus on the latter because it is easier both to recognize and to measure. Investigational drugs have less–well-documented steady-state levels, and the causes of changes in these levels are more difficult to identify than with standard medications. With these fundamental considerations as a background, the following questions—some of which are controversial—may be asked relevant to drug interactions during drug development.

Should observed drug interactions stop drug development? Drug interactions are rarely severe enough to warrant stopping a compound's development solely because of the interaction, especially since drug interactions are common among already marketed antiepileptic agents. Clinicians have learned, for example, that valproate must be very cautiously added to phenobarbital to avoid serious pharmacokinetic interactions. On the other hand, some investigational drugs elicit such a powerful interaction that the viability of the compound as potential drug may be questioned. An example is nafimidone, whose inhibition of carbamazepine metabolism may cause patients to become quite toxic from high carbamazepine levels. Although studies on this drug were not discontinued because of drug interaction, the argument has been made that the interaction is sufficiently severe to render the drug very difficult to use and therefore unmarketable. Counterarguments rest on the assumption that any new, efficacious drug may have a role to play in epilepsy therapy, citing drug interaction as merely one more unfortunate variable that must be learned and considered by the prescribing physician. The consensus at this time seems to favor development of new drugs almost without regard to the degree of interaction. As more drugs are tested, this working thesis may be challenged.

How useful are preclinical data in predicting drug interactions? The effects of combining multiple drugs are usually pharmacokinetic, which explains the fundamental problem in predicting drug interactions in humans. Pharmacokinetic comparisons between species are notoriously difficult because of the dramatic differences in clearance between species. Rats, for example, clear carbamazepine so rapidly that measuring the effect of a new drug on carbamazepine metabolism in this species may be nearly impossible. Although some predictions of human drug interactions may be gleaned from pharmacokinetic studies in animals, the data are neither conclusive nor necessarily quantitative in their comparison. Certain in vitro studies—such as those that utilize liver microsomes—may add to the predictive power of preclinical investigations. In general, most investigators agree that preclinical studies can give strong clues to the nature and extent of drug interaction, but human data are required for definitive observations.

How small can an interaction be and still be significant? In clinical practice, patients and physicians tolerate rather large drug interactions. In clinical trials, however, the tolerance is necessarily much lower. A new compound that causes an increase in the levels of the concomitant drug may, for example, improve the patient but ruin the study. In general, most studies attempt to maintain steady levels of concomitant drugs; fluctuations may influence the variable under study, usually seizure frequency. If some interactions are present, an unblinded monitor may be required to adjust dosages in order to maintain the levels. There are almost certainly interactions that go undetected in clinical trials; the importance of these, of course, remains unknown.

Are better pilot studies needed to evaluate interactions prior to controlled clinical trials? If there is agreement on anything, it is that more investigations are needed prior to initiating a controlled clinical trial. Pilot studies can provide a better definition of drug interactions. In the past, such interactions were thought to be unlikely, and controlled trials were initiated in the hope that such interactions would not occur. However, now that our awareness of the likelihood of significant interactions has been heightened, pilot studies should be performed that at least mimic the pharmacologic setting of the proposed controlled trial. This proposal does not mean that all possibilities of interactions need to be investigated, thus delaying—perhaps for years—the controlled trial. Simple studies, however, can very expeditiously provide clues regarding interaction problems; such human pilot studies are now considered mandatory by most investigators.

Are drug interactions important in the discontinuation of antiepileptic drugs? Appropriate emphasis needs to be placed on the concept of deinduction. Most clinical investigators are concerned with the inhibition of metabolism by one drug or another, but when the inhibitory agent is withdrawn, the patient may be at risk for deinduction and for changes in plasma levels. This interaction differs widely from one patient to another and may be either dose or concentration dependent. The problem is not limited to clinical practice; it may be very troublesome in crossover controlled trials, in which a patient is changed from active to placebo medication.

In summary, the investigation of new antiepileptic drugs requires increasing considerations of drug interactions. Both efficacy and toxicity parameters may be unfavorably altered by failure to identify such interactions and to compensate for them in the clinical trial design.

REFERENCES

1. Porter RJ. New antiepileptic drugs: prospects for improved treatment of seizures. In: Pedley TA, Meldrum BS, eds. *Recent Advances in Epilepsy-4*. London: Churchill Livingstone, 1988:161–79.
2. Porter RJ, White BG. Evaluation in man. In: Meldrum BS, Porter RJ, eds. *Current Problems in Epilepsy: New Anticonvulsant Drugs*. London: John Libbey, 1986:49–61.

III. Mechanistic Aspects of Interactions

11

Carbamazepine Epoxide/Valproic Acid Interaction in Rat, Monkey, and Man

Bradley M. Kerr and René H. Levy

*Department of Pharmaceutics, University of Washington,
Seattle, Washington, U.S.A.*

Carbamazepine-10,11-epoxide (EPO) is a pharmacologically active metabolite of the anticonvulsant carbamazepine (CBZ) that accumulates to measurable concentrations in the plasma of CBZ-treated patients (1). Administration of the anticonvulsant valproic acid (VPA) to CBZ-treated patients has been documented to produce an increase in both EPO plasma levels and in the EPO/CBZ plasma concentration ratio (2–8). The elevations in EPO plasma levels have been reported to be associated with neurological side-effects in patients treated with the CBZ/VPA drug combination (9).

Other anticonvulsant drugs, such as phenobarbital and phenytoin, are also known to increase the EPO/CBZ plasma concentration ratio, with the effect generally attributed to induction of cytochrome P-450 and enhanced formation of EPO from CBZ (2,3,6,10). However, unlike phenobarbital and phenytoin, VPA is not known to induce either cytochrome P-450 or EPO formation clearance. An alternative mechanism by which VPA may elevate EPO plasma levels is by inhibiting the in vivo elimination of EPO.

EPO is almost entirely converted in vivo to CBZ-10,11-transdihydrodiol (DHD) prior to urinary excretion in man (11). This hydrolytic reaction is known to be enzymatically mediated and is believed to be catalyzed by epoxide hydrolase (12–14). It has therefore been speculated that VPA increases EPO plasma levels by inhibiting the in vivo hydrolysis of EPO (6,8), but in vitro investigations have failed to show that VPA inhibits the activity of hepatic microsomal epoxide hydrolase (15–17). The suggestion has been made that perhaps a metabolite of VPA formed in vivo, rather than VPA itself, inhibits the activity of epoxide hydrolase and thereby increases EPO plasma levels (8).

The interaction between VPA and EPO and the effect of VPA on epoxide hydrolase activity has been investigated in our laboratory both in vivo and in vitro, with studies carried out both in man and in lower animal species. The investigations summarized in this chapter have not only led to a better understanding of the mechanism of this unusual drug interaction, but have also led to the development of tools that may be useful for predicting drug interactions involving EPO in epileptic patients.

ELEVATION OF EPO/CBZ PLASMA CONCENTRATION RATIO

The first evidence that VPA affects plasma concentrations of EPO in CBZ-treated patients was provided by McKauge et al. (2). It was noted that patients treated with the CBZ/VPA drug combination had significantly higher plasma concentrations of EPO relative to the dose of CBZ than patients treated with CBZ alone, whereas the plasma levels of CBZ relative to the dose of CBZ did not differ in the two groups. The EPO/CBZ plasma concentration ratio was subsequently shown in several reports to be elevated in patients treated with VPA. The average EPO/CBZ plasma ratio was reported to be approximately 0.10 in adult patients on CBZ monotherapy versus an average ratio of 0.20 in patients treated with CBZ and VPA (3,6). The mean EPO/CBZ plasma ratio in children, which tends to be higher than in adults, was about 0.20 in children receiving CBZ alone versus 0.30 in children treated with the CBZ/VPA drug combination (7). After accounting for the extent to which CBZ and EPO are bound to plasma proteins, Ramsay et al. (4) found that the plasma ratio of unbound EPO to unbound CBZ was 0.27 in CBZ-monotherapy patients, and was elevated to 1.02 in patients treated with CBZ and VPA, indicating that this drug interaction is principally an enzymatic rather than a protein-binding interaction. Two prospective studies have also been carried out in which VPA was added to the drug regimen of patients who were stabilized on CBZ therapy (5,8). The administration of VPA resulted in an increase of the EPO/CBZ plasma ratio in all patients in both studies, with the average increase being approximately 100% in each study.

Investigations in rat and monkey indicate that administration of VPA elevates the EPO/CBZ concentration ratio in these two animal species in addition to man, suggesting that the mechanism by which VPA interacts with EPO may be the same in man, monkey, and rat. Infusion of sodium valproate to steady-state blood concentrations of 0.53 ± 0.24 mM in eight rats increased the EPO/CBZ steady-state concentration ratio from 1.65 ± 0.26 to 2.12 ± 0.23 (18,19). VPA had no effect on the free fractions of CBZ and EPO in the plasma and blood of the rat, indicating that the increased EPO/CBZ ratio in the rat was not the result of a protein-binding interaction (18,19). Displacement of CBZ and EPO from plasma proteins by VPA was found in the rhesus monkey (5). However, the steady-state plasma ratio of unbound EPO to unbound CBZ in the monkey was elevated by VPA, indicating that the interaction of VPA with EPO probably has enzymatic basis. The ratio of unbound EPO to unbound CBZ in the plasma of four monkeys was increased from 0.12 ± 0.03 to 0.24 ± 0.03 by VPA steady-state plasma concentrations of 0.58 ± 0.09 mM, and the ratio was further increased to 0.36 ± 0.05 at VPA concentrations of 1.22 ± 0.19 mM (5).

INHIBITION OF EPO ELIMINATION IN VIVO

The increased EPO/CBZ plasma concentration ratio during VPA administration in man, monkey, and rat suggests that either the formation clearance of EPO from CBZ is enhanced by VPA, or the elimination clearance of EPO is inhibited. The most direct means of distinguishing between these two alternative mechanisms is by evaluating the effect of VPA on the disposition of EPO administered in the absence of CBZ. In view of the similar effects VPA had on the EPO/CBZ plasma ratio in man, monkey, and rat, the hypothesis that VPA is an inhibitor of in vivo EPO metabolism was tested in all three animal species (Table 11-1).

The elimination of an intravenous bolus dose of EPO was inhibited by VPA in eight rats (18,19). Infusion of VPA to steady-state concentrations of 0.34 ± 0.10 mM reduced the systemic clearance of EPO from 4.82 ± 0.94 ml/min/kg to 2.76 ± 0.50 ml/min/kg and prolonged the EPO half-life from 2.64 ± 0.48 h to 4.32 ± 0.43 h. The volume of distribution of EPO was not significantly affected by VPA administration. A similar inhibitory effect of VPA on the disposition of intravenously administered EPO was found in four rhesus monkeys (20). Steady-state VPA blood concentrations of 0.29 ± 0.11 mM reduced the systemic clearance of EPO from 18.1 ± 4.55 ml/min/kg to 9.27 ± 1.59 ml/min/kg, and prolonged to the EPO half-life from 0.78 ± 0.11 h to 1.26 ± 0.21 h. The volume of distribution of EPO appeared to be reduced slightly by VPA administration in the monkey.

The effect of VPA on elimination of EPO in man was evaluated in six healthy, normal male adult volunteers (20,21). An oral dose of EPO, 100 mg, was administered to each subject on two occasions, utilizing the dosing procedure reported by Tomson et al. (11), with a 1-week interval between the two administrations of EPO (20,21). One dose of EPO served as a control, and the other dose was administered while the subject was treated with sodium valproate, 500 mg/day, 250 mg b.i.d. The order of the control and VPA-treatment phases was randomized. Steady-state trough blood levels of VPA were 0.11 ± 0.05 mM during the VPA-treatment phase. These subtherapeutic blood levels of VPA were found to modestly but consistently inhibit the in vivo elimination of EPO in all six volunteers.

Table 11-1. Inhibition of In Vivo Carbamazepine Epoxide Elimination by Valproic Acid in Three Species

Species	N	Epoxide half-life (h)			Epoxide clearance (ml/min/kg)			VPA (mM)
		Control	VPA	% change	Control	VPA	% change	
Rat[a]	8	2.64 ± 0.48	4.32 ± 0.43	+64	4.82 ± 0.94	2.76 ± 0.50	−43	0.34 ± 0.10
Monkey[b]	4	0.78 ± 0.11	1.26 ± 0.21	+62	18.1 ± 4.55	9.27 ± 1.59	−49	0.29 ± 0.11
Man[c]	6	6.27 ± 0.51	7.55 ± 1.22	+20	1.56 ± 0.15	1.30 ± 0.20	−17	0.11 ± 0.05

[a] Data from refs. 18 and 19.
[b] Data from ref. 20.
[c] Data from refs. 20 and 21.

The clearance of EPO was reduced from 1.56 ± 0.15 ml/min/kg to 1.30 ± 0.20 ml/min/kg, and the half-life of EPO was prolonged from 6.3 ± 0.5 to 7.6 ± 1.2 h. The apparent volume of distribution of EPO was not affected by VPA in this study.

The inhibition of EPO in vivo elimination by VPA in the rat, monkey, and man is consistent with the ability of VPA to elevate the EPO/CBZ plasma concentration ratio. However, the mechanism by which VPA inhibits the elimination of EPO requires an understanding of the metabolic disposition of EPO in these animal species.

FORMATION AND ELIMINATION OF DHD

VPA inhibits the in vivo elimination of EPO in man, monkey, and rat, but urinary excretion profiles of EPO and DHD indicate that the metabolism of EPO is quite different among these three animal species (Table 11-2). Therefore, the mechanism by which VPA inhibits EPO metabolism and the role of epoxide hydrolase in the EPO/VPA interaction may also be species-dependent.

The urinary recovery of DHD and unchanged EPO accounts for a small fraction of the administered dose of EPO in the rat (18–20). Urinary excretion of unchanged EPO amounted to $13.2 \pm 3.2\%$ of the EPO dose in the absence of VPA, and was increased to $24.0 \pm 4.5\%$ during administration of VPA (18,19). An increased excretion of unchanged EPO is consistent with the pronounced inhibition of EPO nonrenal clearance by VPA in the rat (18,19). However, inhibition of the nonrenal clearance of EPO is not necessarily equivalent to an inhibition of DHD formation. The percentage of the EPO dose recovered as unconjugated DHD in rat urine was only $1.08 \pm 0.34\%$ in the absence of VPA, and was $1.96 \pm 0.17\%$ during VPA administration (18). Treatment of rat urine with β-glucuronidase indicated that DHD is excreted principally in the unconjugated form (20). Thus, at least 75% of a dose of EPO is apparently converted to unidentified metabolites in the rat.

The low urinary recovery of DHD following administration of EPO in the rat may result because formation of DHD is a minor metabolic pathway of EPO, or perhaps DHD is a major metabolite that undergoes extensive secondary metabolism to unidentified products. DHD was administered as an intravenous bolus to four rats for the purpose of establishing whether or not DHD undergoes extensive secondary metabolism, but $64 \pm 3\%$ of the administered DHD was recovered unchanged in β-glucuronidase-treated urine (20). In contrast, only about 1% of an intravenous dose of EPO is recovered as DHD in β-glucuronidase–treated rat urine (20). These results indicate that the low recovery of DHD in rat urine following administration of EPO is due to extensive metabolism of EPO to alternative unidentified metabolites. It is unlikely that the inhibition of

Table 11-2. Effect of Valproic Acid on Urinary Recovery of Carbamazepine Epoxide and Carbamazepine-10,11-Trans-Dihydrodiol After Administration of Carbamazepine Epoxide in Three Species

Species	N	% epoxide dose recovered unchanged			% epoxide dose recovered as trans-dihydrodiol[a]		
		Control	VPA	% change	Control	VPA	% change
Rat[b]	5	13.2±0.03	24.0±0.04	+82	1.08±0.34	1.96±0.17	+81
Monkey[c]	4	2.49±0.68	4.70±0.93	+89	12.6±4.16	13.2±3.31	+5
Man[c]	6	4.72±1.58	6.22±1.49	+32	76.0±7.91	72.0±6.01	−5

[a]Monkey and human urine was treated with β-glucuronidase. Rat urine was untreated, but it was later shown that dihydrodiol in rat urine is mostly unconjugated (20).
[b]Data from refs. 18 and 19.
[c]Data from ref. 20.

in vivo EPO elimination by VPA in the rat is due to inhibition of DHD formation from EPO. It is more likely that the overall inhibition of EPO elimination by VPA is principally due to inhibition of unidentified EPO metabolic pathways in the rat.

The recovery of DHD in monkey urine following administration of EPO was greater than that found in rat urine, but together with unchanged EPO it accounted for only about 15% of an EPO dose (20). After intravenous administration of a bolus dose of EPO in four rhesus monkeys, the urinary recovery of DHD was $12.6 \pm 4.2\%$, whereas the recovery of unchanged EPO was $2.5 \pm 0.7\%$ (20). Administration of EPO during treatment with VPA increased the urinary recovery of unchanged EPO to $4.7 \pm 0.9\%$, and the urinary recovery of DHD ($13.2 \pm 3.3\%$) was similar to DHD recovery in the absence of VPA (20). The inability to account for at least 80% of the EPO dose makes it difficult to ascertain whether in vivo DHD formation from EPO is inhibited by VPA in the monkey.

The portion of an oral dose of EPO recovered in human urine as DHD was reported as 73–100% in four healthy volunteers, indicating that the extent to which EPO undergoes in vivo hydrolysis in man is much more extensive than in the rat or monkey (11). The high recovery of DHD in human urine was confirmed in the EPO/VPA interaction study, in which single oral doses of EPO were administered to six healthy volunteers (20,21). The percentage of the EPO dose recovered in β-glucuronidase–treated urine as DHD was $76 \pm 7.9\%$ in the control phase, and $72 \pm 6.0\%$ in the VPA treatment phase (20). An additional $4.7 \pm 1.6\%$ of the EPO dose was recovered unchanged in urine in the control phase and was increased to $6.2 \pm 1.5\%$ in the VPA treatment phase (20).

The single-dose EPO studies indicate that DHD formation is the principal route of EPO elimination in man, and inhibition of in vivo EPO elimination in man is therefore likely to reflect inhibition of DHD formation. The fraction of the EPO dose recovered unchanged in urine was increased by VPA despite no change in the renal clearance of EPO (20). The increased fraction of EPO excreted in the urine during the VPA treatment phase was due to an inhibition of the nonrenal clearance of EPO (20). Although this in vivo interaction study supports the hypothesis that the in vivo biotransformation of EPO to DHD in man is inhibited by VPA, the mechanism of the inhibition and the role of epoxide hydrolase can only be clarified with in vitro studies.

INHIBITION OF EPOXIDE HYDROLASE IN VITRO BY VPA

The hydrolysis of EPO has never been documented to occur in preparations of purified microsomal or cytosolic epoxide hydrolase. However, the enzyme-mediated conversion of EPO to DHD takes place in both rat liver microsomes and human liver microsomes (13), suggesting that EPO is a substrate for microsomal epoxide hydrolase. Therefore, it may be hypothesized that microsomal epoxide hydrolase catalyzes the in vivo hydrolysis of EPO and that inhibition of in vivo EPO elimination by VPA in man is due to inhibition of this enzyme. Pacifici et al. (15–17) investigated the ability of VPA to inhibit the hydrolysis of styrene oxide and benzo[a]pyrene-4,5-oxide in liver microsomes of rhesus monkey and man. Concentrations of VPA up to 10 mM were reported to be ineffective at inhibiting enzymatic hydrolysis of these two epoxides in vitro. These results are of interest in view of the fact that VPA plasma concentrations of less than 1 mM are associated with inhibition of EPO hydrolysis in vivo. In order to clarify the role of microsomal epoxide hydrolase in the EPO/VPA interaction, further in vitro studies were carried out in our laboratory to assess the ability of VPA to inhibit this enzyme (20).

The effect of VPA on the enzyme-catalyzed conversion of EPO to DHD in rat liver microsomes and human liver microsomes was investigated in the presence of VPA concentrations up to 1 mM (20). Incubation conditions with EPO were similar to those described by Tybring et al. (13). The 15-min incubations with EPO were carried out at a pH of 7.4 and 37°C with a protein concentration of 2 mg/ml and 1 mg/ml for rat liver microsomes and human liver microsomes, respectively.

Inhibition of EPO hydrolysis by VPA in rat liver microsomes was found to be dependent on the enzyme induction state of the rat. VPA at a concentration of 1 mM had no inhibitory effect in liver microsomes of uninduced rats, but hydrolysis of EPO was inhibited 10–20% in liver microsomes of rats pretreated with sodium phenobarbital (100 mg/kg i.p.×4 days) or trans-stilbene oxide (400 mg/kg i.p.×4 days) (Table 11-3).

Hydrolysis of EPO in human liver microsomes proceeded at a rate roughly 10- to 20-fold greater than in rat liver microsomes, a result that is consistent with the findings of Tybring et al. (13). VPA at concentrations up to 1 mM were found to inhibit the hydrolysis of EPO in human

Table 11-3. Effect of Valproic Acid on Hydrolysis of Carbamazepine Epoxide 0.25 mM in Liver Microsomes at pH of 7.4, 37°C[a]

		Carbamazepine-10,11-trans-dihydrodiol formation rate (pmol/min/mg)		
Species	Inducing agent	Control	VPA 1 mM	% change
Rat	None	2.58 ± 0.06	2.71 ± 0.07	+5
Rat	Phenobarbital	3.74 ± 0.22	3.24 ± 0.02	−13
Rat	Trans-stilbene oxide	4.38 ± 0.39	3.65 ± 0.08	−17
Human	None	51.0 ± 1.49	21.4 ± 0.96	−58

[a]Data from ref. 20. Mean ± SD of four determinations.

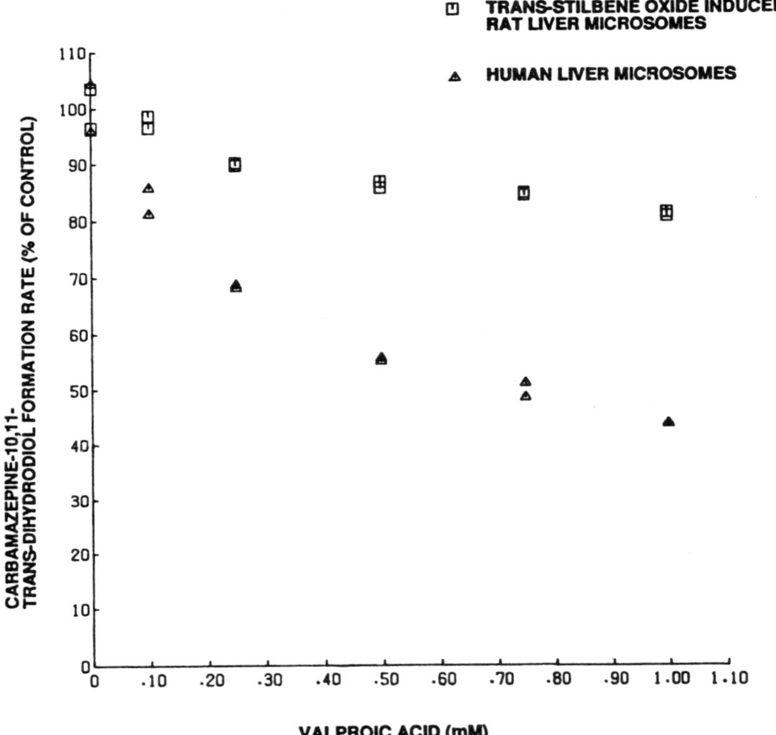

FIG. 11-1. Inhibition of hydrolysis of carbamazepine epoxide 0.25 mM by valproic acid in liver microsomes. Each symbol represents a single determination. Average trans-dihydrodiol formation rates in the control incubations (valproic acid = 0 mM) were 4.70 pmol/min/mg in the rat microsomes and 50.6 pmol/min/mg in the human microsomes.

liver microsomes much more effectively than in rat liver microsomes (Table 11-3, Fig. 11-1). The inhibitory concentration constant (K_I) of VPA was estimated to be 0.55 mM (20). This K_I concentration of VPA is within the range of VPA concentrations typically reported in plasma of patients treated chronically with sodium valproate.

Microsomal epoxide hydrolase was purified to apparent homogeneity from human liver samples on the basis of activity toward benzo[a]pyrene-4,5-oxide (20). The ability of the purified enzyme to catalyze the hydrolysis of EPO was investigated using incubation, extraction, and assay procedures similar to those used for the EPO microsomal incubations, the principal difference being that protein concentration in the incubations with purified enzyme was reduced to 33 μg/ml (20). The preparations of purified enzyme catalyzed the conversion of EPO to DHD at a rate roughly

Table 11-4.   Inhibition of Epoxide Hydrolase In Vitro by Valproic Acid[a]

Substrate	In vitro preparation[c]	Diol formation rate[b]				
		Control	VPA 0.1 mM	% change	VPA 1.0 mM	% change
Carbamazepine epoxide (250 μM)	Microsomes	51.0 ± 1.5	44.6 ± 0.7	−13	21.4 ± 1.0	−58
Carbamazepine epoxide (250 μM)	Epoxide hydrolase	351 ± 65	285 ± 20	−19	194 ± 14	−45
S-styrene oxide (4 μM)	Epoxide hydrolase	40.1 ± 1.3	35.8 ± 2.0	−11	23.7 ± 1.3	−41

[a]Data from ref. 20. Mean ± SD of four determinations.
[b]Units are pmol/min/mg with carbamazepine epoxide as substrate; units are nmol/min/mg with s-styrene oxide as substrate.
[c]Microsomes and pure microsomal epoxide hydrolase were from liver sample of a single human subject.

Table 11-5. Inhibition of Hydrolysis of Styrene Oxide 0.5 μM by Valproic Acid in Human Liver Microsomes[a]

Substrate	Phenylethanediol formation rate (nmol/min/mg)		
	Control	VPA 1 mM	% change
R-styrene oxide	9.99 ± 0.22	3.98 ± 0.09	−60
S-styrene oxide	2.99 ± 0.13	0.63 ± 0.12	−79
R,S-styrene oxide	6.56 ± 0.18	2.22 ± 0.04	−66

[a] Data from ref. 20. Mean ± SD of four determinations.

sevenfold greater than in the microsomal preparations (Table 11-4). VPA concentrations of 0.1 mM and 1.0 mM were found to inhibit the hydrolysis of EPO in the purified epoxide hydrolase preparations. The extent to which hydrolysis of EPO was inhibited by VPA was similar in the purified enzyme preparations and in liver microsomes.

Inhibition of EPO hydrolysis in both human liver microsomes and purified preparations of human liver microsomal epoxide hydrolase occurred at therapeutically relevant VPA concentrations of 1 mM and less. These results conflict with the reports of Pacifici et al. (15–17), in which VPA concentrations of 10 mM failed to inhibit hydrolysis of styrene oxide and benzo[a]pyrene-4,5-oxide in human liver microsomes. In order to resolve this discrepancy, we investigated the inhibition of styrene oxide hydrolysis by VPA in vitro.

Incubations with styrene oxide were carried out according to a procedure similar to that described above for the EPO incubations, the major change being the microsomal protein concentration (20). Styrene oxide is enzymatically hydrolyzed much more rapidly than EPO, and it was necessary to substantially reduce the microsomal protein concentration in the styrene oxide incubations in order to avoid extensive depletion of styrene oxide over the course of the incubation period. The hydrolysis of racemic styrene oxide and the styrene oxide enantiomers was inhibited more than 50% in human liver microsomes in the presence of 1 mM VPA (Table 11-5). The K_I concentration of VPA in human liver microsomes with S-styrene oxide as the epoxide substrate was estimated to be approximately 0.26 mM (20). This K_I concentration is comparable to the VPA K_I concentration of 0.55 mM with EPO as the epoxide substrate, and it is within the range of VPA concentrations typically found in plasma of epileptic patients treated with sodium valproate. Hydrolysis of S-styrene oxide in preparations of purified human liver microsomal epoxide hydrolase was inhibited at VPA concentrations of 0.1 mM and 1.0 mM (Table 11-4). The extent of inhibition was similar to that observed in purified enzyme incubations with EPO as the epoxide substrate.

IN VITRO–IN VIVO CORRELATION

The concentrations of VPA that inhibit the enzymatic hydrolysis of EPO and styrene oxide in vitro are comparable to the VPA plasma levels associated with inhibition of EPO elimination in vivo; the in vitro VPA K_I concentration estimates (0.26 mM and 0.55 mM) are well within the therapeutic range of VPA plasma concentrations (0.3–0.7 mM). Excellent agreement was also found between the extent of inhibition associated with a particular concentration of VPA in vitro and in vivo; the in vivo elimination of EPO and the in vitro hydrolysis of EPO in microsomes and purified enzyme preparations were all inhibited approximately 10–20% at VPA concentrations of 0.1 mM (Tables 11-1 and 11-4).

The finding that purified microsomal epoxide hydrolase catalyzes the hydrolysis of EPO and that there is excellent agreement between the in vitro and in vivo inhibitory potencies of VPA indicate the following: (a) the increased EPO/CBZ plasma concentration ratio in patients treated with VPA results from inhibition of EPO elimination by VPA; (b) in vivo elimination of EPO in man is principally mediated by microsomal epoxide hydrolase; and (c) inhibition of in vivo EPO elimination in man is due to direct inhibition of microsomal epoxide hydrolase by VPA—it is unlikely that metabolites of VPA (e.g., epoxide metabolites) are responsible for the in vivo inhibition of EPO elimination. The documentation that therapeutically relevant concentrations of VPA inhibit the important detoxification enzyme epoxide hydrolysis raises questions about the toxicological consequences of chronic exposure to VPA, especially in epileptic patients concurrently treated with drugs that are biotransformed to reactive arene oxide metabolites.

Extensive in vivo and in vitro studies of the EPO/VPA interaction were carried out both in man and in laboratory animals in order to elucidate the mechanism by which VPA increases EPO plasma levels in CBZ-treated patients. It is interesting that VPA increases the EPO/CBZ plasma concentration ratio and inhibits the in vivo elimination of EPO in man, monkey, and rat, but the similarities of the EPO/VPA interaction in these three animal species are probably coincidental. Urinary metabolite profiles show that the quantitative significance of DHD formation in the overall elimination of EPO varies greatly between the species, indicating that the mechanism by which VPA inhibits in vivo EPO elimination is different in rat and monkey as compared to man.

In vitro studies also support the notion that the mechanism of EPO/VPA interaction is different in man and rat. VPA was observed to be much less potent at inhibiting EPO hydrolysis in rat liver microsomes than in human liver microsomes. Furthermore, inhibition of EPO hydrolysis in rat liver microsomes was only observed when rats were pretreated with enzyme-inducing agents. The reason for the lower VPA inhibitory potency in rat liver microsomes as compared to human liver microsomes is not presently known, but it may be related to species differences in epoxide hydrolase structure and/or differences in overall composition of hydrolytic enzymes and isozymes in the microsomes.

In our studies, the potency with which VPA inhibits human microsomal epoxide hydrolase activity was found to be very similar in vitro and in vivo. However, the ability of VPA at concentrations less than 1 mM to inhibit human liver microsomal epoxide hydrolase in vitro conflicts with published reports of Pacifici et al. (15–17), in which VPA at concentrations up to 10 mM had no effect on the activity of the enzyme toward styrene oxide. It should be noted that the styrene oxide studies conducted in our laboratory were carried out at a physiological pH of 7.4 with a microsomal protein concentration of 2.67 μg/ml and styrene oxide concentrations of 0.5–4.0 μM, whereas the styrene oxide studies of Pacifici et al. (15–17) were conducted at a pH of 8.7 with a microsomal protein concentration up to 1.3 mg/ml and styrene oxide concentrations of 120–2,000 μM. The incubation conditions for the styrene oxide studies conducted in our laboratory were chosen in order to reflect physiological conditions (pH, 7.4), minimize problems of styrene oxide depletion over the course of an incubation period, and avoid saturation of epoxide hydrolase with styrene oxide. The different in vitro incubation conditions is the most likely explanation for the discrepancy in the ability of VPA to inhibit epoxide hydrolase activity in our styrene oxide studies, compared to the studies of Pacifici et al.

The investigations of the EPO/VPA interaction in our laboratory have led to the development of simple methodologies that may be useful for predicting the effects of other drugs on EPO plasma levels in CBZ-treated patients. The good correlation between the ability of VPA to inhibit EPO hydrolysis in vitro and in vivo suggests that human liver microsomes could be used to screen for inhibition of EPO metabolism by other drugs. The ability to predict in vivo inhibition of EPO metabolism through use of simple in vitro methodologies would provide the means to anticipate whether or not administration of a drug to CBZ-treated patients might lead to overaccumulation of EPO and produce neurological side-effects. The effects of other drugs on EPO metabolism can also be easily investigated in vivo through administration of single oral doses of EPO to normal volunteers. It should be noted that, due to species differences in the metabolism of EPO, in vivo drug interaction studies in rat and monkey or in vitro studies in rat liver microsomes are not likely to be useful for predicting the effects of other drugs on EPO disposition in man.

The development of in vitro and in vivo strategies may also be possible for screening enzyme-inhibiting drug interactions among other anticonvulsant agents. In the development of such strategies, it should be recognized that animal models and in vitro incubation conditions need to be appropriately chosen in order to accurately assess or predict inhibitory potency of a drug in man.

REFERENCES

1. Bertilsson L, Tomson T. Clinical pharmacokinetics and pharmacological effects of carbamazepine and carbamazepine-10,11-epoxide. *Clin Pharmacokinet* 1986;11:177–98.
2. McKauge L, Tyrer JH, Eadie MJ. Factors influencing simultaneous concentrations of carbamazepine and its epoxide in plasma. *Ther Drug Monit* 1981;3:63–70.
3. Brodie MJ, Forrest G, Rapeport WG. Carbamazepine-10,11-epoxide concentrations in epileptics on carbamazepine alone and in combination with other anticonvulsants. *Br J Clin Pharmacol* 1983;16:747–50.
4. Ramsay RE, Guterman A, Vasquez D, Percholski R, Wong P. Carbamazepine metabolism in man: the effect of concomitant anticonvulsant therapy. *Epilepsia* 1983;24:254.
5. Levy RH, Moreland TA, Morselli PL, Guyot M, Brachet-Liermain A, Loiseau P. Carbamazepine/valproic acid interaction in man and rhesus monkey. *Epilepsia* 1984;25:338–45.
6. Lindhout D, Höppener RJEA, Meinardi H. Teratogenicity of antiepileptic drug combinations with special emphasis on epoxidation (of carbamazepine). *Epilepsia* 1984;25:77–83.
7. Schoeman JF, Elyas AA, Brett EM, Lascelles PT. Altered ratio of carbamazepine-10,11-epoxide/carbamazepine in plasma of children: evidence of anticonvulsant drug interaction. *Dev Med Child Neurol* 1984;26:749–55.
8. Pisani F, Fazio A, Oteri G, et al. Sodium valproate and valpromide: differential interaction with carbamazepine in epileptic patients. *Epilepsia* 1986;27:548–52.
9. Schoeman JF, Elyas AA, Brett EM, Lascelles PT. Correlation between plasma carbamazepine-10,11-epoxide concentration and drug side-effects in children with epilepsy. *Dev Med Child Neurol* 1984;26:756–64.
10. Eichelbaum M, Tomson T, Tybring G, Bertilsson L. Carbamazepine metabolism in man. Induction and pharmacogenetic aspects. *Clin Pharmacokinet* 1985;10:80–90.
11. Tomson T, Tybring G, Bertilsson L. Single-dose kinetics and metabolism of carbamazepine-10,11-epoxide. *Clin Pharmacol Ther* 1983;33:58–65.
12. Faigle JW, Feldmann KF. Pharmacokinetic data of carbamazepine and its major metabolites in man. In: Schneider H, Janz D, Gardner-Thorpe C, Meinardi H, Sherwin AL, eds. *Clinical Pharmacology of Antiepileptic Drugs* Berlin: Springer-Verlag, 1975:159–65.
13. Tybring G, von Bahr C, Bertilsson L, Collste H, Glaumann H, Solbrand H. Metabolism of carbamazepine and its epoxide metabolite in human and rat liver in vitro. *Drug Metab Dispos* 1981;9:561–4.
14. Bellucci G, Berti G, Chiappe C, Lippi A, Marioni F. The metabolism of carbamazepine in humans: steric course of the enzymatic hydrolysis of the 10,11-epoxide. *J Med Chem* 1987;30:768–73.

15. Pacifici GM, Tomson T, Bertilsson L, Rane A. Valpromide/carbamazepine and risk of teratogenicity. *Lancet* 1985(i):397–8.
16. Pacifici GM, Franchi M, Bencini C, Rane A. Valpromide inhibits human epoxide hydrolase. *Br J Clin Pharmacol* 1986;22:269–74.
17. Pacifici GM, Rane A. Valpromide but not sodium hydrogen divalproate inhibits epoxide hydrolase in human liver. *Pharmacol Toxicol* 1987;60:237–8.
18. Chang S-L. *Mechanism of the interaction between valproic acid and carbamazepine in the rat* [Dissertation]. Seattle, WA: University of Washington, 1983.
19. Chang S-L, Levy RH. Inhibitory effect of valproic acid on the disposition of carbamazepine and carbamazepine-10,11-epoxide in the rat. *Drug Metab Dispos* 1986;14:281–6.
20. Kerr BM. Role of epoxide hydrolase in carbamazepine–epoxide drug interations. Dissertation, University of Washington, Seattle, 1989.
21. Levy RH, Kerr BM, Loiseau P, Guyot M, Wilensky AJ. Inhibition of carbamazepine epoxide elimination by valpromide and valproic acid. *Epilepsia* 1986;27:592.

12

Animal Model Systems for the Study of Antiepileptic Drug Interactions and Their Clinical Implications

Rory P. Remmel and [1]Nina M. Graves

Departments of Medicinal Chemistry and [1]Pharmacy Practice, College of Pharmacy, University of Minnesota, Minneapolis, Minnesota, U.S.A.

Drug interactions among antiepileptic drugs (AEDs) are common and clinically important. Characteristics that predispose AEDs to interactions are extensive metabolism, active metabolites, high protein binding, and the practice of polypharmacy. Since AEDs often have a narrow therapeutic range, the outcome of these interactions has caused many patients to experience unnecessary toxicity or increased seizure frequency. Phenytoin (PHT) displays Michaelis-Menten kinetics, is highly protein-bound, and is subject to both distributional and metabolic interactions (1). Carbamazepine (CBZ) is less susceptible to protein-binding interactions, but it is also extensively metabolized (2). Phenobarbital (PB) has long been recognized as an inducing agent of oxidative metabolism (3) as well as Phase II conjugation reactions (4). All of these compounds are inducers of cytochrome P-450 monoxygenases and thus can affect not only their own metabolism, but also the metabolism of other AEDs (5). In contrast, valproic acid (VPA) has been implicated in the inhibition of the metabolism of several compounds, especially PB (6). VPA is highly protein-bound to albumin and is also subject to displacement interactions (7). Often the discovery and full impact of these interactions are not made until a drug has gone beyond the clinical testing phase and has reached the general population. One approach would be to test for interactions in animal model systems prior to clinical testing of new AEDs. This review will focus on approaches to study metabolic interactions in preclinical animal systems followed by a discussion of clinical study designs that would incorporate the results from these model systems.

Drug interactions can act as confounding variables in AED trials if standard AED concentrations are altered. Stable concentrations are necessary to discern whether a decrease or an increase in seizure frequency is due to the investigational drug or to fluctuations in standard AED concentrations. As an example, interactions between CBZ or PHT and felbamate, an investigational AED that was tested at the Minnesota Comprehensive Epilepsy Program, have been observed. The PHT–felbamate interaction is dramatic, causing a twofold elevation of PHT concentration and resulting in concomitant PHT toxicity (8). Wilensky et al. also found that administration of felbamate increased PHT levels from 9–14 mg/L baseline to 20–30 mg/L treated, resulting in PHT toxicity and subsequent dosage reduction of PHT (9). In the Minnesota clinic, the PHT dosage is routinely reduced 10–30% to prevent toxicity with felbamate. In contrast, CBZ levels were shown to decrease after addition of felbamate to therapy. Carbamazepine-epoxide (CBZ-E) levels either increased or remained stable, such that a significant increase in the CBZ-E/CBZ ratio was observed (8). Wilensky et al. also reported a slight decline in CBZ concentrations in three of four patients (9). These interactions were not fully appreciated until Phase II testing as well underway. Therefore, the results of the safety and efficacy studies may have been compromised. Toxicity secondary to elevations in CBZ-E and efficacy secondary to increased PHT concentrations may have been inappropriately attributed to the investigational drug. If the interactions had been fully defined prior to clinical testing, modifications in the study design may have avoided problems in interpretation of the results.

A second problem that affects clinical trials is dose prediction of a new drug to achieve a desired plasma concentration. This problem is illustrated with lamotrigine. Lamotrigine pharmacokinetics appear to be greatly affected by co-administered standard AEDs (10,11). Normal volunteers had a clearance of 0.60 ± 0.15 ml/min/kg ($t_{1/2} = 24$ h, n = 10) (12), whereas patients on lamotrigine plus VPA had a markedly decreased clearance of 0.27 ± 0.10 ml/min/kg ($t_{1/2} = 58.8$ h, n = 4). In contrast, patients on known metabolic inducers, CBZ and/or PHT and no VPA, had an increased lamotrigine clearance of 1.30 ± 0.37 ml/min/kg ($t_{1/2} = 11.8$ h, n = 12). Patients on VPA and CBZ or VPA and PHT had an intermediate clearance close to normal volunteers of 0.57 ± 0.23 ml/min/kg ($t_{1/2} = 26.4$ h, n = 12). The previous data was obtained from two separate studies at different sites (10,11). The large variability caused by co-medication caused difficulties in obtaining a desired concentration of lamotrigine, and the mechanisms of the interactions are poorly understood. If the interactions were prospectively identified in animal models, the clinical trials could be more efficiently designed to compensate for these significant interactions. Thus, time, expense, and patient suffering would be minimized in these expensive clinical trials. Furthermore, the mechanisms of the interactions can be studied under controlled conditions in animals, a situation that is often impossible in patients due to numerous confounding variables.

PRECLINICAL ANIMAL MODEL SYSTEMS

Several model systems are available that could be used to test for the possibility of drug interactions prior to clinical trials. Liver microsomes, a crude preparation of the endoplasmic reticulum that contains enzymes responsible for oxidative metabolism (cytochrome P-450 mono-oxygenases), and conjugation (UDP-glucuronyl transferases, epoxide hydrolases, and a microsomal glutathione-S-transferase) are the most common in vitro system employed for AED interaction studies. As an example, when VPA is added to a regimen that includes PB, the serum concentrations of PB can increase dramatically, resulting in significant clinical toxicity (5,13). Subsequent studies have shown that VPA is a potent inhibitor of PB metabolism in rat liver microsomes (14). Chronic AED therapy can also induce metabolism. Induction may result in decreased concentrations with a potential for a decrease in seizure control. For example, PB and PHT have been well characterized as enzyme inducers in patients (4) and in microsomal studies (15). Chapter 11 discusses the use of human liver microsomes for AED interaction studies to avoid species differences (16).

Because of the multiplicity of isozymes for each of the major drug metabolizing enzymes, e.g., cytochrome P-450 (17), there has also been interest in the use of purified enzymes for drug interaction studies. The use of a purified enzyme is attractive because detailed mechanistic studies on binding, catalysis, and product release may be performed. However, the purification is technically difficult, and the purified isozymes are not generally available. At this time, little is known about the specific isozymes that catalyze the oxidative metabolism of AEDs. Incubation of each of the AEDs with a collection of isozymes in several species (rat, rabbit, and human are the best studied) will be necessary to employ purified enzymes for interaction studies. In the future, this will continue to be an active and fruitful area of research if specific inhibitors or regulators can be employed to modify the metabolism of drugs to avoid toxic pathways. For example, if a specific inhibitor could be developed that would block the formation of the Δ4-ene metabolite of VPA, a putative hepatotoxic metabolite (18), drug safety could be improved. This approach may also be used to prevent serious interactions.

Unfortunately, most of the AED drugs are not only metabolized by the mono-oxygenases of a microsomal system but also by subsequent or direct conjugation pathways. For example, one of the least recognized pathways of CBZ metabolism is to an *N*-glucuronide (19). PB is metabolized to an unusual N-glucoside in humans and monkeys (20), but not in other species, and the major metabolite of VPA is the glucuronide (21). Unless appropriate co-factors are used in a microsomal system, these pathways will not be activated. Epoxide hydrolase has both cytosolic and microsomal forms, although the conversion of CBZ-E to CBZ-10,11-trans-diol is catalyzed by the microsomal form of epoxide hydrolase in human liver microsomes (see Chapter 11). Furthermore, sulfotransferases and the predominant forms of glutathione-S-transferases are cytosolic enzymes. Consequently, other useful animal-based model systems have been proposed that contain intact metabolic systems in a cellular environment. The two systems that will be discussed in greater detail are freshly isolated or cultured hepatocytes and liver perfusion. Hepatocytes are relatively easy to isolate and contain an intact cell membrane. They may be used to study drug transport processes in detail. For example, the transport of PHT has recently been studied in isolated hepatocytes (22). The isolated perfused liver has been used to study pharmacokinetic models of drug clearance (23–25) and has been used to study the effect of blood flow and protein-binding interactions on the disposition of drugs by this major drug metabolizing organ.

Lastly, one cannot preclude in vivo interactions from an animal model design. Interactions that are identified on a purified enzyme level or in a microsomal model may be masked or enhanced in vivo. Considerations of drug disposition and protein binding can only be adequately described in vivo. Drugs may be extensively metabolized by extrahepatic sites that would not be modeled by any of the above test systems, and renal clearance of drugs is also not considered in the in vitro systems. Another major problem that must be addressed in any animal system is the choice of the appropriate species. It is critical that metabolic disposition data be available for several animal species to select that species that will be most predictive for the human interaction. A classic example of species differences in the AED literature is with PHT, which is metabolized primarily to m-HPPH in dogs (26), but is primarily metabolized to p-HPPH in mice, rats, and humans. If one wishes to use larger species, such as dogs and monkeys, the cost of the in vitro experiments becomes prohibitively expensive.

To develop appropriate models to study drug interactions and their mechanisms, several criteria must be met. The method should be relatively fast, reproducible, technically easy, and inexpensive. An ideal example would be a continuously cultured cell system, thus obviating the use of animals. Unfortunately, when hepatocytes are cultured, they often lose their ability to metabolize drugs unless hormones or other biological modifiers are added. The loss of cytochrome P-450 activity is especially pronounced in rat hepatocytes. Rabbit hepatocytes and human hepatocytes appear to be somewhat more stable in regard to oxidative metabolism (27). Other criteria include the appropriateness of the animal species and the validation of the method. If in vitro systems from animals, such as freshly isolated hepatocytes, are used, then one must determine which animal species is the most appropriate without being prohibitively expensive. For example, diazepam metabolism in rat, rabbit, guinea pig, dog, and human hepatocytes showed markedly different profiles (28). The intrinsic clearance of diazepam was much lower in human hepatocytes than in other species (28), which parallels the in vivo data. Only temazepam and nordiazepam were identified as metabolites in human hepatocytes, whereas additional metabolites were found in other species (4'-OH-diazepam in rat, rabbit, and guinea pig cells, oxazepam in dog and guinea pig hepatocytes). Finally, the method must be validated. First, the in vitro system should correlate with the in vivo results in the animal of choice. Second, and more important, the method to study the interaction should reflect the situation in humans. Thus, it is important initially to correlate the direction and extent of the interaction in the animal models with the interaction in humans. Providing the clinicians with some basic information from the proposed animal studies may improve patient care and improve the efficiency of costly Phase II studies. Analytical techniques and further knowledge concerning the metabolism of these new drugs that are determined in the animal studies may also be beneficial to clinical studies.

An important feature of an animal model is the ability to study the mechanism of the interaction. If the interaction is at the metabolic level, then induction or inhibition of microsomal metabolism may be a good predictor of the clinical interaction. Kapetanovic and Kupferberg have recently used this model to study the effect of nafimidone, a new imidazole AED, on the rat liver microsomal metabolism of PHT (29,30). Other imidazoles such as cimetidine, metronidazole, and ketoconazole are known inhibitors of the cytochrome P-450 mono-oxygenases (31). PHT displays biphasic Michaelis-Menten kinetics in rat liver microsomes; two binding sites have been observed, a high affinity binding site with a low V_{max} and a low affinity binding site with a high V_{max} (15,29). Saturable kinetics of PHT in humans have also been demonstrated (32,33). Nafimidone was shown to inhibit microsomal PHT metabolism of both high-affinity and low-affinity isozymes by a mixed-type inhibition. Kapetanovic and Kupferberg have extended this model for PHT interactions by examining the effects of several other imidazoles and a variety of standard AEDs at a PHT concentration of 15.9 μM in PHT-induced or untreated rat liver microsomes (30). This concentration is near the low-affinity K_m (25.9 μM) and was chosen because the K_m for a large population of epileptic patients based on plasma pharmacokinetics was 22.3 μM (33). This is a simplified approach, however, because the value for K_m in humans is a derived parameter and will be affected by protein binding, extrahepatic sites of metabolism, uptake of drugs into cells, and alternate pathways of metabolism. One might assume that the high-affinity, low-V_{max} isozyme may be primarily responsible for the saturation kinetics observed in vivo.

Although inhibition studies over a series of concentrations require considerably more effort, especially for large numbers of compounds, it is important to examine the inhibitor effect on the high-affinity isozyme. Thus, changes in K_m and V_{max} of both enzymes may be determined, and the mechanism of the inhibition may be delineated. For example, VPA had no inhibitory effect on PHT metabolism in the microsomal system of Kapetanovic and Kupferberg (30), but valproate has been shown to increase unbound PHT levels in humans (corrected for plasma protein displacement). This indicates a decrease in intrinsic (enzymatic) clearance, which may have been missed in the microsomal system because only the low-affinity, high-V_{max} isozyme was studied. Alternatively, a VPA metabolite could be responsible for the inhibition in vivo, thus explaining the lack of inhibition in the in vitro test system. Patsalos et al. have also used microsomes to study the mechanism of inhibition of PHT hydroxylation by four different AEDs. PB and sulthiame were found to be strong competitive inhibitors, ethosuximide was a weak competitive inhibitor, and VPA was a weak noncompetitive inhibitor (34). This data correlated well with clinical data. In particular, sulthiame was known to be a potent inhibitor of PHT clearance in patients (35). Subsequently, Patsalos also was able to demonstrate that co-administration of sulthiame and PHT to rats significantly increase phenytoin plasma concentrations compared to controls (36).

Another important mechanism of AED interactions is induction of metabolism. Induction studies may also be carried out in the microsomal system by pretreatment of rats with the compound of interest prior to isolation of the microsomes. For example, pretreatment of rats with phenobarbital increased PHT metabolism in vitro (29), and this is a documented clinical interaction (5). Kapetanovic and Kupferberg pretreated animals with PHT or nafimidone for 3 days prior to the isolation of microsomes and found that both compounds increased both the high- and low-affinity V_{max} for p-hydroxylation of PHT (30). Carbamazepine is also well known as an inducer of not only other drugs, but also its own metabolism (37). Its active metabolite, CBZ-10,11-epoxide, has been shown to induce a variety of drug-metabolizing enzymes in liver fractions from pretreated rats (38).

Although microsomes are easy to isolate and can be frozen at $-80°C$ for repeated use, they are not reflective of the entire spectrum of metabolism. For instance, epoxide hydrolase, glutathione-S-transferases, and sulfotransferases are primarily cytosolic enzymes, although microsomal forms of epoxide hydrolase and glutathione-S-transferase do exist. Glucuronyl transferases are present in microsomes, but they are only active if the co-factors UDPGA and Mg^{++} is added. This would be important for interaction studies with lamotrigine, because the primary urinary metabolite of lamotrigine in humans is a glucuronide accounting for greater than 60% of the dose and 90% of the urinary metabolites (39). VPA is known to inhibit P-450—dependent metabolism when administered in vivo; thus an effect on glucuronidation by VPA would be a new interaction mechanism. VPA itself is glucuronidated to a large extent, so the interaction with lamotrigine may be a simple competitive process for glucuronyl transferase. Hepatocytes would be an important tool to study this interaction, because metabolic switching could be studied that may not be possible in a microsomal model. Freshly isolated hepatocytes offer a full range of metabolic transformations and hence are much closer to the in vivo conditions. Furthermore, transport of drugs may be studied in hepatocytes by uptake and release experiments. Isolated hepatocytes have not been used widely to study drug interactions, perhaps because the isolation technique is more difficult. In several cases, hepatocyte data has more closely correlated with in vivo data than microsomal data. For example, Yih and van Rossum showed that the in vivo metabolism of a series of barbiturates was comparable in hepatocytes, but did not correlate with 9,000 g fraction (40). PB induces the demethylation of propoxyphene in microsomes; however, no difference in clearance was found in vivo between control rats and induced rats (41). In hepatocytes, the rates were comparable to the in vivo studies (42). PHT metabolism has been studied recently by several groups in hepatocytes (22,43,44). The same spectrum of metabolites has been observed for hepatocytes and in the urine of animals. Species differences in metabolism have recently been investigated in a cultured hepatocyte model with diazepam (28). Hepatocytes should therefore be a useful test system for the study of AED interactions.

Microsomes or hepatocytes may also be obtained from humans. The availability of human liver has improved with the establishment of a human liver bank at the National Institutes of Health (NIH) and the increase in organ transplantation. However, the availability of normal liver is low compared to diseased liver, and livers from patients treated with enzyme inducers such as PHT and CBZ are even rarer. There is little doubt that better correlations should be obtained with human tissue. However, controlled experimental conditions for the more complicated test systems (liver perfusion and in vivo experiments) cannot be done in humans. An appropriate animal model could be verified with human tissue, and this avenue should be explored in the future. An excellent example of this approach for the interaction between valpromide or valproate and CBZ-10,11-epoxide with human liver epoxide hydrolase is presented by Kerr et al. (see Chapter 11).

The isolated perfused liver provides the opportunity to study the disposition, transport, and metabolism of drugs in the major drug-metabolizing organ of the body. Blood flow and protein binding can be controlled in a liver perfusion experiment. Uptake into the organ, release into the perfusate, and excretion into the bile can be studied in this dynamic system. In one of the first interaction experiments with the isolated perfused liver system, induction of CBZ clearance by pretreatment of rats with PB was demonstrated (45). The isolated perfused rat liver has been used to study the interaction of VPA and CBZ (46). VPA significantly decreased the clearance of CBZ-E in this preparation. Drawbacks of liver perfusion experiments are that a high degree of technical expertise is required, the cost is high in terms of animals and perfusate (especially if a single pass system is used), and the longevity of the preparation is short (usually 2–3 h). However, the ability to closely approximate the hepatic clearance in an in vitro system is an exciting prospect.

To validate the results from microsomal, hepatocyte, and perfused liver systems, it is important to study these interactions in the test animal before extrapolating the results to humans. Although obvious interactions may appear at the enzymatic level, the magnitude of the interaction may be affected by other factors such as changes in blood flow, drug distribution, plasma protein binding and tissue binding, extrahepatic metabolism, and renal clearance. Thus, it is critical to evaluate the interaction in vivo, even though these studies are technically more difficult. Numerous studies have published in animals to model drug interactions. The vast majority of these studies are single-dose studies comparing the pharmacokinetics of drugs with and without inhibitor. The recent study of Chang and Levy (47) on the VPA–CBZ interaction is one of the few studies done at steady state. Since AEDs are given on a chronic basis and induction is a well-recognized phenomenon, a steady-state approach more closely approximates the clinical situation. Steady-state levels may be achieved by constant rate infusions in animals with an implanted cannula or by the use of implantable osmotic minipumps in small animals like mice and rats. The latter system has recently been used to study the interaction of VPA and PB in mice (48). PB levels were increased by VPA, whereas VPA concentrations declined due to enzyme induction by PB.

CLINICAL IMPLICATIONS

Assumptions

There are assumptions that must be made prior to proposed clinical implementation of the results of the model. The primary assumption is that the proposed model will be able to predict the direction (induction vs. inhibition) and qualitative extent (strong vs. weak induction or inhibition) of the potential drug interactions as well as some potential mechanisms for the interactions (competitive vs. noncompetitive/protein binding). Although important, the model may not be able to define product inhibition and/or inhibition of protein synthesis. During clinical studies of the safety and efficacy of an investigational AED, there exists the implicit assumption that stable concentrations of the concomitant AEDs will result in more valid conclusions.

Similar preclinical investigations have been used retrospectively with investigational and standard AEDs. Two examples are nafimidone's effect on PHT and CBZ and VPA's effect on PB. Both were studied with a microsomal model after an interaction had been observed in patients. During a clinical trial of nafimidone in patients (49), a significant increase in toxicity and serum concentrations of PHT and CBZ was observed. Kapetanovic and Kupferberg (30,31) demonstrated the interaction in a microsomal system, with the extent of inhibition by nafimidone and its metabolite almost identical to the decrease in PHT elimination seen in the clinical trial. Since the interaction was not predicted *a priori,* serum concentrations were drawn only every 24 h during the clinical trial. Therefore, patients were exposed to toxicity, and the interaction was left relatively undefined in patients. The microsomal model was not used to study the CBZ interaction in detail, despite even larger decreases in CBZ elimination in the patients.

The situation is analogous with VPA and PB. The inhibition of PB elimination by VPA was noted clinically (5) and then confirmed using rat hepatic microsomes, indicating VPA acts as a competitive inhibitor of PB p-hydroxylation (6). Again, the extent of inhibition in the microsomal model closely correlated with the extent of inhibition observed in humans.

Continuum of the Interactions

The first step in utilizing the results from a preclinical model is to define where the investigational AED falls on a continuum of interactions. On one end of the continuum is the ideal situation in which the investigational AED exhibits no drug–drug interactions. On the other end is the worst situation, in which the investigational drug affects the pharmacokinetics and/or the pharmacodynamics of the standard drugs, and the standard drugs affect the investigational drug. In between there is a continuum where standard drugs may affect investigational drugs and vice versa (Fig. 12-1). These interactions can be minimal or produce dramatic results.

Preliminary investigations with stiripentol indicate that it may fall in the category of "bad" interactions, whereas gabapentin appears to provide the more favorable profile. Nafimidone's effect on PHT and CBZ, VPA's effect on PB, and most other investigational AEDs fall somewhere in between (Fig. 12-1).

Stiripentol is nonlinear in its elimination, it dramatically decreases the

```
                      HIGH                                              LOW

Invest. drug          10---------8-----------6---------------------------------------1
effects on            STP-----FBM------VPA---------------------------------------GBP
standard drugs        NAF                                                     LAM


Standard drugs        10---------8-----------------------------------3-------------1
effects on            STP----NAF-----------------------------------VPA---------GBP
invest. drug          LAM                                                     FBM
```

FIG. 12-1. Continuum of drug interactions.

elimination of concomitant AEDs, and concomitant AEDs dramatically increase its elimination (50). No preclinical investigation of possible drug interactions were conducted. Therefore, the interactions and nonlinearity were detected through trial and error. Patients were given stiripentol, and serum concentrations of the investigational and standard drugs were monitored. Patients exhibited toxicity, serum concentrations of the standard drugs increased, and the interaction was verified. In all likelihood, this affected the safety and efficacy evaluation of stiripentol. In addition, stiripentol elimination was increased 300% in the patients receiving enzyme inducers compared to normal volunteers (50). Although there were significant effects on the standard drugs, detailed pharmacokinetic determinations on these drugs were not done. No conclusions of efficacy could be made due to the short exposure to stiripentol and to the wide fluctuations in the serum concentrations of the standard drugs. Further efficacy trials will require strict attention to maintenance of serum concentrations. This will involve extensive dosage manipulation with its concomitant practical problems of binding. If a preclinical model had predicted these dramatic interactions, clinical investigations would have been designed to assess the interactions in a more detailed manner, thereby allowing more definition of the drug–drug interactions (Table 12-1).

Gabapentin appears to be on the opposite end of the spectrum of interactions. It is minimally protein bound and is significantly renally excreted (51). Therefore, significant drug–drug interactions among AEDs would not be expected, and few, if any, clinically important interactions have been detected. Therefore, the drug is far easier to evaluate for safety and efficacy (Table 12-1) and will be relatively easy to use if it is eventually marketed.

Our own experience with felbamate also illustrates interactions that are intermediate in nature. Felbamate strongly inhibits PHT elimination and weakly induced CBZ elimination (8). During the first clinical study (9),

Table 12-1. Recommended Actions

| | Efficient————————————————————————————————Time-consuming | | | | | | |
| | Inexpensive————————————————————————————————Expensive | | | | | | |
	Routine evaluation	Close Cp monitoring	Extensive Cp evaluation	Extensive protocol considerations	Poly Rx ok	Mono Rx preferred	Mono Rx required
No interactions							
(e.g., spectrum = 2)							
Phase I-pts	X					X	
Phase II-pts	X				X		
Phase III	X				X		
Weak interaction							
(e.g., spectrum ≤ 10)							
Phase I-pts		X				X	
Phase II-pts		X				X	
Phase III		X			X		
Strong interaction							
(e.g., spectrum ≈ 20)							
Phase I-pts			X	X			X
Phase II-pts			X	X			X
Phase III		X				X	

significant increases in PHT serum concentrations and slight decreases in CBZ concentrations were observed in pilot studies prior to ADD program study. Design modifications required to accommodate the PHT interaction were implemented (see Chapter 7). PHT doses were automatically decreased with the addition of felbamate, and PHT doses and serum concentrations were blinded to the principal investigators. These changes caused long delays in the implementation of the protocol. Since the felbamate/CBZ interaction was not as obvious, the study design did not incorporate blinding techniques for the CBZ dose. Since CBZ concentrations had to be maintained, the required increases in CBZ dose led to a threat of the blind. If the interactions had been predicted prior to clinical studies, the initial clinical studies could have been designed to obtain pharmacokinetic parameters of PHT and CBZ before and after the addition of felbamate, thus defining the interactions prior to the large-scale clinical trial. Therefore, protocol design and implementation for the safety and efficacy study may have proceeded more smoothly. Further refinement in the extent of the interactions and definition of the patients most at risk could have been accomplished with more detailed serum concentration collections, possibly using stable isotope technology. Despite over 70 patients receiving the drugs in combination, we still do not know the mechanism of the interaction, or the extent, or if it is dose-related to felbamate. There is no information on a possible interaction with VPA, which may lead to a decreased felbamate clearance. Also, it is not known if the increase in PHT led to the decrease in CBZ. Therefore, further Phase III studies will be needed to clarify these interactions prior to marketing, so that clinicians will be able to use felbamate appropriately in their patient population. The aforementioned studies on lamotrigine is another important example of a drug intermediate in the continuum that presented problems in the dose prediction of a new agent when added to standard therapy.

Proposal

We propose the following scheme to investigate drug interactions among AEDs (see Table 12-1): (a) preclinical determination of protein binding and metabolic pathways to be performed by the sponsoring drug company (enables definition of appropriate in vitro model); (b) initiation of a preclinical model for drug interactions; (c) submission of IND; (d) initiation of Phase I studies in normal volunteers; (e) conclusion of preclinical model for drug interactions; (f) design of subsequent clinical trials based on the following predictions from the preclinical model: No interactions predicted (e.g., gabapentin)—conduct preliminary pharmacokinetic trials in patients on concomitant AEDs with minimal monitoring of serum concentrations of all AEDs [e.g., single area under the curve (AUC), compare results to the normal volunteer studies]; if a lack of interactions is verified in above, design safety and efficacy trials with blinding needed only for investigational drug and serum concentrations monitored primarily for compliance purposes. Weak interactions predicted (e.g., felbamate, lamotrigine)—determine preliminary pharmacokinetics in patients on concomitant AEDs with AUC determinations of standard and investigational drugs on first and subsequent exposures to the investigational AED; based on above investigation, design Phase II safety and efficacy trials with appropriate dosing and blinding of all AEDs (probably unnecessary to make *a priori* changes in doses of drugs; changes will be needed only in the event serum concentrations of standard AEDs fall out of some predetermined range). Strong interactions predicted (e.g., stiripentol, nafimidone)—determine preliminary pharmacokinetics in patients on specific AEDs with extensive determination of pharmacokinetic parameters of standard and investigational drugs. This will require AUC measurements on first exposure to various doses of the investigational drug and extensive serum concentration sampling during any extended phase of the study. The investigators should be prepared to make changes in the doses of the drugs to enable maintenance of stable serum concentrations. To enable extrapolation into Phase II studies, a larger number of patients will be required than in either of the above situations. Stratification based on doses, changes in serum concentrations observed, and dose changes required will be needed. Based on the predictions from the above, the Phase II safety and efficacy trials can be designed. Appropriate *a priori* dose changes will probably be required, as will blinding of all involved AEDs, both standard and investigational. Further investigation as to the mechanism and extent of the interactions should be incorporated into the Phase II study design. This may involve using stable isotope technology.

REFERENCES

1. Perucca E, Richens A. Drug interactions with phenytoin. *Drugs* 1981;21:120–37.
2. Lertratanangkoon K, Horning MG. Metabolism of carbamazepine. *Drug Metab Dispos* 1981;10:1–10.
3. Conney AH. Pharmacologic implication of microsomal enzyme induction. *Pharmacol Rev* 1967;19:317–66.
4. Ullrich D, Bock KW. Glucuronide formation of various drugs in liver microsomes and in isolated hepatocytes from phenobarbital and 3-methylcholanthrene treated rats. *Biochem Pharmacol* 1984;33:97–101.
5. Perucca E. Clinical consequences of microsomal enzyme-induction by antiepileptic drugs. *Pharmacol Ther* 1978;2:285–314.
6. Henriksen O, Johannessen SI. Clinical and pharmacokinetic observations on sodium valproate. A 5-year follow-up study in 100 children with epilepsy. *Acta Neurol Scand* 1982;65:504–23.

7. Perucca E, Hebdige S, Frigo GM, Gatti G, Lecchini S, Crema A. Interaction between phenytoin and valproic acid: plasma protein binding and metabolic effects. *Clin Pharmacol Ther* 1980;28:779–89.

8. Fuerst RH, Graves NM, Leppik IM, Remmel RP, Rosenfeld WE, Sierzant TL. A preliminary report of the alteration of carbamazepine and phenytoin metabolism by felbamate. *Drug Intell Clin Pharm* 1986;20:465–6.

9. Wilensky AJ, Friel PN, Ojemann LM, Kupferberg HJ, Levy RH. Pharmacokinetics of W-554 (ADD 03055) in epileptic patients. *Epilepsia* 1985;26:602–6.

10. Binnie CD, Van Emde Boas W, Kasteleijn-Nolste-Trenite DGA, et al. Acute effects of lamotrigine (BW430C) in persons with epilepsy. *Epilepsia* 1986;27:248–54.

11. Jawad S, Yuen WC, Peck AW, Hamilton MJ, Oxley JR, Richens A. Lamotrigine: single dose pharmacokinetics and initial 1 week experience in refractory epilepsy. *Epilepsy Res* 1987;1:194–201.

12. Cohen AF, Fowle ASE, Land GS, Bye A. BW430C—a new anticonvulsant. Pharmacokinetics in normal man. *Epilepsia* 1985;25:656.

13. Patel IH, Levy RH, Cutler RE. Phenobarbital-valproic acid interaction. *Clin Pharmacol Ther* 1980;27:515–21.

14. Kapetanovic IM, Kupferberg HJ. Inhibition of microsomal phenobarbital metabolism by valproic acid. *Biochem Pharmacol* 1981;30:1361–63.

15. Kutt H, Fouts JR. Diphenylhydantoin metabolism by rat liver microsomes and some of the effects of drug or chemical pretreatment on diphenylhydantoin metabolism by rat liver microsomal preparations. *J Pharmacol Exp Ther* 1971;176:11–26.

16. Kerr BM, Levy RH. Carbamazepine epoxide/valproic acid interaction in rat, monkey, and man. In: Pitlick WH, ed. *Antiepileptic Drug Interactions*. New York: Demos Publications, 1989:165–79.

17. Guengerich FP, Dannan GA, Wright ST, Martin MV, Kaminsky LS. Purification and characterization of liver microsomal cytochromes P-450: electrophoretic, spectral, catalytic, and immunochemical properties and inducibility of eight isozymes isolated from rats treated with phenobarbital or β-naphthoflavone. *Biochemistry* 1982;21:6019–30.

18. Rettenmeier AW, Prickett KS, Gordon WP, Bjorge SM, Chang SL, Levy RH, Baillie TA. Studies on the biotransformation in the perfused rat liver of 2-n-propyl-4-pentenoic acid, a metabolite of the antiepileptic drug valproic acid. Evidence for the formation of chemically reactive intermediates. *Drug Metab Dispos* 1985;13:81–96.

19. Bauer JE, Gerber N, Lynn RK, Smith R, Thompson RM. A new N-glucuronide metabolite of carbamazepine. *Experientia* 1976;32:1032–3.

20. Tang BK, Kalow W, Grey AA. Metabolic fate of phenobarbital in man. N-glucoside formation. *Drug Metab Dispos* 1979;7:315–8.

21. Granneman GR, Wang SI, Machinist JM, Kesterson JW. Aspects of the metabolism of valproic acid. *Xenobiotica* 1984;14:375–87.

22. Morais JA, Wagner JG. A model describing the disposition of phenytoin in isolated rat hepatocytes. *Biopharm Drug Dispos* 1984;5:357–76.

23. Pang KS, Rowland M. Hepatic clearance of drugs. II. Experimental evidence for the acceptance of the "well-stirred" model over the "parallel tube" model

using lidocaine in the perfused rat liver in situ preparation. *J Pharmacokinetic Biopharm* 1977;5:655–80.

24. Roberts MS, Rowland M. Correlation between in-vitro microsomal enzyme activity and whole organ hepatic elimination kinetics: analysis with a dispersion model. *J Pharm Pharmacol* 1986;38:177–81.

25. Grey MR, Tam YK. The series compartment model for hepatic elimination. *Drug Metab Dispos* 1987;15:27–31.

26. Butler TG, Dudley KH, Johnson D, Roberts SB. Studies of the metabolism of 5,5-diphenylhydantoin relating principally to the stereo-selectivity of the hydroxylation reactions in man and dog. *J Pharmacol Exp Ther* 1976;199:82–92.

27. Le Bigot JF, Begue JM, Kiechel JR, Guillouzo A. Species differences in metabolism of ketotifen in rat, rabbit and man: demonstration of similar pathways in vivo and in cultureded hepatocytes. *Life Sci* 1987;40:883–90.

28. Chenery RJ, Ayrton A, Oldham HG, Standring P, Norman SJ, Seddon T, Kirby R. Diazepam metabolism in cultural hepatocytes from rat, rabbit, dog, guinea pig, and man. *Drug Metab Dispos* 1987;15:312–7.

29. Kapetanovic IM, Kupferberg HJ. Nafimidone, an imidazole anticonvulsant, and its metabolite as potent inhibitors of microsomal metabolism of phenytoin and carbamazepine. *Drug Metab Dispos* 1984;12:560–4.

30. Kapetanovic IM, Kupferberg HJ. Inhibition of microsomal phenytoin metabolism by nafimidone and related imidazoles. Potency and structural considerations. *Drug Metab Dispos* 1985;13:430–7.

31. Wilkinson CF, Hetnarski K, Cantwell GP, DiCarlo FJ. Structure-activity relationships in the effects of 1-alkylimidazoles on microsomal oxidation in vitro and in vivo. *Biochem Pharmacol* 1974;23:2377–86.

32. Gerber N, Wagner JG. Explanation of dose dependent decline of diphenylhydantoin plasma levels by fitting to the integrated form of the Michaelis-Menten equation. *Res Commun Chem Pathol Pharmacol* 1972;3:455–66.

33. Patsalos PN, Lascelles PT. In vitro hydroxylation of diphenylhydantoin and its inhibition by other commonly used anticonvulsant drugs. *Biochem Pharmacol* 1977;26:1929–33.

34. Grasela TH, Sheiner LB, Rambeck B, et al. Steady-state pharmacokinetics of phenytoin from routinely collected patient data. *Clin Pharmacokinet* 1983;8:355–64.

35. Houghton GW, Richens A. Inhibition of phenytoin metabolism by sulthiame in epileptic patients. *Br J Clin Pharmacol* 1974;1:59–66.

36. Patsalos PN, Lascelles PT. Metabolic interactions of phenytoin in the rat: effect of coadministration with the anticonvulsant drugs sodium valproate, sulthiame, ethosuximide, or phenobarbital. *Gen Pharmacol* 1985;15:7–12.

37. Bertilsson L, Hojer B, Tybring G, Osterloh J, Rane A. Autoinduction of carbamazepine metabolism in children examined by a stable isotope technique. *Clin Pharmacol Ther* 1980;27:83–8.

38. Jung R, Bentley P, Oesch F. Influence of carbamazepine-10,11-oxide on drug metabolizing enzymes. *Biochem Pharmacol* 1980;29:1109–12.

39. Parsons DN, Miles DW. Metabolic studies with BW430C, a novel anticonvulsant. *Epilepsia* 1984;25:656.

40. Yih TD, van Rossum JM. Isolated rat hepatocytes and 9000 g rat liver super-

natant as metabolic systems for the study of the pharmacokinetics of barbiturates. *Xenobiotica* 1977;7:573–82.

41. McMahon RE, Ridolfo AS, Culp HW, Wolen RL, Marshall FJ. The fate of radiolabeled propoxyphene in rat, dog, and human. *Toxicol Appl Pharmacol* 1971;19:417–44.

42. Billings RE, McMahon RE, Ashmore J, Wagle SR. The metabolism of drugs in isolated rat hepatocytes. *Drug Metab Dispos* 1977;5:518–26.

43. Billings RE. Sex differences in rats in the metabolism of phenytoin to 5-(3,4-dihydroxy)-5-phenylhydantoin. *J Pharmacol Exp Ther* 1983;225:630–6.

44. Inaba T, Umeda T, McMahon WA, Ho J, Jeejeebhoy KN. Isolated rat hepatocytes as a model to study drug metabolism: dose-dependent metabolism of diphenylhydantoin. *Life Sci* 1975;16:1227–32.

45. Rane A, Shand DG, Wilkinson GR. Disposition of carbamazepine and its 10,11-epoxide metabolite in the isolated perfused rat liver. *Drug Metab Dispos* 1977;5:179–84.

46. Chang S-L, Levy RH. Inhibition of epoxidation of carbamazepine by valproic acid in the isolated perfused rat liver. *J Pharmacokinet Biopharm* 1985;13:453–66.

47. Chang SL, Levy RH. Inhibitory effect of valproic acid on the disposition of carbamazepine and carbamazepine-10,11-epoxide in the rat. *Drug Metab Dispos* 1986;14:281–6.

48. Kuhnz W, Zierer R, Nau H. A new method for kinetic studies of drug interactions in experimental animals during steady state. *Arzneimittelforsch* 1983;33:1579–82.

49. Treiman DM, Ben-Menachem E, Barber KO. Inhibition of carbamazepine and phenytoin metabolism by nafimidone, a new antiepileptic drug. *Epilepsia* 1987;28:699–705.

50. Levy RH, Loiseau P, Guyot M, Blehaur HM, Tor J, Moreland TA. Stiripentol kinetics in epilepsy: nonlinearity and interactions. *Clin Pharmacol Ther* 1984;36:661–9.

13

Time Courses of Interaction

Allen A. Lai and Nancy C. James

Burroughs Wellcome Co.,
Research Triangle Park, North Carolina, U.S.A.

Many drug–drug interactions have a pharmacodynamic basis, whereas others have a pharmacokinetic basis. The purpose of this chapter is to review briefly the time courses of pharmacokinetic drug–drug interactions commonly encountered in antiepileptic drug therapy. While the epilepsy literature contains many studies in which the underlying mechanisms and clinical significance of these interactions are discussed and elaborated, there have been few well-designed studies in which the time courses of some of these interactions are investigated and pharmacokinetically modeled.

A pharmacokinetic drug–drug interaction in vivo is demonstrated by measurable changes in drug concentrations in the systemic circulation following the addition of a second drug to the dosage regimen. Hence, the changes in systemic drug concentration as a function of time should reflect the activities at the molecular level. Thus, in the investigation of the time course of a specific pharmacokinetic drug–drug interaction, it becomes vital to identify in the whole scheme one or more molecular events that actually control the onset and the subsequent time course of the changes in systemic drug concentration. In the best of circumstances, it should be feasible to develop a pharmacokinetic model based on this relationship for the prediction of the time course and extent of the interaction. In this chapter, the time courses of four types of drug–drug interactions with pharmacokinetic bases, for which examples are available in the epilepsy literature, will be discussed. It will be shown that the onset of the interaction, as indicated by commencement of changes in the plasma drug level, is dependent on its temporal relationship to the underlying mechanism. However, the subsequent time course is governed by the rate of elimination of the drug, which directly or indirectly may have been modified by the underlying mechanism. In some instances, the elimination of the agent causing the interaction becomes the rate-limiting step and dictates the subsequent time course.

DISPLACEMENT FROM BINDING SITES

Displacement interactions may take place at plasma binding sites, tissue binding sites, or both. For the purpose of this chapter, displacement from plasma protein-binding sites is assumed, since such a phenomenon can be easily verified by studies in vitro. Note that several conditions must be met before displacement from protein-binding sites takes place. They include: (a) a high percentage of drug bound to binding sites, (b) a displacing drug with a high affinity for the same binding site, and (c) a displacing drug present at a concentration that will occupy the majority of binding sites. It must be emphasized that the displacement interaction is a two-step process. The first step involves the establishment of a new equilibrium between the bound and unbound drugs following the introduction of the displacer. The second step involves the eliminating organs in their function of extracting drug following abrupt changes in total and unbound drug concentrations.

Perhaps the easiest way to appreciate a displacement interaction is to simulate the time course of the steady-state plasma concentration profile of the displaced drug following the introduction of the displacer via an intravenous loading dose along with a simultaneous constant rate infusion (1). For drugs with low extraction ratios—most antiepileptic agents are drugs with low extraction ratios—the onset of the displacement interaction is extremely rapid. As soon as the displacer is introduced, the total concentration of the displaced drug falls and the unbound concentration rises abruptly. Subsequently, the total concentration decays from the depressed level to a lower steady state, and on a parallel time frame, the unbound concentration decays from the elevated level to its original steady state.

The initial fall of total plasma concentration reflects rapid movement of some drug molecules (formerly bound to plasma protein) into the tissue compartment. The simultaneous increase in unbound concentration reflects the fact that some of the displaced drug molecules remain in the systemic circulation. The subsequent decay of total and unbound concentrations to their respective steady states can be explained by two basic pharmacokinetic relationships:

$$\text{Rate of elimination} = \text{Cu}\cdot\text{Cl}_u = \text{C}\cdot\text{Cl} = \text{C}\cdot\text{fu}\cdot\text{Cl}_u \tag{1}$$
$$\text{Zero-order infusion rate} = \text{Cu}_{ss}\cdot\text{Cl}_u = \text{C}_{ss}\cdot\text{Cl} \tag{2}$$

where Cu, C, Cu_{ss}, and C_{ss} are the unbound concentration, the total concentration, the steady-state unbound concentration, and the steady-state concentration, respectively, and Cl_u and Cl are the unbound and total clearances, respectively, and fu is the fraction unbound. Note total clearance is the product of fu and Cl_u and therefore increases as fu increases. The decay of C to an even lower steady state is due to an increase in fu. The concurrent return of Cu to the original steady state is due to the fact that the infusion rate now is exceeded by the elimination rate of the unbound drug ($Cu \cdot Cl_u$), since Cu now has been elevated by the displacer. The time required by both C and Cu to achieve their respective steady states depends on the half-life of the drug in the presence of the displacer. Often the half-life ($0.7\ V_d/Cl$) is shortened slightly due to an increase in C.

During antiepileptic therapy, there are few occasions that a displacing agent is added to an existing dosage regimen via a loading intravenous dose along with a simultaneous infusion. However, there are examples in which high doses of a displacer with a short half-life (relative to the half-life of the displaced drug) are administered frequently. Under these circumstances, the displacement interaction can be easily observed if C and Cu are monitored.

A well-documented displacement interaction in epilepsy is the interaction between phenytoin and valproic acid, although this interaction is confounded by enzyme inhibition. Phenytoin is approximately 90% bound to plasma proteins, has one binding site on serum albumin, and has an affinity constant (K_a) of 1.3×10^4 L/mole. Valproic acid has two binding sites on serum albumin and has a K_a of 2.7×10^4 L/mole (2). Valproic acid exhibits concentration-dependent binding to serum albumin, with relative saturation of binding sites occurring at a plasma concentration of approximately 80 μg/ml (3). Valproic acid has been shown, in vitro and in vivo, to displace the more loosely bound phenytoin from binding sites (2).

Total plasma phenytoin concentration decreased within 2 h after valproic acid was added to the dosage regimen (4,5). This decrease was maintained for at least 10 weeks (6) but was not present after several months (7,8). The observation that the lowered total phenytoin concentration was not maintained was attributed to inhibition of phenytoin metabolism by valproic acid (8). The free concentration and free fraction of phenytoin were shown to increase after valproic acid administration and were reported to remain elevated up to 19 weeks (4,8,9). At least one group of investigators attributed the observation of free phenytoin concentration failing to return to its original level to valproic acid mediated inhibition (8).

ENZYME INDUCTION

The most frequently observed drug–drug interactions during antiepileptic therapy are due to enzyme induction. Several antiepileptic agents (e.g., carbamazepine) are potent enzyme inducers. They have the ability to derepress the expression of genes for certain cyctochrome P-450 isozymes. As a result, inducers apparently stimulate the metabolism of concurrently administered drugs (heteroinduction) and in some cases their own metabolism (autoinduction). In epileptic patients, enzyme induction is demonstrated by decreases in plasma concentrations of the induced drugs, which sometimes can lead to loss of seizure control.

Due to the high occurrence rate and the potential seriousness of the result of this interaction, much effort has gone into identifying interactions caused by various inducers, assessing the clinical significance, documenting the time courses, and developing recommendations for therapeutic drug monitoring and dosage management. For a long time, a pharmacokinetic model for describing both the time course and extent of interaction due to enzyme induction was lacking. About a decade ago, Levy and co-workers (10) proposed a general theory to predict both the rate and extent of hetero- and autoinduction. Their theory is based on a model developed by Berlin and Schimke for describing the change of intracellular protein/enzyme levels upon the introduction of an inducer to the system (11).

The scheme that Levy and co-workers followed in relating the Berlin-Schimke model for changes in enzyme level to changes in plasma concentration of an induced drug is depicted in Fig. 13-1. The enzyme level in a cell remains constant in the absence of any perturbation, because enzyme synthesis (k_s) is zero order and enzyme degradation is first order (k_I). An inducer causes an immediate increase in the synthesis rate from k_s to $k_{s'}$. The time course of the rise in enzyme level from basal level (k_s/k_I) to a higher plateau ($k_{s'}/k_I$) as depicted in Fig. 13-1 is analogous to that which occurs to the plasma concentration of a drug as it climbs from a lower steady state to a higher one upon the increase in the infusion rate. The climb of the enzyme level is therefore governed by the enzyme degradation rate constant, k, and it will take five half-lives ($5 \times 0.7/k_I$) for the enzyme to achieve the higher plateau.

In pharmacokinetics, the first-order elimination constant is a direct indicator of enzyme level if the drug has a low extraction ratio and exhibits linear pharmacokinetics. When enzyme level is not perturbed, the elimination constant remains at a fixed value. Induction causes the enzyme level to increase, and accordingly the elimination constant also increases, climbing from its original value (K_E^o) to a higher value (K_E^∞). The time course for increase of the elimination constant parallels that for increase in enzyme level (Fig. 13-1). Both time courses are governed by the degradation constant for the enzyme. Mathematically, the increase in elimination constant as a function of time is given by the following expression:

$$K_E(t) = K_E^\infty - (K_E^\infty - K_{E_o})\, e^{-k_I t} \qquad (3)$$

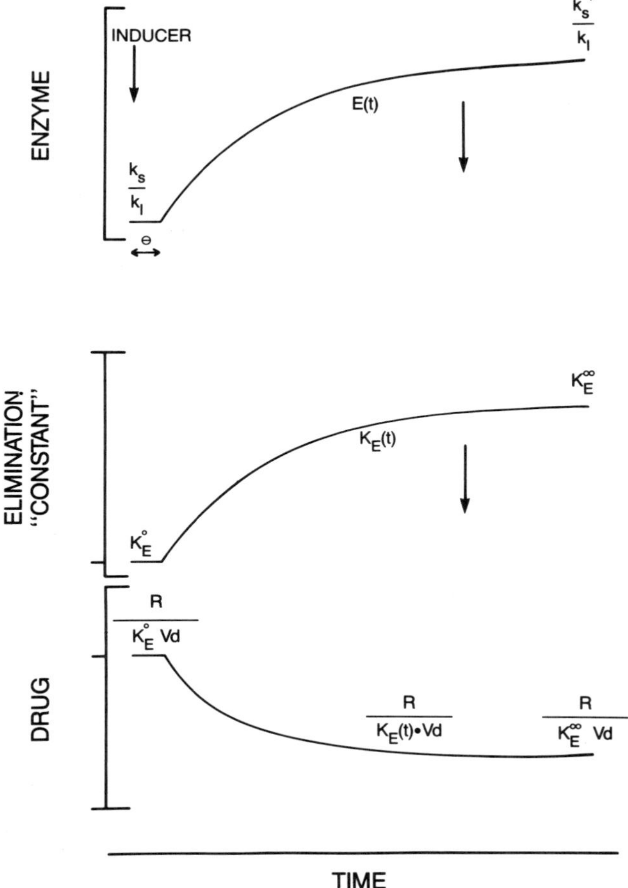

FIG. 13-1. Temporal relationships between enzyme level, elimination "constant," and plasma drug concentration following the addition of an enzyme inducer.

The steady-state plasma level of a drug (which is equal to the ratio between infusion rate and clearance) is inversely proportional to the elimination constant. During induction, plasma drug concentration decreases as the elimination constant increases (Fig. 13-1). Hence, the time course for plasma drug concentration decaying from its original steady state to a lower one moves in opposite direction when compared to the respective time courses for the change in the elimination constant and enzyme level. Note that the degradation constant for the enzyme still governs the change in steady-state drug level, as shown in the expression below:

$$C(t) = \frac{R}{K_E(t) \cdot V_d} \tag{4}$$

where R is the zero-order infusion rate of the induced drug and V_d is its volume of distribution. The induction model assumes that the half-life of the inducer is substantially shorter than the turnover half-life of the enzyme. Otherwise, slow achievement of effective inducer concentration and/or slow elimination of the inducer will confound the interpretation of the time courses of the induced drug in induction studies (12).

In the pharmacokinetic model for hetero- and autoinduction, Levy and co-workers also introduced a new parameter: induction lag time (θ), which is the time from the addition of an enzyme inducer to the dosage regimen to the commencement of decrease in plasma drug level (Fig. 13-1). A lag time generally is observed, because inducers act in transcriptional events that precede enzyme synthesis.

The applicability of the induction model was tested in a number of experimental studies. First, a direct relationship between changes in cytochrome P-450 and clearance of an induced drug was demonstrated by Wedlund and co-workers (13). They showed that, in monkeys, carbamazepine clearance increased from 0.88 ± 0.17 to 1.35 ± 0.34 L/h/kg following autoinduction while the hepatic cyctochrome P-450 level went up from 0.26 ± 0.04 to 0.44 ± 0.14 nmol/mg of protein ($p < 0.05$).

Second, in an interaction study in rhesus monkeys (14), steady-state concentrations of clonazepam were achieved by constant rate intravenous infusion prior to addition of the inducer (carbamazepine). Use of Eq. 4 to analyze the decay in plasma clonazepam concentration successfully yielded estimates for the enzyme turnover half-life, the basal half-life, and the induced half-life of clonazepam. The induction model also predicts that upon the withdrawal of the inducer, the decrease in enzyme level is to be reflected by an exponential increase in plasma drug concentration until the original steady state has been achieved. This prediction was verified via the modeling of observed plasma clonazepam concentrations in monkeys following the withdrawal of carbamazepine (14).

Furthermore, the induction model also was tested in human studies (15–17). In these studies, both the inducer (carbamazepine) and the induced drugs (clonazepam, valproic acid, and ethosuximide) were administered orally, and a pharmacokinetic model for induction during multiple dosing (18) was applied in the regression analysis. As in the monkey studies, estimates for both the basal and induced half-lives of the drug and the turnover half-life of enzyme were obtained.

ENZYME INHIBITION

From a biochemical viewpoint, enzyme inhibition is broadly classified into two types: irreversible and reversible. Irreversible inhibition usually involves the modification or destruction of the enzyme by the substrate (e.g., via covalent bonding). Reversible inhibition can further be classified into subtypes: competitive and noncompetitive. In competitive inhibition, the inhibitor competes with the substrate for the same active binding site on the enzyme. In noncompetitive inhibition, the inhibitor binds at a locus on the enzyme other than the substrate binding site. In studies in vitro, the time courses of these two subtypes of inhibition can be monitored via real-time measurement of metabolite formation in an isolated system. Lineweaver-Burke plots then are constructed for the purpose of distinguishing the mechanism that the inhibitor follows in exerting its effect.

It is more difficult to investigate the time course of enzyme inhibition in vivo for a number of reasons. First, the inhibitor sometimes acts via multiple mechanisms, and the resultant inhibition has more than one component. Second, a patient is more complex than a purified enzyme system isolated in a cell, and there can be concurrent events (e.g., induction effected by one of the two interacting drugs) that can confound the interpretation of changes in plasma level of the inhibited drug. In drug biotransformation, Phase I metabolism is mediated mostly by Cytochrome P-450s. To date, at least three types of P-450 inhibitors have been identified: (a) reversible inhibitors that mimic substrate binding, (b) moieties, such as imidazoles, which coordinate with the heme ion atom of P-450s, and (c) suicide substrate inhibitors that covalently attach to the heme. Phase II metabolism involves conjugation and is mediated by various transferases, which are less complex enzyme systems when compared to the P-450s. Most inhibitors for these transferases are of the competitive type.

A general scheme that depicts the time course of competitive inhibition in vivo could be developed based on known behavior in vitro, and clinical reports of elevation of plasma level by a second drug, and similarity of metabolic pathways between the two agents. In competitive inhibition in vivo, the plasma level of the drug (whose metabolism is being inhibited) begins to rise as soon as the competitive inhibitor is presented to the hepatic microsomal enzymes in adequate concentration to effect the inhibition. From a pharmacokinetic viewpoint, total body clearance of the inhibited drug is reduced, its elimination half-life is prolonged, and a higher steady state is achieved after five half-lives of the drug in the presence of the inhibitor. Sometimes, these changes are accompanied by clinical signs of drug intoxication. Competitive inhibition in vivo is reversible upon the withdrawal of the inhibitor. The plasma level of the inhibited agent begins to return to its original level as soon as the inhibitor is removed from the dosage regimen. The time the drug takes to return to its original steady state, of course, depends on its elimination half-life in the absence of the inhibitor. There is at least one antiepileptic drug (phenytoin) whose metabolism is inhibited by another agent in a competitive fashion. Phenytoin is an obvious case, since it exhibits dose-dependent pharmacokinetics even at moderate therapeutic doses. Thus, it is not surprising that there are many reports of common therapeutic agents (e.g., dicoumarol) having the capability of raising plasma phenytoin levels and causing drug intoxication. Any drug that utilizes the same site on the enzyme system for metabolism should be a reasonable competitive inhibitor.

The time courses of inhibitions other than the competitive type should be more varied because it depends on the chain of events which take place following the addition of a noncompetitive inhibitor to the dosage regimen. In some cases, commencement of changes in the plasma level of the inhibited drug is extremely rapid while in others, changes in plasma drug levels are delayed. The inhibition of carbamazepine metabolism by erythromycin is an interesting example. Generally, after three or more days of erythromycin therapy, many patients maintained on carbamazepine develop the classic symptoms of carbamazepine intoxication, and measurement of carbamazepine levels would yield values above 15 μg/ml (19,20). There is evidence that a metabolite of erythromycin inhibits carbamazepine metabolism. Recently, it was demonstrated that erythromycin is oxidized by cytochrome P-450 and the metabolite forms a stable, inactive complex with the heme of the reduced cytochrome, causing a decrease in the activity of selective mono-oxygenases (21).

ABSORPTION INTERACTION

There are many mechanisms for drug interactions that affect drug absorption. These mechanisms can be classified into two major categories: (a) indirect actions that occur as a result of the pharmacological action of the drug [e.g., changes in gastrointestinal (GI) blood flow, GI motility, gastric emptying] and (b) direct actions that result from direct effects of one drug on the other (e.g., adsorption, chelation). Although many of these mechanisms are of theoretical importance, antiepileptic drugs are, in general, less affected by drug absorption interactions than most other classes of drugs.

Drug absorption interactions can affect the extent of absorption, the rate of absorption, or both. For most drugs, a significant change in the extent of absorption will have a major effect on the therapeutic efficacy. A change in the rate of absorption, in most cases, will not be of clinical significance since antiepileptic drugs are administered chronically.

In the case of direct action of one drug on another, the interaction commences within a short time in the gastrointestinal tract following concurrent ingestion of the two drugs, and changes in the blood levels of the affected drug can be observed within hours. In the case of indirect action of one drug on another, there might be a slightly longer time lag before changes in the blood levels of the affected drug are observed. However, in either case, the time required to achieve a new steady-state concentration will be dependent on the elimination half-life of the affected drug.

A review of the literature shows very few clinically significant drug interactions that affect absorption of antiepileptic drugs. One of the most widely discussed is the effect of antacids on phenytoin absorption. Since phenytoin exhibits dose-dependent kinetics, small changes in the extent of absorption may result in large changes in the plasma phenytoin concentration. Several studies reported that phenytoin bioavailability was reduced in the presence of aluminum hydroxide with magnesium hydroxide or magnesium trisilicate (22–24). While this effect was not found in all studies, there have been significant differences in study design, including the dose of antacid administered, the time of antacid administration, and the duration of treatment (25,26). A decrease in plasma phenytoin concentration could be observed within 2 h following antacid administration in some subjects (24). The study conducted by Kulshrestha et al. demonstrated that the decreased plasma phenytoin concentrations were present 5 days after the initiation of the antacid therapy. It was suggested that antacids could alter both the rate and extent of absorption of phenytoin (24).

Perhaps a better example of the time course of absorption interaction is the effect of activated charcoal on the GI absorption of carbamazepine. The greatest effect on absorption was observed when the charcoal was administered within 5 min following ingestion of phenytoin, whereas no effect was observed if charcoal was administered 10–48 h after phenytoin (27). The inhibitory effect of charcoal on the absorption of carbamazepine and other drugs also was dependent on the amount of charcoal administered. The effects of charcoal were not limited to the absorption phase. Repeated charcoal doses decreased the elimination half-life of carbamazepine, probably by adsorbing drug secreted into the intestine from the bile or other routes (27).

CONCLUSIONS

Over the past 20 years, tremendous progress has been made in our understanding of the time courses of drug–drug interactions with pharmacokinetic bases. The time courses for absorption interactions are relatively simple, because the underlying mechanisms for the situations encountered in the field of epilepsy appear to be physicochemical processes. In the case of interactions due to displacement from binding sites, the in vivo time courses often can be predicted, to a fair extent, based on results of in vitro equilibrium dialysis experiments and prior knowledge of respective pharmacokinetic characteristics of the displacing and displaced agents. In the case of enzyme induction, our understanding of the time course has been helped by the work of many researchers outside the field of pharmacokinetics. In the case of enzyme inhibition, much remains to be learned since there are many locations (perhaps including the locus for suppression of cytochrome P-450 genes) at which an inhibitor can elicit its action. However, the future of research in this area is bright. There is now a battery of compounds that can modulate expression of cytochrome P-450 genes. Furthermore, the techniques for harvesting and purifying cytochrome P-450 isozymes have been refined, and our understanding of the metabolism of various antiepileptic drugs are more thorough. It is highly feasible that within the next decade the mechanisms, and hence the time courses, for some of the unusual interactions (e.g., inhibition followed by induction elicited by valproic acid) will be solved.

Acknowledgment: The authors acknowledge the assistance of Karen Brady in the preparation of this manuscript.

REFERENCES

1. Rowland M, Tozer TN. *Clinical Pharmacokinetics.* Philadelphia: Lea and Febiger, 1980.
2. Patel IH, Levy RH. Valproic acid binding to human serum albumin and determination of free fraction in the presence of anticonvulsants and free fatty acids. *Epilepsia* 1979;20:85–90.
3. Cramer JA, Mattson RH. Valproic acid: *in vitro* plasma protein binding and interaction with phenytoin. *Ther Drug Monit* 1979;1:105–16.
4. Perucca E, Hebdige S, Frigo GM, Gatti G, Lecchini S, Crema A. Interaction between phenytoin and valproic acid: plasma protein binding and metabolic effects. *Clin Pharmacol Ther* 1980;28:779–89.
5. Monks A, Richens A. Effect of single doses of sodium valproate on serum phenytoin levels and protein binding in epileptic patients. *Clin Pharmacol Ther* 1980;27:89–95.
6. Wilder BJ, Willmore LJ, Bruni J, Villareal HJ. Valproic acid interaction with other anticonvulsant drugs. *Neurology* 1978;28:892–6.
7. Bruni J, Wilder BJ, Willmore LJ, Barbour B. Valproic acid and plasma levels of phenytoin. *Neurology* 1979;29:904–5.
8. Bruni J, Gallo JM, Lee CS, Perchalski RJ, Wilder BJ. Interactions of valproic acid with phenytoin. *Neurology* 1980;30:1233–6.
9. Haidukewych D, Rodin EA. Serial free and plasma valproic acid and phenytoin monitoring and drug interactions. *Ther Drug Monit* 1981;3:303–7.
10. Levy RA, Lai AA, Dumain MS. Time-dependent kinetics: IV: pharmacokinetic theory of enzyme induction. *J Pharm Sci* 1979;68:398–9.
11. Berlin CM, Schimke RT. Influence of turnover rates on the responses of enzymes to cortisone. *Mol Pharmacol* 1965;1:149–56.
12. Abramson EP. Kinetic models of induction: I. Persistence of the inducing substance. *J Pharm Sci* 1986;75:223–8.
13. Wedlund PJ, Nelson SD, Nickerson S, Levy RH. Linear relationship between cyctochrome P-450 and carbamazepine clearance in rhesus monkey. *Drug Metab Dispos* 1982;10:480–5.
14. Lai AA, Levy RH. Pharmacokinetic description of drug interaction by enzyme

induction: carbamazepine-clonazepam in monkeys. *J Pharm Sci* 1979;68:416–21.

15. Lai AA, Levy RH, Cutler RE. Time-course of interaction between carbamazepine and clonazepam in normal man. *Clin Pharmacol Ther* 1978;24:316–23.

16. Warren JW, Benmaman JD, Wannamaker BB, Levy RH. Kinetics of a carbamazepine–ethosuximide interaction. *Clin Pharmacol Ther* 1980;28:646–51.

17. Bowdle TA, Levy RH, Cutler RE. Effects of carbamazepine on valproic acid kinetics in normal subjects. *Clin Pharmacol Ther* 1979;26:629–34.

18. Levy RH, Dumain MS, Cook JL. Time-dependent kinetics: V. Time course of drug levels during enzyme induction (one compartment model). *J Pharmacokinet Biopharm* 1979;7:557–78.

19. Wong YY, Ludden TM, Bell RD. Effect of erythromycin on carbamazepine kinetics. *Clin Pharmacol Ther* 1983;33:460–4.

20. Pippenger CE. Clinically significant carbamazepine drug interactions: an overview. *Epilepsia* 1987;28:S71–S76.

21. Mao SCH, Tardrew PL. Demethylation of erythromycin by rabbit tissues in vitro. *Biochem Pharmacol* 1965;14:1049–58.

22. Kutt H. Interactions of antiepileptic drugs. *Epilepsia* 1975;16:393–402.

23. Kulshrestha WK, Thomas M, Wadsworth J, Richens A. Interactions between phenytoin and antacids. *Br J Clin Pharmacol* 1978;6:177–9.

24. Carter BL, Garnett W, Pellock JM, Stratton MA, Howell JR. Effect of antacids on phenytoin bioavailability. *Ther Drug Monit* 1981;3:333–40.

25. O'Brien LS, Orme ML, Breckenridge AM. Failure of antacids to alter the pharmacokinetics of phenytoin. *Br J Clin Pharmacol* 1978;6:176–7.

26. Chapron DJ, Kramer PA, Mariano SL, Hohnadel DC. Effect of calcium and antacids on phenytoin bioavailability. *Arch Neurol* 1979;36:436–8.

27. Neuvonen PJ, Elonen E. Effect of activated charcoal on absorption and elimination of phenobarbitone, carbamazepine, and phenylbutazone in man. *Eur J Clin Pharmacol* 1980;17:51–7.

14

Antiepileptic and Neurotoxic Interactions Between Antiepileptic Drugs

Blaise F.D. Bourgeois and [1]W. Edwin Dodson

Department of Neurology, Section of Epilepsy and Clinical Neurophysiology, The Cleveland Clinic Foundation, Cleveland, Ohio, and [1]The Malinckrodt Department of Pediatrics and the Department of Neurology and Neurological Surgery (Neurology), Washington University School of Medicine and St. Louis Children's Hospital, St. Louis, Missouri, U.S.A.

Single-drug therapy of epilepsy has been increasingly advocated in recent years (1). Arguments in favor of monotherapy of epilepsy are based on the observation that a reduction in the number of antiepileptic drugs often reduces the incidence of undesirable side-effects without a corresponding loss in seizure control (2–7) and that the additional seizure reduction achieved with drug combinations is often modest when seizure control has not been achieved with one drug (8). It is nevertheless likely that patients whose seizures are not controlled by various antiepileptic drugs given alone will continue to receive two or more drugs simultaneously. The theoretical, experimental, and clinical background for the practice of combining antiepileptic drugs has received relatively little attention. Thus, the pharmacokinetic interactions between antiepileptic drugs are much better known than the pharmacodynamic interactions. Reasons for combining antiepileptic drugs might be the following: First, a wider antiepileptic spectrum might be achieved, i.e., the combination protects against two or more seizure types that cannot be prevented by one single drug. Second, the combination might have a better efficacy/toxicity ratio, i.e., the increase in antiepileptic effect could exceed the increase in overall toxicity. In the latter case, when the dose of the two drugs is pushed to the limit of toxicity, the antiepileptic effect would be greater than for either drug alone. A supra-additive (potentiated) antiepileptic interaction has been suggested as evidence in favor of a drug combination. However, the interactions with regard to both the antiepileptic and the toxic effects have to be considered. If toxicity is potentiated to the same extent as the anticonvulsant effect, the efficacy/toxicity ratio, or therapeutic index, of the combination cannot be superior to the corresponding ratio for each of the drugs when tested alone. Clinically, it is possible to study the antiepileptic spectrum of single or combined drugs, but it would be extremely difficult to study the efficacy/toxicity ratio, because this requires a quantitative assessment of the antiepileptic effect and of the neurotoxic side-effects of each drug alone and of a given combination of drugs in a homogeneous population of patients with epilepsy. Therefore, the basic pharmacological question of the effect of combining antiepileptic drugs on their therapeutic index has been addressed by using an experimental model in animals and will be the subject of the present review.

METHODS

All studies under consideration were carried out in mice. Drugs were administered either by transesophageal gavage or intraperitoneally (i.p.). Seizure protection was measured either against maximal electroshock (MES) or against pentylenetetrazole (PTZ), depending on the drug or pair of drugs to be studied (9,10). Neurological toxicity was assessed by the roto-rod toxicity test (11); the ability to remain on the rotating rod for at least 10 min in the first trial was defined as absence of neurotoxicity. For each drug studied, the time interval between administration and testing was constant, whether the drug was tested alone or in combination with another drug. After the tests, the animals were killed immediately by decapitation, and the brains were obtained for the determination of drug concentrations.

In the studies to be reviewed, brain concentrations of drugs were determined either by high-performance liquid chromatography (HPLC), gas chromatography (GC) or gas chromatography–mass spectrometry (GC–MS). Concentrations were expressed in μg/g or μmol/kg wet brain weight. All results were expressed in terms of brain concentrations in order to eliminate any possible pharmacokinetic interactions that might affect the analysis if results are expressed in terms of doses. Based on the brain concentrations in a group of animals, a quantitative assessment of drug potency was made. The anticonvulsant potency was expressed as either the median effective brain concentration (EC50) or as the minimal effective brain concentration (MEC) against MES or PTZ. The neurotoxic potency was expressed correspondingly as either the median toxic brain concentration (TC50) or as the minimal toxic brain concentration (MTC). The therapeutic index (TI) was defined as the ratio TC50/EC50 or MTC/MEC, respectively.

The quantitative assessment of pharmacodynamic drug interactions was based on two methods: the isobolographic analysis (12,13) in a modified form (14) and the fractional effective concentration (FEC) index (15). A value of 1.0 for the FEC index indicates a strictly additive interaction, whereas values of less than 0.7 are indicative of a supra-additive effect, and values above 1.3 indicate an infra-additive interaction (16). Details of the methods for the assessment of the drug potency and pharmacodynamic interactions are presented in the original studies included in this review.

RESULTS AND DISCUSSION

Interaction Between Phenytoin and Phenobarbital

Both phenytoin (PHT) and phenobarbital (PB) are widely used antiepileptic drugs that have been frequently combined (17,18). Results of experiments on efficacy and neurotoxicity of PHT and PB alone and in combination are summarized in Fig. 14-1 (14). This modified graphic representation of the isobolographic analysis indicates a purely additive effect of PHT and PB against MES, since the EC50 value for the sum of their

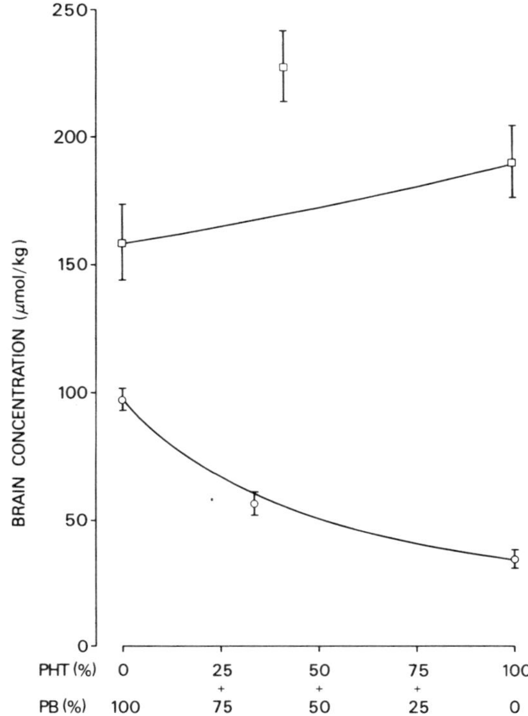

FIG. 14-1. Median effective brain concentration against MES (EC50, circles) and median toxic brain concentration (TC50, squares) for PB alone (left) and PHT alone (right), as well as for the sum of PB + PHT combined. The abscissa represents the relative concentration of the two drugs, and the ordinate represents the brain concentrations. Solid lines represent values for a purely additive interaction, and vertical bars indicate the 95% confidence limits. The antiepileptic effect is purely additive, whereas there is antagonism with regard to the neurotoxic effect. [Reproduced from Bourgeois (14) with permission.]

Table 14-1.   Fractional Effective Concentration (FEC) and FEC Indices of PB and PHT

Test	FEC[a]	FEC index[b]
MES		
PB	$\dfrac{40.2}{97.1} = 0.41$	
		0.92
PHT	$\dfrac{17.1}{33.8} = 0.51$	
ROTOROD		
PB	$\dfrac{129.4}{157.9} = 0.82$	
		1.34
PHT	$\dfrac{98.8}{189.2} = 0.52$	

[a] FEC = EC_{50} or TC_{50} in combination/EC_{50} or TC_{50} alone.
[b] FEC index = sum of FEC values for PB and PHT. A value of 1.0 ± 0.3 indicates an additive interaction, values below 0.7 being indicative of a supra-additive interaction and values above 1.3 indicating an infra-additive interaction.
Reproduced with permission from ref. 14.

concentrations coincides with the expected value for an additive interaction. In contrast, the TC50 of the combination is well above the expected value for an additive interaction, indicating an infra-additive or antagonistic interaction. These results are confirmed by the determination of the FEC index (Table 14-1). An FEC index of 0.7–1.3 suggests additive interaction, lower values being indicative of a supra-additive effect and higher values indicating an infra-additive effect (16). Thus, in this model, for a combination of PHT and PB in which PHT accounts for 30–40% of the total drug concentration in the brain, the efficacy/toxicity ratio is 1.46 times (1.34/0.92) higher than expected if both the antiepileptic and the neurotoxic interactions were purely additive.

An additive anticonvulsant interaction against MES based on brain concentrations of PHT and PB in rats had been reported by Leppik and Sherwin (19). Previous reports based on the analysis of doses had suggested a supra-additive interaction (20–23). This discrepancy between results based on brain concentrations and results based on doses can be explained by the observation that the ratio between the brain concentration and the dose of PHT increases when PHT is administered acutely together with PB (14,19). Thus, the antiepileptic pharmacodynamic interaction in the strict sense appears to be additive for PHT and PB.

FIG. 14-2. Median effective brain concentration against MES (EC50, circles) and median toxic brain concentration (TC50, squares) for PB alone (left) and CBZ alone (right), as well as for the sum of PB + CBZ combined. The abscissa represents the relative concentration of the two drugs, and the ordinate represents the brain concentrations. Solid lines represent values for a purely additive interaction, and vertical bars indicate the 95% confidence limits. Both the antiepileptic effect and the neurotoxic effect are purely additive. [Reproduced from Bourgeois and Wad (25) with permission.]

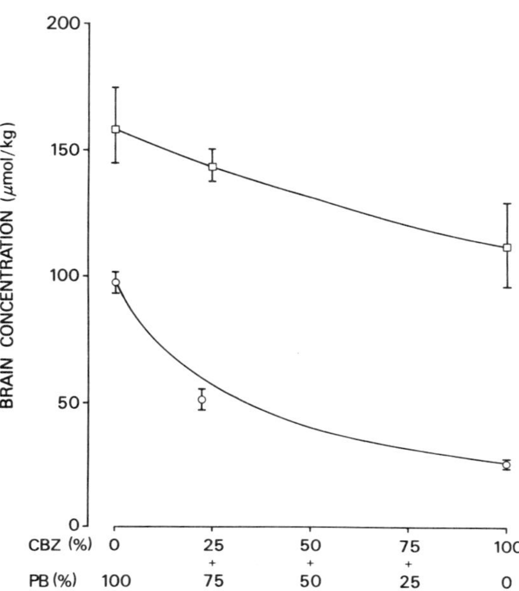

Interaction Between PHT and Carbamazepine

Carbamazepine (CBZ) and PHT are equipotent in preventing MES-induced seizures in mice after i.p. administration (24). Given singly, the TI values for PHT and CBZ are 5.2 and 4.6, respectively, based on doses. However, based on brain concentrations, the TI values of the individual drugs are 4.8 and 2.9, respectively. In brain, the FEC index for combined PHT + CBZ was 0.89, and the FTC index was 1.04, both in the range of additive interactions. This indicates that both efficacy and toxicity of this combination are additive. Therefore, the analysis suggests no advantage for this combination relative to either drug given alone.

Interaction Between CBZ and PB

Figure 14-2 shows individual and combined efficacy and neurotoxicity of CBZ and PB (25). The concentration ratio between the two drugs after combined administration was selected according to their potency against MES, and PB was thus in excess of CBZ due to its lower potency. The analysis reveals that both the anticonvulsant and the neurotoxic interaction were purely additive. Accordingly, the FEC index of the combination was 0.86 against MES and 1.0 for the rotorod test. Therefore, the combination of CBZ and PB in this experimental model is not beneficial with regard to the efficacy/toxicity ratio.

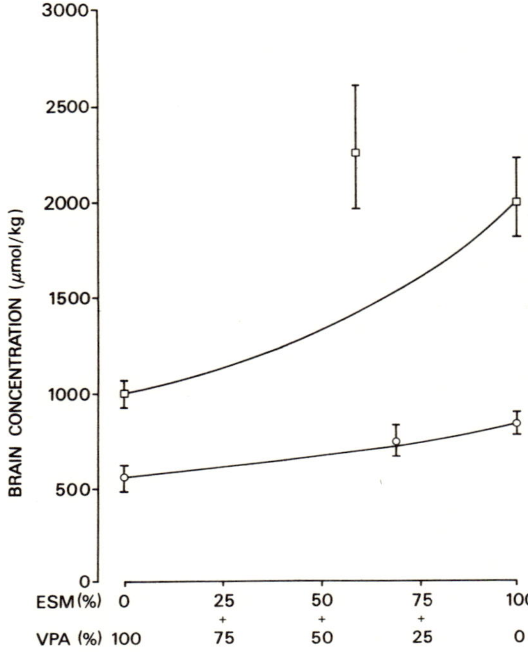

FIG. 14-3. Median effective brain concentration against PTZ (EC50, circles) and median toxic brain concentration (TC50, squares) for VPA alone (left) and ESM alone (right), as well as for the sum of VPA + ESM combined. The abscissa represents the relative concentration of the two drugs, and the ordinate represents the brain concentrations. Solid lines represent values for a purely additive interaction, and vertical bars indicate the 95% confidence limits. The antiepileptic effect is purely additive, whereas there is antagonism with regard to the neurotoxic effect. [Reproduced from Bourgeois (30) with permission.]

Interaction Between Valproate and Ethosuximide

Both ethosuximide (ESM) and valproate (VPA) are effective in the treatment of absence seizures. The combination of the two drugs has been recommended in patients whose seizures are not fully controlled by ESM or VPA alone (26–29). The pharmacodynamic interaction between the two drugs with regard to protection against PTZ-induced seizures and neurotoxicity by the rotorod test in mice is represented in Fig. 14-3 (30). The antiepileptic effect of the drug combination is again purely additive, whereas there is a clearly infra-additive neurotoxic interaction. Correspondingly, the FEC index for the antiepileptic interaction was 1.02, indicating a strictly additive interaction, and the FEC index for the neurotoxic interaction was 1.6, indicating it was in the infra-additive range. Thus, combining the two drugs in this model increased the efficacy/toxicity ratio by a factor of 1.6.

Interaction Between VPA and PB

The association of VPA and PB has been reported to be more effective than either drug alone in patients with the Lennox-Gastaut syndrome (31). An experimental study of the pharmacodynamic interaction between the two drugs in mice revealed an FEC index of 0.9 against PTZ-induced seizures and an index of 1.05 for neurotoxicity (32). Since both interactions are additive, this combination is not associated with an increase in the efficacy/toxicity ratio in this model.

Interaction Between VPA and CBZ

Both VPA and CBZ are now widely used drugs and, since they appear to have relatively little sedative effect, they are also combined in the treatment of epilepsy (33–35). In mice, the FEC index for the combination of VPA with CBZ was found to be 0.94 against MES seizures and 1.43 for the neurotoxic effect (32). The association of an additive antiepileptic interaction with an infra-additive neurotoxic interaction in this experimental model accounted for a relative gain in efficacy vs. toxicity by a factor of 1.52.

Results of a previous study on the interaction between VPA and CBZ were based on doses and suggested a supra-additive anticonvulsant interaction and additive acute toxicity (36). A separate study suggested that VPA, when administered with CBZ, increased the area under concentration vs. time curve for CBZ and for its active epoxide metabolite (37). This pharmacokinetic interaction would fully explain the discrepancy between results obtained from the analysis of doses and results obtained from the analysis of brain concentrations.

Interaction Between Antiepileptic Drugs and Active Metabolites

Primidone (PRM) and CBZ both have active metabolites that can be measured in plasma during chronic therapy. Most of the therapeutic effect of PRM is derived from its conversion to PB. The interaction between PB and PRM was found to be supra-additive for the anticonvulsant effect and infra-additive for the neurotoxic effect (38,39). In the same study, the interaction between PB and phenyl-ethyl-malonamide (PEMA), the other active metabolite of PRM, was found to be supra-additive for both the antiepileptic and the neurotoxic effect. The active epoxide metabolite of CBZ interacted additively with CBZ with regard to both the antiepileptic activity and the neurotoxicity (40).

CONCLUSIONS

As can be seen in Table 14-2, which summarizes the various pharmacodynamic interactions included in this review, the great majority of antiepileptic interactions are characterized by a purely additive effect and not by synergism or potentiation. An anticonvulsant potentiation could be shown only for PRM and PB and for PB and PEMA, all of which belong

Table 14-2. Summary of Pharmacodynamic Antiepileptic Drug Interactions

	Interaction	
Drug pair[a]	Antiepileptic	Neurotoxic
PHT + PB	Additive	Infra-additive
PHT + CBZ	Additive	Additive
CBZ + PB	Additive	Additive
VPA + ESM	Additive	Infra-additive
VPA + PB	Additive	Additive
VPA + CBZ	Additive	Infra-additive
CBZ + CBZ-E	Additive	Additive
PRM + PB	Supra-additive	Infra-additive
PB + PEMA	Supra-additive	Supra-additive

[a]CBZ, carbamazepine; CBZ-E, carbamazepine-epoxide; ESM, ethosuximide; PB, phenobarbital; PEMA, phenyl-ethyl-malonamide; PHT, phenytoin; PRM, primidone; VPA, valproate.

to the barbiturate compounds whose clinical use has been declining. The interactions are more variable with regard to the neurotoxic effect, as measured by the rotorod test in mice. Approximately one-half of the drug pairs studied display an additive combined neurotoxic activity, whereas for the remainder of the combinations the toxicity is infra-additive. In case of additive antiepileptic interaction, the neurotoxic interaction must be infra-additive if the combination is to have a better efficacy/toxicity ratio than each drug given alone. Combinations with an infra-additive neurotoxic interaction were PB + PHT, PB + PRM, VPA + ESM, and VPA + CBZ. The therapeutic index of PB alone is relatively low, in patients as well as in the experimental model. Although the combined neurotoxicity of PB + PHT and PB + PRM was infra-additive, the relatively high neurotoxicity of PB could not be compensated for, and the efficacy/toxicity ratio of these two combinations was still lower than that of PHT alone or PRM alone. Thus, of all antiepileptic drug interactions included in the present review, only two drug pairs were advantageous: VPA + ESM and VPA + CBZ.

The results presented in this review were obtained after single doses in a standardized animal model, and two aspects must be considered regarding their interpretation. First, they cannot necessarily be extrapolated to patients with epilepsy and, second, the results after single doses might differ from those obtained during chronic administration of the drugs. Also, because of the complexities involved in the quantitative assessment of pharmacodynamic interactions, toxicity was evaluated by the rotorod test alone, whereas the clinical spectrum of toxic side-effects in patients varies among different antiepileptics. However, the side-effects that will most commonly determine the maximal tolerated dose of any antiepileptic drug in patients are motor incoordination and sedation, both of which are assessed by the rotorod test. Although most animal models of neurological toxicity reflect motor incoordination, it might be of interest to use other tests such as the effect on learned behavior. Nevertheless, since antiepileptic and toxic pharmacodynamic interactions of antiepileptic drugs are very difficult to assess in a quantitative manner in epileptic patients, the animal model presented is an attempt to objectively address the question of pharmacodynamic antiepileptic drug interactions.

Acknowledgment: Part of this work was supported by grant 3.946-0.85 from the Swiss National Science Foundation.

REFERENCES

1. Reynolds EH, Shorvon SD. Single drug or combination therapy for epilepsy? *Drugs* 1981;21:374–82.
2. Fischbacher E. Effect of reduction of anticonvulsants on wellbeing. *Br Med J* 1982;285:423–4.
3. Bennett HS, Dunlop T, Ziring P. Reduction of polypharmacy for epilepsy in an institution for the retarded. *Dev Med Child Neurol* 1983;25:735–7.
4. Schmidt D. Reduction of two-drug therapy in intractable epilepsy. *Epilepsia* 1983;24:368–76.
5. Theodore WH, Porter RJ. Removal of sedative-hypnotic antiepileptic drugs from the regimen of patients with intractable epilepsy. *Ann Neurol* 1983;13:320–4.
6. Lesser RP, Pippenger CE, Lüders H, Dinner DS. High-dose monotherapy in treatment of intractable seizures. *Neurology* 1984;34:707–11.
7. Albright P, Bruni J. Reduction of polypharmacy in epileptic patients. *Arch Neurol* 1985;42:797–9.
8. Schmidt D. Two antiepileptic drugs for intractable epilepsy with complex partial seizures. *J Neurol Neurosurg Psychiatry* 1982;45:1119–24.
9. Swinyard EA, Brown WC, Goodman LS. Comparative assays of antiepileptic drugs in mice and rats. *J Pharmacol Exp Ther* 1952;106:319–30.
10. Krall RL, Penry JK, White BG, Kupferberg HJ, Swinyard EA. Antiepileptic drug development: II. Anticonvulsant drug screening. *Epilepsia* 1978;19:409–28.
11. Dunham NW, Miya TS. A note on a simple apparatus for detecting neurological deficit in rats and mice. *J Am Pharmacol Assoc* 1957;46:208–9.
12. Loewe S. The problem of synergism and antagonism of combined drugs. *Arzneimittelforsch* 1953;3:285–90.
13. Hewlett PS. Measurement of the potencies of drug mixtures. *Biometrics* 1969;25:477–87.
14. Bourgeois BFD. Antiepileptic drug combinations and experimental background: the case of phenobarbital and phenytoin. *Naunyn Schmiedebergs Arch Pharmacol* 1986;333:406–11.

15. Elison GB, Singer S, Hitchings GH. Antagonists of nucleic acid derivatives: VIII. Synergism in combinations of biochemically related antimetabolites. *J Biol Chem* 1954;208:477–88.

16. Kerry DW, Hamilton-Miller JMT, Brumfitt W. Trimethoprim and rifampicin: in vitro activities separately and in combination. *J Antimicrob Chemother* 1975:1:417–27.

17. Schmidt RP, Wilder PJ. *Epilepsy.* Oxford: Blackwell Scientific Publications, 1968:172–3.

18. Morselli PL, Rizzo M, Garattini S. Interaction between phenobarbital and diphenylhydantoin in animals and in epileptic patients. *Ann NY Acad Sci* 1971;179:88–107.

19. Leppik IE, Sherwin AL. Anticonvulsant activity of phenobarbital and phenytoin in combination. *J Pharmacol Exp Ther* 1977;200:570–5.

20. Chen G, Ensor CR. A study of the anticonvulsant properties of phenobarbital and dilantin. *Arch Int Pharmacodyn Ther* 1954;100:234–48.

21. Weaver LC, Swinyard EA, Woodbury LA, Goodman LS. Studies on anticonvulsant drug combinations: phenobarbital and diphenylhydantoin. *J Pharmacol Exp Ther* 1955;113:358–70.

22. Wallin RF, Blackburn WH, Napoli MD. Pharmacological interactions of albutoin with other anticonvulsant drugs. *J Pharmacol Exp Ther* 1970;174:276–82.

23. Consroe P, Wolkin A. Cannabidiol-antiepileptic drug comparisons and interactions in experimentally induced seizures in rats. *J Pharmacol Exp Ther* 1977;201:26–32.

24. Morris JC, Dodson WE, Hatlelid JM, Ferrendelli JA. Phenytoin and carbamazepine alone and in combination: anticonvulsant and neurotoxic effects. *Neurology* 1987;37:1111–8.

25. Bourgeois BFD, Wad N. Combined administration of carbamazepine and phenobarbital: effect on anticonvulsant activity and neurotoxicity. *Epilepsia* 1988;29:482–7.

26. Jeavons PM, Clark E. Sodium valproate in the treatment of epilepsy. *Br Med J* 1974;2:584–6.

27. Porter RJ. General principles: clinical efficacy and use of antiepileptic drugs. In: Woodbury DM, Penry JK, Pippenger CE, eds. *Antiepileptic Drugs.* New York: Raven Press, 1982:167–75.

28. Rowan AJ, Meijer JWA, de Beer-Pawlikowski N, van der Geest P, Meinardi H. Valproate-ethosuximide combination therapy for refractory absence seizures. *Arch Neurol* 1983;40:797–802.

29. Tassinari CA, Bureau M. Epilepsy with myoclonic absences. In: Roger J, Dravet C, Bureau M, Dreifuss FE, Wolf P, eds. *Epileptic Syndromes in Infancy, Childhood and Adolescence.* London: John Libbey, 1985:121–9.

30. Bourgeois BFD. Combination of valproate and ethosuximide: antiepileptic and neurotoxic interaction. *J Pharmacol Exp Ther* 1988;247:1128–32.

31. Vassella F, Rüdeburg A, da Silva V, et al. Doppeltblind-Untersuchung über die antikonvulsive Wirkung von Phenobarbital und Valproat beim Lennox-Syndrom. *Schweiz Med Wochenschr* 1978;108:713–6.

32. Bourgeois BFD. Anticonvulsant potency and neurotoxicity of valproate alone

and in combination with carbamazepine or phenobarbital. *Clin Neuropharmacol* 1988;11:348–59.

33. Covanis A, Gupta AK, Jeavons PM. Sodium valproate: monotherapy and polytherapy. *Epilepsia* 1982;23:693–720.
34. Henriksen O, Johannessen SI. Clinical and pharmacokinetic observations on sodium valproate—a 5-year follow-up study in 100 children with epilepsy. *Acta Neurol Scand* 1982;65:504–23.
35. Fröscher W, Stoll KD, Hoffmann F. Kombinationsbehandlung mit Carbamazepin und Valproinsäure bei Problemfällen einer Epilepsie-Ambulanz. *Drug Res* 1984;34:910–4.
36. Schmutz M. Carbamazepine: drug interactions. In: Frey HH, Janz D, eds. *Antiepileptic Drugs*. Berlin: Springer-Verlag, 1985:496.
37. Schuetz H, Feldmann KF, Faigle JW: Animal model to study the influence of drugs on the metabolism of carbamazepine in vivo. *Eighth European Workshop on Drug Metabolism*, Liege, 1982 (cited by Schmutz 1985 in ref. 36).
38. Bourgeois BFD, Dodson WE, Ferrendelli JA. Primidone, phenobarbital and PEMA: I. Seizure protection, neurotoxicity and therapeutic index of individual compounds in mice. *Neurology* 1983;33:283–90.
39. Bourgeois BFD, Dodson WE, Ferrendelli JA. Primidone, phenobarbital and PEMA: II. Seizure protection, neurotoxicity and therapeutic index of varying combinations in mice. *Neurology* 1983; 33:291–5.
40. Bourgeois BFD, Wad N. Individual and combined antiepileptic and neurotoxic activity of carbamazepine and carbamazepine-10,11-epoxide in mice. *J Pharmacol Exp Ther* 1984;231:411–5.

15

Stereoselective Considerations in the Study of Drug Interactions

William F. Trager

Department of Medicinal Chemistry, University of Washington, Seattle, Washington, U.S.A.

The phenomenon of stereoselective differences in the biologic activity elicited by the enantiomers of chiral drugs has long been recognized. However, only in recent years has the pervasiveness and importance of the effect begun to be appreciated and studied as a matter of routine. The fact that the enantiomers of a chiral molecule have identical physical and chemical properties in an achiral environment is undoubtedly the primary cause of the slow development of the field. But the recent development of relatively simple methodologies for separating and quantitating enantiomeric mixtures has changed the picture dramatically.

Prior to considering specific examples of stereoselective effects in drug interactions, it may be worthwhile to consider why stereoselective differences occur at all. As stated above, the enantiomers of a racemic mixture are, in general, indistinguishable from each other unless they interact with a chiral medium. The building blocks of the human body, such as amino acids, carbohydrates, and phospholipids, are almost exclusively chiral molecules of a singlehandedness. This means, of course, that the proteins, enzymes, nucleic acids, lipids, and other macromolecules that form the human body are also asymmetric. In addition, at a higher organizational level, new asymmetries result from the bending and folding of these elements to produce α and β helicles, β-turns, and unique three-dimensional structures. Thus, the human body and indeed all living organisms are highly asymmetric systems. If we symbolize the chirality of the human body as being (R), then in its interaction with the two enantiomers of a chiral drug diastereomeric complexes will be generated.

$$\text{(R) body} + \text{(R,S) racemic drug} \quad \begin{array}{l} \nearrow \quad \text{(R) body·(R) drug} \\ \\ \searrow \quad \text{(R) body·(S) drug} \end{array}$$

Since diastereoisomers are inherently different physical and chemical entities, the basic criterion for stereoselective differentiation is met.

IN VIVO STEREOSELECTIVE DIFFERENCES

In vivo stereoselective differences are possible at a number of different levels, several of which are enumerated below:

Stereoselective Absorption

Even though membranes are asymmetric, they are generally porous enough to allow the ready passage of both enantiomers of small chiral molecules by passive diffusion. There may be, and probably are, stereoselective differences in initial rates of absorption, but these are soon compensated for by an enhanced rate of absorption of the more slowly absorbed enantiomer as its relative concentration increases with time. Thus, insofar as the author is aware, there is no documentation in the literature of stereoselective differences in absorption in which passive diffusion is the operative mechanism. By contrast, stereoselective absorption in active processes have been documented, e.g., L-Dopa, and it is likely that the phenomenon is generally important for such compounds.

Stereoselective Distribution

Differences in the chemical composition of the cellular components of various tissues and organs can lead to differences in the binding affinity of the two enantiomers of a chiral drug to such structures. Hence, their relative distribution throughout the body may vary. While not a great deal of work has been done in this area, there are some significant examples in the literature. For example, it has been shown that (S)-propranolol selectively accumulates in the rat heart (1) and that (S)-α-methydopa selectively accumulates in rat brain (2).

Stereoselective Plasma Protein Binding

In principle the phenomenon governing stereoselective plasma protein binding is no different than that governing stereoselective distribution. It is just that the system is a little more well defined in that what is being considered is stereoselective differences in binding to albumin or α-1-glycoprotein. What is biologically significant about plasma protein binding is that it effectively moderates the concentration of free drug reaching the end receptor. This is particularly true for highly protein-bound drugs where small changes in the free fraction can reflect large changes in relative plasma concentration. For example, if a drug is bound to the extent of 99% in one individual versus 99.5% in another, a 100% difference in potentially free drug concentration for redistribution to other sites exists between the two.

End Receptor

Stereoselective differences between enantiomers in eliciting a given pharmacologic response are exceedingly well documented and range from a measurable difference to an all-or-none response (i.e., single enantiomer possesses all of the biological activity). In general, the more potent a given drug, the greater the difference one will find in the relative activities of their enantiomers. Since such effects are common and well understood, they will not be explored further in this chapter.

Stereoselective Biotransformation

Since the biotransformation of any drug involves enzymatic reactions, it is not surprising that such reactions tend to be stereoselective. Indeed, this is found to be the case and numerous stereoselective oxidations by the cytochrome P-450s; stereoselective conjugations by the glucuronyl transferases and other drug metabolizing systems have been documented (3). What is particularly important about these processes is that they tend to govern drug elimination and are therefore as important to overall drug action as the inherent activity of the parent drug itself.

Thus, the pharmacokinetic analysis of a racemic drug, particularly one in which the two enantiomers have differing degrees of biological activity, becomes meaningless or even misleading unless one is able to independently monitor the kinetics of the two individual enantiomers (4). If drug interactions are to be studied, the situation becomes even more complex. If an interaction arises through interference of the metabolism of a chiral drug by a secondary medication, the secondary drug may not affect the metabolism of the two enantiomers of the primary drug identically. Indeed, just the opposite situation would be the general expectation.

DISCUSSION

Two examples, warfarin–sulfinpyrazone and mephenytoin–mephobarbital, will be considered that highlight different aspects of the importance of stereochemical considerations in assessing drug interactions.

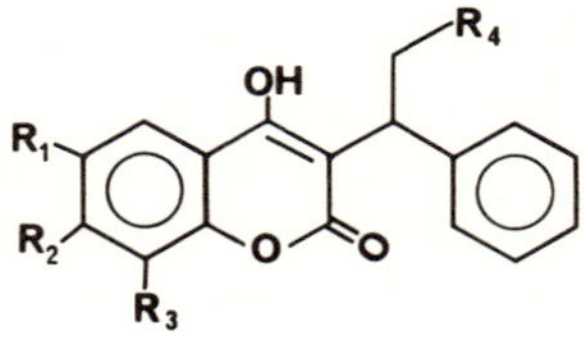

	R₁	R₂	R₃	R₄
WARFARIN	H	H	H	COCH₃
6 OH	OH	H	H	COCH₃
7 OH	H	OH	H	COCH₃
8 OH	H	H	OH	COCH₃
A1(RS,SR)	H	H	H	CHOHCH₃
A2(RR,SS)	H	H	H	CHOHCH₃

FIG. 15-1. Structure of warfarin and its metabolites. Symbols A1 and A2 refer to the two diastereomeric warfarin alcohol metabolites.

Warfarin–Sulfinpyrazone

The first example is the interaction between the oral anticoagulant warfarin (Fig. 15-1) and the uricosuric agent sulfinpyrazone. Many reports have appeared in the chemical literature that document the fact that a therapeutic regimen of sulfinpyrazone invariably augments the anticoagulant effect of warfarin but that no correlation seems to exist between warfarin plasma concentration and anticoagulant response. That is, in some cases an increased biologic effect is apparent, even though there is no significant change in the plasma clearance of warfarin, whereas in others, clearance increases rather than decreases relative to what it was in the absence of sulfinpyrazone. Since the plasma concentration of a drug is generally believed to be directly related to biologic effect, an increased effect coupled to a decreased plasma concentration is perplexing and seemingly inexplicable. One possible answer to the dilemma might lie in stereoselective effects associated with the metabolism of warfarin. Although the drug is clinically available only as the racemate, it is known that the (S) enantiomer is three to five times as potent as the (R) enantiomer. If sulfinpyrazone exerted differential effects on the elimination of the two enantiomers, then it is possible that a given plasma concentration, although less than that measured at a corresponding time and dose in the absence of sulfinpyrazone, could be enriched in the more potent enantiomer. If true, the effect would never have been detected because only total warfarin [(R) plus (S)] was measured in the clinical studies.

To determine whether or not stereoselective effects are involved in an interaction that is based in metabolic effects, and to be certain of the mechanism of the effect, two conditions must be met. First, the independent pharmacokinetic behavior of the two enantiomers in the presence of each other must be determinable and, second, total drug must be accounted for. We undertook such a study in six healthy volunteers (5). To meet the first condition, pseudoracemic warfarin was prepared in which one of the enantiomers was selectively labeled with ^{13}C. This allowed the two enantiomers of the drug to be readily quantified in the presence of each other by mass spectrometry. Moreover, since the label is not lost by metabolic transformation, stereoselective effects in the various metabolic pathways were also provided by the experiment. To attain mass balance, one of the individuals also received a tracer dose of 10 μCi ^{14}C warfarin incorporated into the pseudoracemic dose. Stool was collected for 15 days along with urine and plasma. Daily prothrombin times were determined on all subjects during the course of study to provide a measure of biologic response. In all individuals, sulfinpyrazone dramatically increased the hypothrombinemic response of a standard (1.5 mg/kg) single dose of pseudoracemic warfarin relative to the same dose of pseudoracemic warfarin administered alone in the same individual in a different time period. Of particular relevance to the present discussion are the results obtained from subjects J.A. and D.C. In the presence of sulfinpyrazone, subject J.A. showed a 58% increase in elimination half-life of total warfarin, a result consistent with the observed enhanced anticoagulant effect. By contrast, subject D.C. showed a 25% decrease in the elimination half-life of total warfarin, a result consistent with earlier reports in the literature but one that is inconsistent with the enhanced anticoagulant response. If, however, the half-lives for the individual enantiomers are considered, the paradox is resolved. In subject J.A., the half-life of (S)-warfarin increased from 18.2 to 49.5 h, whereas that for the (R) enantiomer decreased from 46.2 to 38.5 h with sulfinpyrazone dosing. In the case of subject D.C., the half-life of (S)-warfarin also increased (49.5 to 57.7 h), whereas that of (R)-warfarin so greatly decreased in the presence of sulfinpyrazone (86.8 to 25.4 h) that the total warfarin measured was less than the control. These data clearly illustrate that if the enantiomers of a racemic drug have different potencies, it is impossible to correlate the plasma concentration of the racemate to biologic effect. Such a correlation requires knowledge of the pharmacokinetic behavior of the individual enantiomers.

In all six individuals, sulfinpyrazone decreased the clearance of (S)-warfarin and increased the clearance of (R)-warfarin. On first analysis, the overall interaction would seem to be due to inhibition of the metabolism of the biologically more potent (S)-enantiomer coupled to an enhanced elimination of the less active (R)-enantiomer. However, to be certain of the mechanism of the interaction, the fate of total administered dose must be known. In Table 15-1, the metabolic profile obtained from K.M. is presented, since he was the individual who received the tracer radioactive dose and since his profile is representative of the group. Inspection of

Table 15-1. Percentage of the Warfarin Dose Excreted in Urine and Feces as Metabolites or as Unchanged Warfarin Before and with Sulfinpyrazone Dosing During ^{14}C Study in Subject K. M.

| | Control | | | | With sulfinpyrazone | | | |
| | R | | S | | R | | S | |
	Urine	Feces	Urine	Feces	Urine	Feces	Urine	Feces
Warfarin	1.00	7.00	0.90	4.50	1.40	12.50	1.30	12.90
6-Hydroxylation	9.40	1.00	8.10	0.62	7.00	1.00	5.50	1.00
7-Hydroxylation	4.60	0.72	32.40	1.30	2.50	0.88	19.10	2.10
8-Hydroxylation	7.00	0.31	0.14	ND	7.10	0.36	ND	ND
Alcohol 1	8.10	0.82	ND	ND	2.30	0.33	ND	ND
Alcohol 2	0.01	ND	1.30	ND	ND	ND	2.30	ND
Cumulative % excreted	39.91		49.24		35.40		44.21	
		89.15				79.61		
Expected % based on ^{14}C mass balance		96.40				92.60		

ND, not detected.
Reproduced from Toon et al. (5) with permission.

Table 15-1 reveals that the metabolism of warfarin is highly stereoselective but that the stereoselectivity varies widely depending on which metabolite is being considered. For example, 7-hydroxylation favors (S)-warfarin by better than a 6:1 ratio over (R)-warfarin. Conversely, 8-hydroxylation favors (R)-warfarin by a 50:1 ratio. In the presence of sulfinpyrazone, the 6- and 7-hydroxylation of both warfarin enantiomers appear to be inhibited, but the major effect is seen with the 7-hydroxylation of (S)-warfarin. Since 7-hydroxylation is the primary mode of inactivation of (S)-warfarin (approximately 70% of the dose), inhibition of this pathway of metabolism provides an explanation for the biologic effect of the interaction. The data, however, do not explain the increased clearance of (R)-warfarin in the presence of sulfinpyrazone. Since the clearance of a highly plasma protein-bound drug like warfarin is directly related to its free plasma concentration, the effect of sulfinpyrazone on protein-bound warfarin had to be evaluated. The study was carried out (6), and it was found that sulfinpyrazone selectively displaced (R)-warfarin from its plasma protein-binding sites. Sulfinpyrazone increased the unbound fraction of (R)-warfarin by approximately 50% while increasing the unbound fraction of (S)-warfarin by approximately 10%. With these data, the unbound clearances of (R)- and (S)-warfarin (CL_{un}) as well as the unbound formation clearance (CL_{unf}) of the metabolites were calculated and are listed in

Table 15-2. CL_{un} (L/h) of the Warfarin Enantiomers and CL_{unf} of Their Respective Metabolites During the ^{14}C Study in Subject K. M.[a]

	R		S	
	Control	With sulfinpyrazone	Control	With sulfinpyrazone
Warfarin	17.34	17.04	36.87	20.89
6-Hydroxylation	3.61	2.73	6.43	2.72
7-Hydroxylation	1.84	1.16	24.85	8.86
8-Hydroxylation	2.53	2.57	0.11	0.005
Alcohol 1	3.09	0.89	ND	ND
Alcohol 2	0.001	ND	0.96	0.96

[a]The CL values for (R)- and (S)-warfarin in this subject were 147.4 and 195.4 ml/h in the control studies and 214.7 and 117.0 ml/h in the sulfinpyrazone studies.
ND, not detected.
Reproduced from Toon et al. (5) with permission.

Table 15-2. Inspection of these data clearly establishes that sulfinpyrazone inhibits the oxidative pathways (primarily 7-hydroxylation) associated with the metabolism of (S)-warfarin. Inhibition of the metabolic pathways (except 8-hydroxylation) of (R)-warfarin is also seen, but to a lesser extent. However, this inhibition is more than counterbalanced by the increased unbound fraction of (R)-warfarin resulting from selective plasma protein-binding displacement, such that an increase in clearance (but not unbound clearance) is observed. Thus, accounting for the pharmacokinetic behavior of the individual warfarin enantiomers leads to a natural explanation for the overall interaction and serves to highlight the importance of stereoselective considerations when studying racemic drugs.

Mephenytoin–Mephobarbital

The second example that will be considered is the mephenytoin-mephobarbital interaction. In 1981 Kupfer et al. (7) reported that the metabolism of the anticonvulsant mephenytoin (Fig. 15-2) in man is highly stereoselective. The (S)-enantiomer is almost stereospecifically hydroxylated in the 4 position of the aromatic ring, e.g., better than 90% of the initial dose of (S)-mephenytoin administered as the racemate was recovered in the urine after 24 h as the glucuronide. In contrast, (R)-mephenytoin is slowly eliminated (clearance approximately 30–40 ml/min) and slowly metabolized primarily by N-demethylation to generate phenylethylhydantoin (PEH). Since the rate of PEH elimination is even slower (2–4 ml/h) than its rate of production, it accumulates with chronic dosing. This creates the unusual situation in which, after 11 days of chronic mephenytoin dosing,

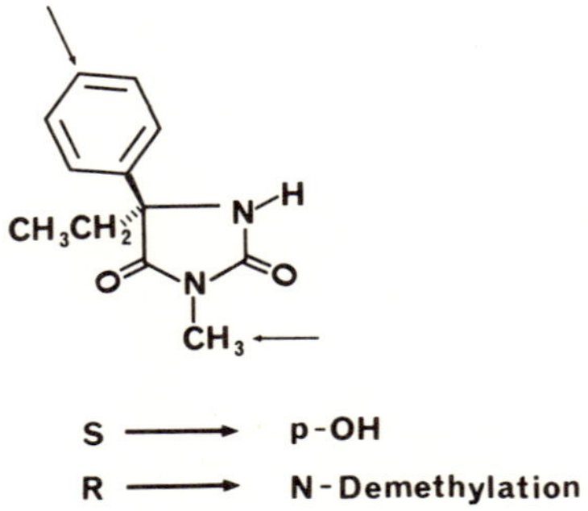

FIG. 15-2. Structure of mephenytoin and its metabolites.

the plasma concentration of active hydantoin is essentially all (10:1 PEH/(R)-mephenytoin) PEH derived from (R)-mephenytoin. Thus the primary therapeutic agent is a metabolite of essentially a single enantiomer of a drug administered as a racemate.

Subsequently (8) it was found that the 4-hydroxylation of (S)-mephenytoin was subject to genetic polymorphism. Moreover, this polymorphism is independent, i.e., it involves an enzyme of cytochrome P-450 different from those involved in the polymorphic oxidation of debrisoquine/sparteine or nifedipine. Since the 4-hydroxylation pathway effectively controls half a racemic dose of mephenytoin, and since both enantiomers of mephenytoin have anticonvulsant activity, it suggests that secondary medication that can specifically inhibit this process should give rise to a significant interaction. In this regard, Küpfer and Branch (9) found that metabolism of the anticonvulsant, mephobarbital, co-segregates with the 4-hydroxylation of mephenytoin, whereas Jacqz et al. (10) report that mephobarbital is an effective inhibitor of mephenytoin metabolism in vivo. Recently, this same research group reported (11) that the interaction can be modeled in vitro, since mephobarbital is an effective inhibitor (K_i 39 μM) of the 4-hydroxylation of (S)-mephenytoin by human liver microsomes. Thus, one can expect to observe a significant drug interaction if these two drugs, mephenytoin and mephobarbital, are co-administered to extensive metabolizers of mephenytoin in which 4-hydroxylation is a major route of deactivation and elimination, but little effect if they are administered to poor metabolizers in which 4-hydroxylation is not important in modifying anticonvulsant response.

Historically, stereochemical considerations have not been important to the clinical efficacy of anticonvulsants primarily because the major anticonvulsants in therapeutic use, e.g., phenobarbital, diphenylhydantoin, valproic acid, and others, are achiral molecules. However, as new anticonvulsants are developed and tested, it is likely that chirality will occur in at least some of these agents. If it is, then clearly stereochemical considerations will be of primary importance in evaluating their potential efficacy and may provide new insight into their mode of activity.

REFERENCES

1. Kawashima K, Levy A, Spector S. Stereospecific radioimmunoassay for propranolol isomers. *J Pharmacol Exp Ther* 1976;196:517–23.
2. Ames MA, Melmon KL, Castagnoli N Jr. Stereochemical course in vivo of alpha methyldopa decarboxylation in rat brains. *Biochem Pharmacol* 1977;26:1757–62.
3. Trager WF, James JP. Stereochemical considerations in drug metabolism. In: Bridges JW, Chasseaud LF, Gibson GG, eds. *Progress in Drug Metabolism,* vol. 10. London: Taylor and Frances Ltd., 1987.
4. Ariens EJ. Stereochemistry, a basis for sophisticated nonsense in pharmacokinetics and clinical pharmacology. *Eur J Clin Pharmacol* 1984;26:663–8.
5. Toon S, Low LK, Gibaldi M, Trager WF, O'Reilly RA, Motley CH. The warfarin-sulfinpyrazone interaction: stereochemical considerations. *Clin Pharmacol Ther* 1986;39:15–24.
6. Toon S, Trager WF. Pharmacokinetic implications of stereoselective changes in plasma-protein binding: warfarin/sulfinpyrazone. *J Pharm Sci* 1984;73:1671–3.
7. Küpfer A, Roberts RK, Schenker S, Branch RA. Stereoselective metabolism of mephenytoin in man. *J Pharmacol Exp Ther* 1981;218:193–9.
8. Küpfer A, Preisig R. Pharmacogenetics of mephenytoin: A new drug hydroxylation polymorphism in man. *Eur J Clin Pharmacol* 1984;26:753–9.
9. Küpfer A, Branch RA. Stereoselective mephobarbital hydroxylation cosegregates with mephenytoin hydroxylation. *Clin Pharmacol Ther* 1985;38:414–8.
10. Jacqz E, Hall SD, Branch RA, Wilkinson GR. Polymorphic metabolism of mephenytoin in man: pharmacokinetic interaction with a co-regulated substrate, mephobarbital. *Clin Pharmacol Ther* 1986;39:646–53.
11. Hall SD, Guengerich FP, Branch RA, Wilkinson GR. Characterization and inhibition of mephenytoin 4-hydroxylase activity in human liver microsomes. *J Pharmacol Exp Ther* 1987;240:216–22.

Mechanistic Aspects of Interactions: Summary

René H. Levy

Department of Pharmaceutics, University of Washington, Seattle, Washington, U.S.A.

The previous sections of this monograph have underlined the clinical relevance of interactions among major antiepileptic drugs. The problems posed by drug interactions during the various phases of drug development indicate that the phenomenon of drug interactions will accompany the new generation of antiepileptic drugs. Will it be possible, in the future, to achieve a certain degree of prediction? The only hope of realizing such an objective is to replace the descriptive approach to the study of drug interactions with a more mechanistic one. This section includes four distinct directions that can be used to probe the various mechanisms of drug interactions.

The area of pharmacodynamic interactions has received little attention, even though it can provide information essential to access the relative merits of monotherapy versus polytherapy. The study of pharmacodynamic interactions in epileptic patients is fraught with limitations. The judicious use of animal models can allow a distinction between additive and synergistic effects. Furthermore, one must consider separately additivity of anticonvulsant effects and additivity of neurotoxic effects. Animal models provide quantitative measures of potentiation (i.e., supra-additive effects) and of the therapeutic index (efficacy/toxicity ratio). Anticonvulsants must be studied individually and in pairs in a systematic fashion. Such studies using a mouse model are described in the chapter by Bourgeois and Dodson.

The three preceding chapters covered different facets of pharmacokinetic drug interactions. Whereas most treatments of this topic cover the steady-state situation, Lai and James examined the time course of various types of pharmacokinetic interactions: protein-binding displacement, enzyme induction and inhibition, and absorption interactions. Time courses of various interactions cannot be rationalized without a clear understanding of the molecular events and adequate pharmacokinetic models.

Most antiepileptic drugs are achiral molecules, i.e., they do not contain a center of asymmetry. As a result the notion of stereochemical considerations in the study of interactions among antiepileptic drugs has not been established. However, recent studies with mephenytoin have illustrated the profound differences that exist in the disposition of two enantiomers of a drug marketed as a racemate. The two enantiomers of mephenytoin have distinct metabolic fates and, as a result, the concentration of active hydantoin in plasma at steady state is essentially made up of the metabolite of one enantiomer (R-mephenytoin). Furthermore, since the 4-hydroxylation of S-mephenytoin is subject to genetic polymorphism that cosegregates with mephobarbital, the mephenytoin–mephobarbital interaction is visible in extensive metabolizers but not in poor metabolizers of mephenytoin. These studies, and particularly those with warfarin, demonstrate that drug interactions involving racemates cannot be understood without considering each enantiomer as a separate pharmacokinetic and pharmacodynamic entity.

The first chapter of this section illustrated how human liver microsomes and purified enzyme from human liver were used to explain the mechanism of the interaction between valproic acid and carbamazepine-10,11-epoxide, an active metabolite of carbamazepine. Purified epoxide hydrolase was used to prove that it catalyzes the hydrolysis of carbamazepine epoxide and that investigation of the mechanism of interaction should focus on that enzyme system. Most importantly, it was found that the degree of inhibition of epoxide hydrolase associated with therapeutic concentrations of valproate (0.3–0.7 mM) was the same in vivo, in human liver microsomes, and in purified enzyme preparations. These findings suggest that it will be possible to develop in vitro strategies to screen for enzyme inhibition drug interactions.

IV. Predictability and Scale-up: From the Bench to Man

Drug–Drug Interactions Arising from Changes in the Activities of Hepatic Xenobiotic Metabolizing Enzymes

Michael R. Franklin

Department of Pharmacology and Toxicology, University of Utah, Salt Lake City, Utah, U.S.A.

The long periods of time over which anticonvulsant drugs are given in humans make them of prime concern for possible drug interactions occurring when other pharmacologically unrelated drugs are administered. Whereas dosing adjustments can be made for any self-inhibition or self-induction of their metabolism, the effects of a second drug given only occasionally can produce unexpected changes in the effectiveness of the anticonvulsant.

In an experimental situation, a dose of 20 mg/kg of phenytoin protected 50% of the rats against maximal electroshock-induced seizures 2 h later (Fig. 17-1). A second drug, clotrimazole, which had no anticonvulsant activity, was able to increase the protection to 60% at 2 h, and, whereas with phenytoin alone only 10% were protected 6 h later, 90% were protected when clotrimazole had been co-administered. Most noticeable, however, was the extension of protection above the 50% value from the single phenytoin dose for up to 30 h.

The potentiation of phenytoin anticonvulsant activity is due to the inhibition of its oxidative metabolism to a pharmacologically inactive hydroxylated product (1). Inhibition of cytochrome P-450 catalyzed oxidations can occur by a number of mechanisms. Since cytochrome P-450 has broad substrate selectivity, one of the most common mechanisms is that of mutual competition for the active site, which results in slowed metabolism of each substrate, although the cytochrome may still be working at its full capacity. A widely used drug that is often found to inhibit in a

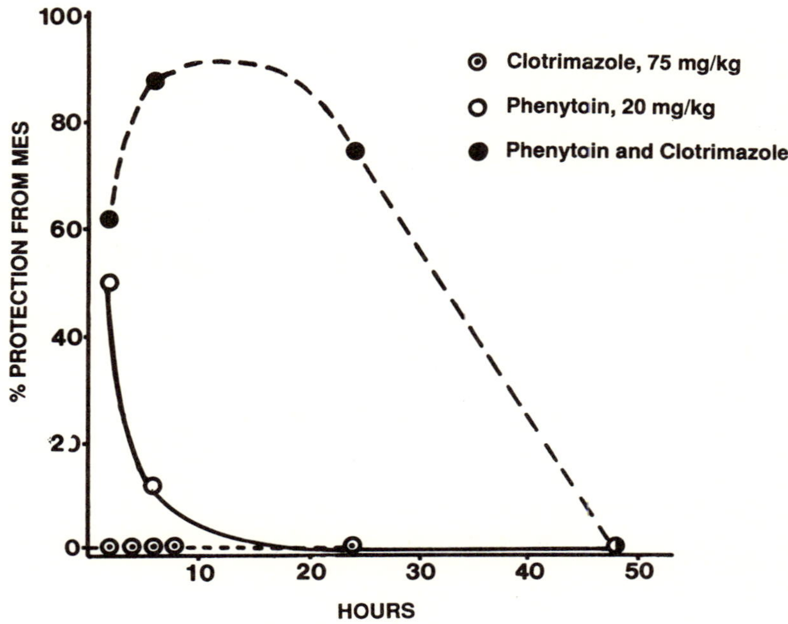

FIG. 17-1. Protection against maximal electroshock seizures (MES) by phenytoin and clotrimazole. At the times indicated, groups of eight rats were tested for protection against maximal electroshock-induced seizures as described by Swinyard and Woodhead (14). Clotrimazole and phenytoin were given as a suspension in 0.5% methylcellulose.

competitive manner and result in many drug interactions is cimetidine (2). Most of the common anticonvulsant drugs inhibit the metabolism of each other by this mechanism (Table 17-1) (3). Cytochrome P-450 possesses another site for inhibition in addition to the drug binding site: the oxygen binding site or heme iron. Inhibition at this site shows no competition with the drug and appears to be noncompetitive. A good example of a group of drugs that inhibits at this site is the antifungal N-substituted imidazole agents (4). A third mechanism of inhibition is in reality a combination of the previous two and requires initial metabolism to produce an intermediate product, which then binds at the heme site. The inhibition first appears competitive, but becomes noncompetitive when the metabolic-intermediate (MI) complexes with the heme (5). Some compounds with anticonvulsant properties can inhibit by this mechanism, but the range of compounds extends into numerous chemical and pharmacological classes (6).

In addition to having inhibitory properties, many of the agents are also able to induce hepatic cytochrome P-450, although the extent to which

Table 17-1. Anticonvulsant Agents and Their Effects on Hepatic Cytochrome P-450

Agent	Anticonvulsant activity (ED_{50}) in Mice[a]		In vitro inhibition (mechanism)	In vivo induction	
	MES	PTZ		% of control	Dosing (mg/kg × days)
Proadifen (SKF 525-A)	135[b]	—	Comp/MI	400	80 × 4
Phenobarbital	22	13	Comp	250	80 × 4
Ethosuximide	>1,000	130	Comp	230	260 × 7
Nafimidone[c]	25	—	Mixed	133	50 × 1
Nafimidone alcohol[c]	—	—	Mixed	205	100 × 4
Piperonyl butoxide	457	443	Comp/MI	150	160 × 3
Phenytoin	10	∞	Comp	112	30 × 7
Felbamate[d]	50	148	—	100	238 × 7

MES = maximal electroshock seizure; PTZ = pentylenetetrazol seizure; comp = competitive; mixed = competitive and noncompetitive; MI = metabolic-intermediate complex.

[a] Data reproduced from ref. 7, unless otherwise indicated by superscript.
[b] Data reproduced from ref. 8.
[c] Data reproduced from ref. 9.
[d] Data reproduced from ref. 10.

the induction occurs is extremely variable between agents (Table 17-1). Induction by agents, which can inhibit through the formation of cytochrome P-450 MI complexes (Table 17-2), is dependent on whether such complexes are formed in vivo (i.e., can be detected in microsomes isolated from animals treated with the compounds). Thus, for example, the amphetamine and oxidized alkylamine classes of agents, although they show extensive complex formation under in vitro incubations using microsomes isolated from either uninduced rats or rats induced with phenobarbital, do not appear to form such complexes in vivo and do not induce. Once formed, the MI complexes are long-lived and resist displacement and degradation, providing effective long-term inhibition of cytochrome P-450. This provides the rationale for the use of methylenedioxybenzene derivatives as insecticide synergists.

Although they do not form MI complexes, the N-substituted imidazoles also provide potent inhibition of a variety of cytochrome P-450 catalyzed oxidations in microsomes from untreated animals and animals induced with dexamethasone or phenobarbital (Table 17-3). The concentrations required for 50% inhibition ranged from around 0.5 (stoichiometric bind-

Table 17-2. Cytochrome P-450 Metabolic-Intermediate (MI) Complex Formation in Vitro and In Vivo

Class of MI complex	Substrate investigated in vitro/in vivo	Maximum extent (%) of cytochrome complexation in rat liver		Inducing agent?
		In vitro con:PB[a]	In vivo con:PB	
Methylenedioxybenzene	Piperonylbutoxide/iso-safrole	$21 < 32$	$18 > 7$	Yes
Amphetamine	Norbenzphetamine	$26 < 59$	0	No
Oxidized alkylamine	N-hydroxyamphetamine	$84 = 83$	0	No
SKF 525-A	SKF 8742-A/SKF 525-A	$40 = 37$	$29 = 25$	Yes
Arylamine	p-chloroaniline	$16 < 39$	—	—
Hydrazine	N-aminopiperidine	$25 < 53$	—	—
Macrolide	Troleandomycin	$0 < 12$	$9 < 22$	Yes

[a]Con = untreated; PB = phenobarbital induced.

Table 17-3. In Vitro Inhibition and In Vivo Induction of Rat Hepatic Cytochrome P-450 by Substituted Imidazoles

	In vitro inhibition (IC-50/cytochrome P-450) of the oxidation of				In vivo induction of cytochrome P-450	
Agent	P-nitroanisole[a]	Ethylmorphine[b]	Trimetrexate[c]	Erythromycin[d]	% control	Dosing (mg/kg × days)
Clotrimazole	0.46, 0.33	0.50, 0.40	0.41	0.32	410	75×3
N-benzylimidazole	— —	— —	—	—	1-	75×3
Miconazole	1.32, 0.85	2.00, 150	0.82	1.00	.50	150×3
Tioconazole	0.75, 0.45	1.17, 0.86	—	0.63	131	150×3
Ketoconazole	0.75, 0.36	2.00, 1.82	0.53	0.80	128	150×3
Cimetidine	— —	— —	189.00	—	99	350×3

[a] In uninduced (cytochrome P-450 = 1.02 nmoles/mg) and dexamethasone-induced (cyt P-450 = 2.15 nmoles/mg) microsomes.
[b] In phenobarbital-induced (cyt P-450 = 1.48 nmoles/mg) and dexamethasone-induced (cyt P-450 = 1.87 nmoles/mg) microsomes.
[c] In phenobarbital-induced (cyt P-450 = 1.72 nmoles/mg) microsomes. Data from Heusner et al. (11).
[d] In dexamethasone-induced (cyt P-450 = 2.01 nmoles/mg) microsomes.

Table 17-4. Animal Pretreatment and Phenytoin[a] Protection Against Maximal Electroshock Seizures

Pretreatment	% Protected[b] 3 h after phenytoin (22 mg/kg)
None	75
Clotrimazole (75 mg/kg × 3 days)	0
None	50
Nafimidone (75 mg/kg × 3 days)	0
N-benzylimidazole (75 mg/kg × 3 days)	14

[a] Administered 72 h after final pretreatment dose.
[b] n = 8, except nafimidone (n = 5) and N-benzylimidazole (n = 7).

ing) to 2.0 (four inhibitor molecules for every cytochrome P-450 molecule). Cimetidine, a 4,5-disubstituted imidazole, with an IC-50/cytochrome P-450 value of 189, is shown for comparison purposes. It was one hundredfold less effective as an inhibitor than the N-substituted derivatives.

The much less inhibitory cimetidine also differentiated itself from the other agents by not exhibiting inductive properties. However, the similar inhibitory potencies of all the N-substituted imidazoles did not result in similar inductive properties when given in high daily doses for 3 days. Two agents, clotrimazole and N-benzylimidazole, were remarkable for their high-magnitude (over 300%) induction of cytochrome P-450. This degree of induction rendered a 22 mg/kg dose of phenytoin almost ineffective in protecting against maximal electroshock seizures (Table 17-4). Based on the outcome of the in vivo observation, it appears that nafimidone is a similarly effective cytochrome P-450 inducer. How much induction is required to render the phenytoin ineffective within 3 h requires experimental determination, especially since it is known that selective induction of forms or isozymes of cytochrome P-450 with differing substrate selectivities occurs with clotrimazole and N-benzylimidazole. Clotrimazole induces activities associated with isozymes b and p to the greatest extent, whereas N-benzylimidazole predominantly induces those associated with isozyme (Table 17-5). However, both agents induce b, p, and c activities to some degree. Whether all three forms metabolize phenytoin or whether only a small amount of induction of a particular isozyme is needed to make the phenytoin ineffective by 3 h has not yet been elucidated.

Induction is not restricted to cytochrome P-450 but extends to many drug-metabolizing enzymes. Accompanying the changes in microsomal cytochrome P-450, microsomal UDP-glucuronosyltransferase enzymes are often induced. However, induction of the two enzymes is not directly linked. For some N-substituted imidazoles (e.g., tioconazole), large changes in

Table 17-5. Differential Cytochrome P-450 and UDP-glucuronosyltransferase Isozyme Induction[a]

Inducing agent	% of control activity of cytochrome P-450 (isozyme/substrate)				% of control activity of UDP-glucuronosyltransferase (isozyme/substrate)	
	"b"/pentoxy-resorufin	"p"/erythro-mycin	"j"/dimethyl nitrosamine	"c"/ethoxy-resorufin	"GT$_1$"/1-naphthol	"GT$_2$"/morphine
Phenobarbital	7,500	520	160	450	112	392
Clotrimazole	5,100	1,202	118	441	124	188
N-benzylimidazole	1,600	200	36	5,600	250	272
N-me-naph-imidazole[b]	400	155	48	4,040	308	250
Nafimidone[c]	—	—	—	3,000	110	96
Miconazole	—	216	97	145	139	95
Tioconazole	—	142	89	100	213	331
Ketoconazole	—	179	129	234	109	174
Imidazole	—	109	161	—	100	123

[a] Data reproduced from refs. 12 and 13 and unpublished observations.
[b] N-(2-methylnaphthyl) imidazole.
[c] Data from Rush et al. (9) after 50 mg/kg × 4 days of nafimidone (cytochrome P-450 changes) or nafimidone alcohol (UDP-glucuronosyltransferase changes). GT$_1$ and GT$_2$ were assayed with 4-methylumbelliferone and 4-hydroxybiphenyl, respectively.

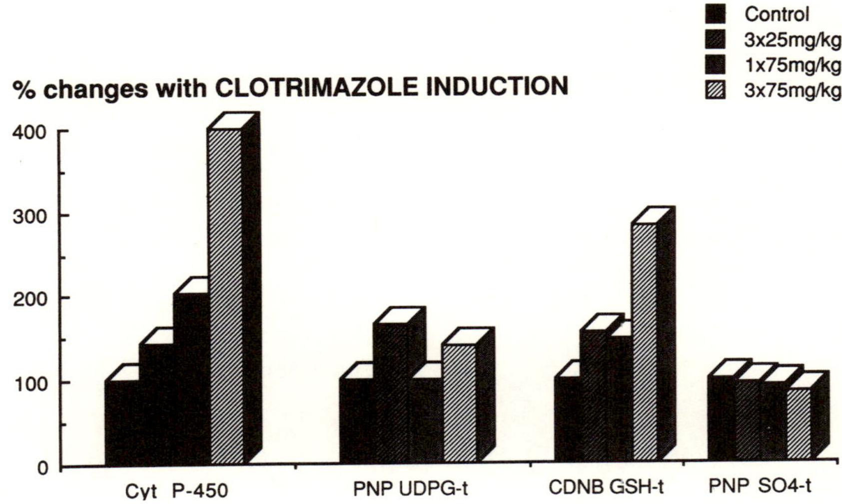

FIG. 17-2. Effect of different dosing protocols on clotrimazole induction of rat hepatic drug metabolizing enzymes. Clotrimazole was administered by intragastric intubation as a 20% PEG 400 suspension. Animals were killed 48 h after the final dose, and hepatic microsomal and cytosolic fractions were prepared. Microsomes were analyzed for cytochrome P-450 content and UDP-glucuronosyltransferase activity toward p-nitrophenol (PNP UDPG-t). The cytosol was analyzed for glutathione transferase activity toward 1-chloro-2, 4-dinitrobenzene (CDNB GSH-t) and sulfotransferase activity toward p-nitrophenol (PNP SO$_4$-t).

glucuronosyltransferase activities can occur without major induction of cytochrome P-450. The tioconazole induction of glucuronosyltransferases is greater than that seen with clotrimazole, although the predominance of the isozymes induced is the same (GT1 < GT2). Both N-benzylimidazole and N-(2-methylnaphthyl)-imidazole induce the two isozymes to a similar extent. These changes in glucuronosyltransferases could be of great importance in the consideration of drug interactions in which the pharmacological effect of one or both drugs is terminated by glucuronidation.

An aspect of induction that has escaped serious consideration is the dosing regimen required to trigger the inductive response and whether the same parameters trigger all the responses that are going to occur. The answer to the last question appears to be "no" (Fig. 17-2). The inductive effect of three dosing regimens of clotrimazole (75 mg/kg as a single dose or as a divided dose, and 225 mg as a divided dose) were investigated. The period of administration (3 days vs. 1 day) appears to be more important than the total dose for induction of UDP-glucuronosyltransferase activity toward p-nitrophenol, whereas the total dose (225 mg/kg vs. 75 mg/kg), whether administered as divided or single doses, appears more

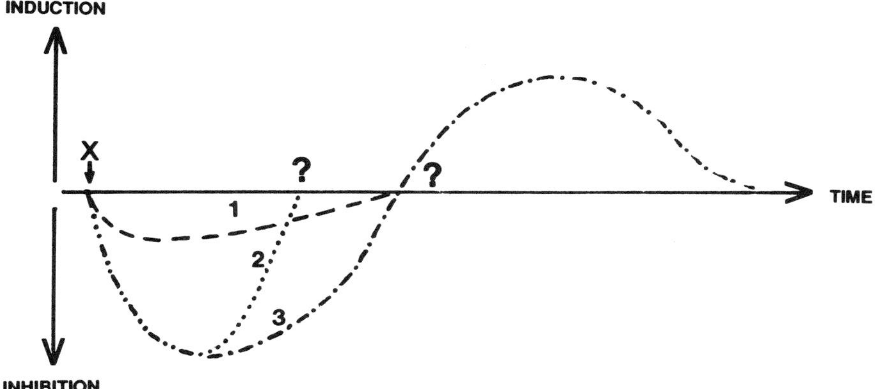

FIG. 17-3. Possible temporal interrelationship between inhibition and induction of drug metabolizing enzymes.

important in determining the degree of induction of the cytosolic conjugating enzyme, glutathione-S-transferase. Both total dose and time period appear to modulate the cytochrome P-450 response. Another cytosolic conjugation enzyme, phenol sulfotransferase, was not induced by any treatment investigated.

The possible links between cytochrome P-450 induction and inhibition are avenues of needed research before we will be able to move far into predicting on a rational basis drug–drug interactions arising from changes in drug-metabolizing enzymes. By empirical observation, it appears that if cytochrome P-450 reactions are inhibited to a sufficient extent and for an extended period of time, the animal responds with induction (Fig. 17-3, curve 3). It is not known whether the extent of inhibition rather than the duration is the important determinant (e.g., Fig. 17-3, curve 2) or whether less extensive inhibition for the same duration (e.g., Fig. 17-3, curve 1) will evoke the same response.

Acknowledgment: This work was supported in part by NINCDS contract: N01-NS-1-2347.

REFERENCES

1. Glazko, AJ. Diphenylhydantoin metabolism: a prospective review. *Drug Metab Dispos* 1972;1:711–4.
2. Gerber MC, Tejwani GA, Gerber N, Bianchine JR. Drug interactions with cimetidine: an update. *Pharmacol Ther* 1985;27:353–70.
3. Netter KJ. Inhibition of oxidative drug metabolism in microsomes. *Pharmacol Ther* 1980;10:515–35.

4. Murray M. Mechanisms of the inhibition of cytochrome P-450–mediated drug oxidation by therapeutic agents. *Drug Metab Rev* 1987;18;55–81.

5. Franklin MR. The inhibition of hepatic oxidative xenobiotic metabolism by piperonyl butoxide. *Biochem Pharmacol* 1972;21:3287–99.

6. Franklin MR. Inhibition of mixed-function oxidations by substrates forming reduced cytochrome P-450 metabolic-intermediate complexes. In: Schenkman JB, Kupfer D, eds. *International Encyclopedia of Pharmacology and Therapeutics: Section 108: Hepatic Cytochrome P-450 Monooxygenase System.* Oxford: Pergamon Press, 1982:763–83.

7. Ater SB, Swinyard EA, Tolman KG, Franklin MR. Anticonvulsant activity and neurotoxicity of piperonyl butoxide in mice. *Epilepsia* 1984;25:551–5.

8. Swinyard EA, Madsen JA, Goodman LS. The effect of β-diethylaminoethyl-diphenylpropylacetate (SKF No. 525A) on the anticonvulsant properties of antiepileptic drugs. *J Pharmacol Exp Ther* 1954;111:54–63.

9. Rush WR, Smith SA, Mulvey JH, Graham DJM, Chaplin MD. Inhibition and induction of hepatic drug metabolism in rats and mice by nafimidone and its major metabolite nafimidone alcohol. *Drug Metab Dispos* 1987;15:571–8.

10. Swinyard EA, Woodhead JH, Franklin MR, Sofia RD, Kupferberg HT. The effect of chronic felbamate administration on anticonvulsant activity and hepatic drug-metabolizing enzymes in mice and rats. *Epilepsia* 1987;28:295–300.

11. Heusner JJ, Franklin MR. Inhibition of metabolism of the "non-classical" antifolate, TMQ (2,4-diamino-5-methyl-6-[(3,4,5-trimethoxyanilino)methyl] quinazoline) by drugs containing an imidazole moiety. *Pharmacology* 1985;30:266–72.

12. Ritter JK, Franklin MR. Induction and inhibition of rat hepatic drug metabolism by N-substituted imidazole drugs. *Drug Metab Dispos* 1987;15:335–43.

13. Papac DI, Franklin MR. N-Benzylimidazole, a high magnitude inducer of rat hepatic cytochrome P-450 exhibiting both polycyclic aromatic hydrocarbon- and phenobarbital-type induction of Phase I and Phase II drug metabolizing enzymes. *Drug Metab Dispos* 1988;16:259–64.

14. Swinyard EA, Woodhead JH. Experimental detection, quantification and evaluation of anticonvulsant. In: Woodbury DM, Penry JK, Pippenger CE, eds. *Antiepileptic Drugs.* New York: Raven Press, 1982:111–26.

18

Use of Response Surface Methodologies in Understanding Drug Interactions

[1,2] R.A. Carchman, [2] C. Gennings, [3] E.A. Swinyard, and [1,2] W.H. Carter, Jr.

[1] *Departments of Pharmacology and Toxicology and* [2] *Biostatistics, Medical College of Virginia/Virginia Commonwealth University, Richmond, Virginia, and* [3] *Department of Pharmacology and Toxicology, University of Utah, Salt Lake City, Utah, U.S.A.*

Using preclinical paradigms, we have analyzed drug combination data on both anticonvulsant and neurotoxic effects of felbamate (FBT)/Dilantin (DLTN) and FBT/carbamazapine (CBZ) respectively. Classically, these types of studies have been designed and analyzed using isobolographic procedures (1–5). The information provided from these studies have been useful in guiding researchers in their efforts to identify antiepileptic treatment strategies.

Isobolographic procedures assume that the drug's relationship to each other follows a dose addition model. Deviations from this render this analysis useless (6). In addition, statistical analysis of drug combination data using isobolographic procedures has been attempted (7–11). Recently, the use of isobolographic analysis for more than two drugs in combination studies has been documented in a statistically valid manner (12). Certain of the issues raised above concerning isobolographic design and analysis of drug combination studies have or are being dealt with (12), but others remain unresolved. In an attempt to enhance our understanding of this problem, we have therefore applied response surface methodologies (RSM). RSM is a well-established (13–18) technique that combines experimental design components and regression analysis to handle a wide variety of data. Using this technique, rigorous statistical standards can be applied, drug optima determined, and the nature of drug interactions inferred. No theoretical limit is placed on the number of drugs to be studied. These techniques also allow for the generation of hypotheses that can be experimentally validated.

MATERIALS AND METHODS

Animal Study and Design

The animals used in the examples provided in this chapter, as well as the procedures and endpoints measured, are described in Chapter 19.

Model Description

Many Phase I and Phase II studies of anticonvulsant compounds involve the analysis of binary (response/no response) outcomes. These data are often recorded as the number of "responses" out of a fixed denominator at specified treatment levels. The classical regression models for the analysis of this type of data are based on the probit (19) model or the logistic (20) model. In what follows, the use of the logistic model is developed in the context of the analysis of a combination of two compounds, e.g., Drug 1 and Drug 2. In general, the constraint on the number of compounds considered in combination is a practical one and not a theoretical one.

The complex three-dimensional relationship between Drug 1 (e.g., FBT) and Drug 2 (e.g., CBZ) and the probability of response (e.g., a neurotoxic response) is approximately modeled by the logistic model:

$$P(response) = \frac{1}{1 + exp^{-f(x)}} \tag{1}$$

where

$$f(x) = \beta_0 + \beta_1 \chi_1 + \beta_2 \chi_2 + \beta_{12} \chi_1 \chi_2$$

X_1 is the dose of Drug 1; X_2 is the dose of Drug 2; β_0 is an unknown parameter associated with untreated responders; β_1 is an unknown parameter associated with the effect on the response of Drug 1; β_2 is an unknown parameter associated with the effect on the response of Drug 2; and β_{12} is an unknown parameter associated with the interaction of Drug 1 and Drug 2.

The model parameters can be estimated from the experimental data by the method of maximum likelihood and are commonly denoted with "^", i.e., $\hat{\beta}_0$, $\hat{\beta}_1$, $\hat{\beta}_2$, $\hat{\beta}_{12}$. With this model, positive coefficients are associated with agents or effects that tend to increase the probability of response, whereas negative coefficients are associated with agents or effects that tend to decrease the probability of response.

Once the model parameters are estimated, predicted responses (PRED) can be evaluated from the fitted model at specified treatment levels as:

$$PRED(X) = 1/(1 + exp(-(\hat{\beta}_0 + \hat{\beta}_1 X_1 + \hat{\beta}_2 X_2 + \hat{\beta}_{12} X_1 X_2))). \tag{2}$$

Comparison of observed versus predicted (expected) responses are useful in ascertaining how well the model describes the data. Table 18-1 is an example of such a comparison. A goodness of fit statistic is evaluated as:

$$X^2 = \sum_{i=1}^{g} \frac{(o_i - p_i)^2}{p_i(1 - p_i)} \tag{3}$$

where o_i is the observed response for the ith treatment group, $1 \leq i \leq g$; p_i is the predicted response for the ith treatment group; and g is the number of treatment groups. The significance of this statistic can be evaluated by comparing X^2 to a chi-square distribution with $g - 4$ degrees of freedom. If X^2 is less than or equal to the tabular, $X^2_{1-\alpha;g-4}$, the data are adequately described by the model.

Analysis of Contours of Constant Response

Once the model parameters are estimated, the fitted regression equation can be used to estimate contours of constant response. For a single-dose–response relationship, for example, an ED_{100p} is an estimate for the dose that yields $100p\%$ response. Based on the fitted model with two independent variables, an estimate for the ED_{100p} for Drug 1 alone is given by:

$$\hat{X}1_{ED100p} = \frac{log[p/(1-p)] - \hat{\beta}_0,}{\hat{\beta}_1} \tag{4}$$

and similarly for Drug 2 alone,

$$\hat{X}2_{ED100p} = \frac{log[p/(1-p)] - \hat{\beta}_0.}{\hat{\beta}_2} \tag{5}$$

The dose of Drug 1 on the estimated contour of constant $100p\%$ response at a specified nonzero dose of Drug 2 (X_2) is given by:

$$\hat{X}_1(ED_{100p}X_2) = \frac{log(p/(1-p)) - \hat{\beta}_0 - \hat{\beta}_2 X_2,}{\hat{\beta}_1 + \hat{\beta}_{12} X_2} \tag{6}$$

Table 18-1. Neurotoxicity Screening: Combination Treatment of Felbamate (FBT) and Carbamazapine (CBZ) with Experimentally Observed (OBS) and Model-Predicted (PRED) Responses[a]

Dose (mg/kg)		Time							
		0.25 h		0.5 h		1 h		2 h	
FBT	CBZ	OBS	PRED[b]	OBS	PRED[c]	OBS	PRED[d]	OBS	PRED[e]
0	50	1	0.44						
0	75	3	2.24						
0	100	6	5.77						
0	150	8	7.93						
158	19	0	0.14	0	0.11	0	0.49	0	1.08
210	25	1	0.34	1	0.40	3	1.73	4	2.94
263	31	2	0.77	1	1.33	4	4.53	5	5.75
315	37.5	1	1.69	4	3.58	8	7.02	8	7.45
122	41	0	0.57	0	0.70	1	2.12	0	1.71
162	54	2	1.81	2	3.22	4	5.99	3	4.76
203	68	6	4.41	7	6.75	7	7.76	7	7.35
243	81	6	6.61	8	7.80	8	7.98	8	7.92
199	12	0	0.11	0	0.08	0	0.41	0	1.27
232	14	0	0.17	0	0.16	1	0.76	1	2.14
265	16	0	0.25	0	0.30	3	1.39	5	3.37
300	18	0	0.38	0	0.57	2	2.46	5	4.86
300	18	2	0.38	3	0.57	5	2.46	8	4.86
65	38	0	0.30	0	0.25	0	0.72	0	0.52
80	47	0	0.64	2	0.77	3	1.84	1	0.98
94	55	1	1.24	1	1.87	4	3.66	2	1.75

and similarly for Drug 2 at a specified dose of Drug 1. Using these results, the complete contour of constant $100p\%$ response can be estimated for Drug 1 and Drug 2. Figure 18-1 includes an example of the estimated 50% contour for FBT and DLTN.

Isobolographic techniques are often used to describe an additive, synergistic, or antagonistic relationship between compounds of interest. The line of additivity is the theoretical line that connects the point estimates of the ED_{50}s for each of two compounds. If the 50% contour falls below the line of additivity, a synergism is concluded. If the estimated contour falls above the line of additivity, an antagonism is concluded. Finally, if the contour is not different from the theoretical line of additivity, an additive relationship seems to exist. Figure 18-2h includes the estimated 50% contour for FBT and CBZ at 2 h post-treatment. The contour falls below the theoretical line that connects the two ED_{50} point estimates for FBT and CBZ, i.e., the line of additivity. Therefore, a synergism seemingly exists

Table 18-1. *(cont'd)*

Dose (mg/kg)		Time							
		0.25 h		0.5 h		1 h		2 h	
FBT	CBZ	OBS	PRED[b]	OBS	PRED[c]	OBS	PRED[d]	OBS	PRED[e]
107	63	2	2.19	3	3.72	7	5.65	5	2.92
250	7	0	0.11	0	0.09	0	0.43	2	1.71
315	9	1	0.21	1	0.26	1	1.15	3	3.60
394	11	0	0.44	1	0.83	3	3.04	5	6.11
473	13.5	0	0.91	1	2.38	4	5.74	7	7.49
43	53	0	0.75	0	0.89	0	1.62	0	0.54
50	62	1	1.44	2	2.14	2	3.15		
57	70	3	2.40	5	3.91	6	4.87	2	1.29
62	76	2	3.31	6	5.30	7	6.00		
200	0							0	0.61
300	0							4	1.75
400	0							5	3.92
600	0							6	7.35

[a]Over a two hour time course.

[b]The p value associated with the goodness of fit statistic given in Eq. 3 is equal to 0.549.

[c]The p value associated with the goodness of fit statistic given in Eq. 3 is equal to 0.293.

[d]The p value associated with the goodness of fit statistic given in Eq. 3 is equal to 0.248.

[e]The p value associated with the goodness of fit statistic given in Eq. 3 is equal to 0.171.

between FBT and CBZ. However, the procedure discussed thus far does not take into account the biological variability of the data, hence the estimated contour. A more appropriate test that does consider the variability of the data is the test for the significance of the interaction term, i.e., β_{12}. If β_{12} is positive and significant, it can be shown (12) that a statistically significant synergism exists between Drug 1 and Drug 2; if β_{12} is negative and significant, an antagonism is said to exist; if β_{12} is not significant, then the relationship is said to be additive.

RESULTS

The initial study presented analyzed the use of FBT and DLTN in an anticonvulsant screen (i.e., maximal electroshock). Table 18-2 presents the doses of the drugs used (mg/kg), the number of animals responding (x/8), and the expected response rate based on the predictive model. In gen-

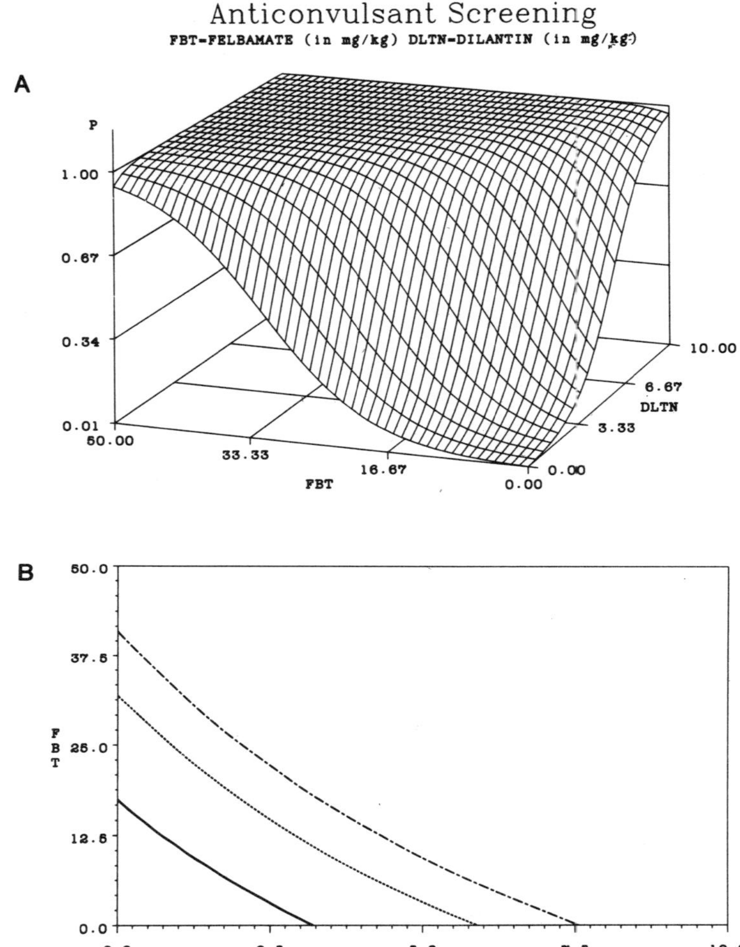

FIG. 18-1. Three-dimensional representation (A) and contour plot (B) of the probability of no convulsion (P axis) as a function of felbamate (FBT) and dilantin (DLTN) doses.

eral, visual inspection comparing the observed versus expected shows good agreement. A statistical evaluation of the goodness of fit of the predictive equation indicates the appropriateness of the model. A plot of the residuals (data not shown) does not indicate any systematic deviations between the observed and predicted data, further supporting the appropriateness of this model. Table 18-3 provides the parameter estimates (i.e., regression coefficients) for each single drug (i.e., FBT and DLNT) and the drug

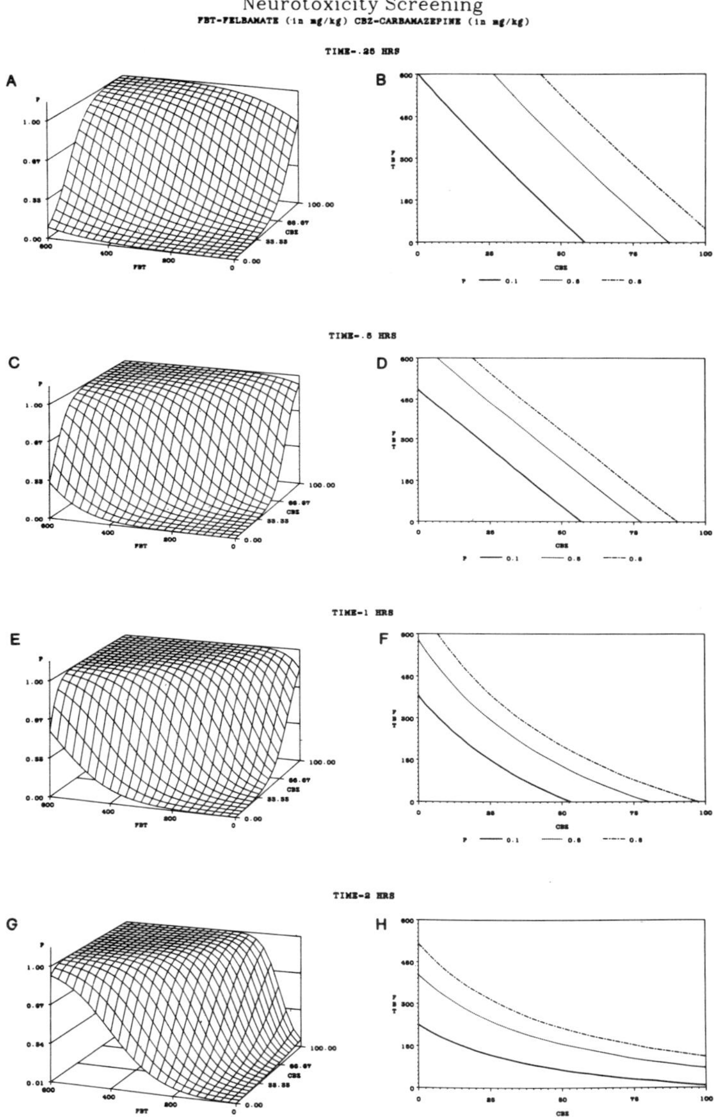

FIG. 18-2. Three-dimensional representations and associated contour plots of the probability of neurotoxicity (P-axis) as a function of felbamate (FBT) and carbamazepine (CBZ) doses at specified time (post-treatment). **A,B:** Time = 0.25 h; **C,D:** Time = 0.5 h; **E,F:** Time = 1h; **G,H:** Time = 2h.

Table 18-2. Anticonvulsant Screening: Combination Treatment of Felbamate (FBT) and Dilantin (DLNT) with Experimentally Observed (OBS) and Model-Predicted (PRED) Responses

Group	FBT (mg/kg)	DLTN (mg/kg)	OBS	PRED[a]
1	20.0	0.0	1	1.13
2	30.0	0.0	4	3.44
3	40.0	0.0	6	6.21
4	50.0	0.0	7	7.52
5	0.0	3.5	1	0.98
6	0.0	5.0	3	2.61
7	0.0	7.5	6	6.33
8	0.0	10.0	7	7.74
9	20.3	0.6	0	2.03
10	23.7	0.7	3	3.18
11	27.0	0.8	6	4.49
12	30.5	0.9	7	5.77
13	11.8	0.8	0	0.76
14	17.7	1.2	2	2.40
15	20.6	1.4	3	3.75
16	23.5	1.5	7	4.97
17	9.8	1.2	1	0.81
18	14.6	1.7	3	2.39
19	19.5	2.3	5	5.32
20	29.2	3.4	6	7.84
21	8.6	2.6	1	2.06
22	10.1	3.1	4	3.43
23	11.5	3.5	6	4.77
24	12.9	3.9	6	5.98
25	3.8	2.2	0	0.71
26	5.7	3.3	1	2.19
27	6.6	3.8	3	3.33
28	7.5	4.3	7	4.64
29	3.0	3.8	2	2.02
30	3.5	4.4	2	3.10
31	4.0	5.0	6	4.36
32	4.5	5.7	6	5.72

[a]The p value associated with the goodness of fit statistic given in Eq. 3 is equal to 0.0482. The statistic is inflated due to group 20, which accounts for 52% of the overall chi-square. For this group, the model predicted 7.84 out of 8 would respond, and six of eight responses were observed. Therefore, the authors feel the data are adequately described by the model.

Table 18-3. Anticonvulsant Screening: Estimated Regression Coefficients for Modeling the Efficacy of Felbamate (FBT) and Dilantin (DLTN) as an Anticonvulsant Combination Treatment[a]

Coefficient	Parameter estimate	SE	p value
Intercept	−4.8441	0.7013	<0.0001
FBT[b]	0.1522	0.0245	<0.0001
DLTN[c]	0.8234	0.1370	<0.0001
FBT*DLTN	0.0150	0.0103	0.1454

[a] See Eq. 1 for definitions.
[b] Estimated ED_{50} for FBT is 31.84 with a 95% confidence interval of (27.29, 36.38).
[c] Estimated ED_{50} for DLTN is 5.88 with a 95% confidence interval of (5.01, 6.76).

combinations. (Under these experimental conditions, each drug alone exhibits a statistically significant ($p < 0.0001$) dose response curve (including a positive sign); as the treatment dose increases, so does the drug's anticonvulsant activity. The size of the parameter estimate(s) can be used to describe the rate at which the above relationship occurs. The interaction of FBT and DLNT (FBT × DLNT) is not statistically significant ($p = 0.1454$), indicating that the interaction parameter (0.0150) cannot be distinguished from zero. An important conclusion based on this analysis is that FBT and DLNT, when used in combination under these experimental conditions, exhibit a strictly additive response (e.g., no synergism or antagonism). Figure 18-1 is a graphical depiction of the response surface of the FBT and DLNT combination study. The individual drug dose responses can be seen by viewing either edge of the response surface along the appropriate drug dose axis. The surface itself describes the effects of all possible drug combinations within the experimental region. Figure 18-2 presents three contours of constant response (i.e., isobols) for 10%, 50%, and 80%. Since β_{12} is not significantly different from zero, it can be concluded that neither of these isobols differs significantly from the theoretical line of additivity, thereby supporting the conclusion that these drugs interact in an additive fashion in this study.

Table 18-1 presents the results from a neurotoxicity study in which FBT and CBZ were administered alone and in combination. The doses of the two drugs (mg/kg), the observation times (0.25, 0.5, 1, and 2 h) and the experimental observations (OBS) (the number of responders out of eight) and the PRED responses are given. As in the case of the anticonvulsant analysis, there is no indication of model inadequacy. The observed and predicted values compare favorably, and a plot of the residuals of these values (data not shown) is unremarkable. Interpretation of these results suggests that the observation time represents an important experimental variable for both single drugs and for the drug combinations. Table 18-4 provides the parameter estimates for single drugs and combinations at the various time points, as well as their statistical significance. At the earliest time point measured (0.25 h), CBZ but not FBT demonstrates a significant dose response. CBZ dose responsiveness is evident at 0.25, 0.5, and 1 h but is absent at the 2-h observation period. FBT, on the other hand, only exhibits a significant dose response when observed following the 0.25-h period, and this response is still significant at the 2-h period. An interaction between CBZ and FBT occurs only at the 2-h observation period. These data strongly suggested that a synergistic interaction takes place with respect to the neurotoxicity of the combination of these drugs and that this interaction is time related. Finally, this interaction occurs at a time (i.e., 2 h) when only FBT is exhibiting a significant neurotoxic response. Figure 18-2 **(A,C,E,G)** are the response surfaces at 0.25, 0.5, 1, and 2 h for FBT and CBZ. The changes in the single drug responses as a function of time are evident by viewing the edge of the response surface at each observation time **(A,C,E,G).** In addition, the overall change in the response surface as a function of time reflects the change in the nature of the interactions of the two drugs. (Figure 18-2 **(B,D,F,H)** are the contours of constant response (i.e., isobols) for this neurotoxicity study at the various observation points. The change in curvilinearity as one goes from Fig. 18-2 **(B,D,F,H)** reflects the change in the interaction and is associated with the same interpretation (i.e., synergism) as the standard isobolographic procedure.

DISCUSSION

We have briefly described here the use of a series of procedures that have the ability to enhance our understanding of drug combination studies. The examples we have used in this chapter were for two useful endpoints in the development of drugs as antiepileptics (i.e., anticonvulsant activity and neurotoxicity). The value of these statistical procedures, which we have explored here for the first time in these kinds of studies, could also include more efficient experimental designs requiring fewer animals and treatment groups [e.g., (21)], the use of more than a two-drug combination (22,23), determination of combination dose and time optima (24,25), experimental validation (18), hypothesis generation [e.g., (18,22,23)], and the evaluation of drugs with dissimilar dose response curves (22,23). There are a number of situations in which the above issues have been addressed in other test/therapeutic situations and have been shown to be of value (14–16,18,22,23,26,27).

As stated earlier, in the past we have attempted to use the RSM analysis as a hypothesis generator (e.g., 15, 16, 22, 23). In the present study, this might take the form of a series of speculations that, if deemed significant, could result in further study. In viewing the synergistic neurotoxic re-

Table 18-4. Neurotoxicity Screening: Estimated Regression Coefficients for Modeling the Efficacy of Felbamate (FBT) and Carbamazapine (CBZ) as a Combination Treatment For Neurotoxicity at Specified Times (in Hours)[a]

Time (h)	Coefficient	Parameter estimate	SE	p value
0.25	Intercept	−6.6313	1.1693	<0.0001
	FBT[b]	0.0073	0.0038	0.0535
	CBZ[c]	0.0758	0.0158	<0.0001
	FBT*CBZ	0.00001	0.0001	0.8283
0.5	Intercept	−8.3719	1.5578	<0.0001
	FBT[d]	0.0127	0.0044	0.0039
	CBZ[e]	0.1081	0.0250	<0.0001
	FBT*CBZ	0.00001	0.0001	0.9175
1	Intercept	−6.5303	1.1493	<0.0001
	FBT[f]	0.0113	0.0036	0.0017
	CBZ[g]	0.0813	0.0199	<0.0001
	FBT*CBZ	0.0002	0.0001	0.1430
2	Intercept	−4.9642	0.9077	<0.0001
	FBT[h]	0.0123	0.0027	<0.0001
	CBZ[i]	0.0238	0.0184	0.1955
	FBT*CBZ	0.0002	0.0001	0.0084

[a] See Eq. 1 for definitions.

[b] Estimated TD_{50} for FBT at 0.25 h is 906.45 with a 95% confidence interval of (232.4, 1,580).

[c] Estimated TD_{50} for CBZ at 0.25 h is 87.43 with a 95% confidence interval of (76.0, 98.8).

[d] Estimated TD_{50} for FBT at 0.5 h is 661.21 with a 95% confidence interval of (409.3, 913.1).

[e] Estimated TD_{50} for CBZ at 0.5 h is 77.47 with a 95% confidence interval of (65.3, 89.6).

[f] Estimated TD_{50} for FBT at 1 h is 578.0 with a 95% confidence interval of (371.3, 784.8).

[g] Estimated TD_{50} for CBZ at 1 h is 80.34 with a 95% confidence interval of (62.6, 98.1).

[h] Estimated TD_{50} for FBT at 2 h is 403.1 with a 95% confidence interval of (338.8, 467.4).

[i] Estimated TD_{50} for CBZ at 2 h is 208.08 with a 95% confidence interval of (0, 468.1).

sponse between CBZ and FBT, which occurred only at 2 h and at a point in which only one of the test drugs demonstrated a significant dose response, a number of possible scenarios could exist. CBZ exhibited an earlier dose response and may have sensitized the neurotoxic targets to a subsequent drug exposure. In addition, a CBZ metabolite, inactive by itself, may be generated that can facilitate FBT toxicity, and/or the reverse may be true. These represent testable speculations based on this analysis. Furthermore, one might consider altering the dosing schedule in such a way as to minimize this neurotoxic interaction, which is an experimental option of RSM. In those clinical situations in which the therapeutic (e.g., anticonvulsant) combination is additive and the neurotoxic responses are synergistic, one can predict the impact of what may appear to be an unfavorable combination, so as to give a more informed approach to issues such as this.

The theoretical basis for the use of isobolographic procedures has been stated in reviews a number of times (6, 9, 11). The underlying assumptions associated with this technique are that a drug cannot interact with itself. A combination effect could therefore be obtained by doses of the individual drugs whose proportions, relative to the other single drug dose that achieves the combination effect, adds up to 1 (6). Where the individual drugs exhibit dissimilar slopes, this procedure cannot be used (9) since contradictory predictions can result. The procedure we have employed in this study is not restricted by the assumption of dose addition (28). As the number of drugs to be studied increases, the mathematical terms reflecting them are introduced into this model. The values of the regression coefficients are derived from the experimental data, and their statistical significance is given. This procedure can provide the same conclusions as the dose addition model, but it is not restricted to analyzing drugs with similar dose response curves (15, 16, 23). There are other advantages to this procedure that are reviewed in (29), which are beyond the scope of this chapter.

Investigators interested in studying drug combinations should be cognizant of the procedures, models, and assumptions that underlie their use. Sometimes the biological information available will assist the investigators in deciding the best way to proceed; at other times it may require using several different procedures. The selection of any procedure should be based on objective (statistical and experimental) information. The experimental validation and testing of the proposed model are critically important in establishing its utility. We have successfully validated the use of RSM in modeling combinations of genotoxic drugs (18). Nonparametric procedures are often useful when there is uncertainty about the form of the dose–response relationship and/or the distribution of the data. One such procedure, kernel estimation, has been applied and, at least within the context of the systems studied, has provided some significant benefits (30). An appealing feature of this technique is that there are fewer underlying stated assumptions and that the procedure is data- and not model-driven (30). We are currently exploring the usefulness of these techniques in describing multidimensional dose response relationships.

With respect to the use of RSM to the examples provided in this chapter, it should be helpful to the investigator to have both quantitative and qualitative descriptions of these drugs and responses. We have to date only attempted to validate the neurotoxicity studies (FBT/CBZ) by performing a separate study, testing doses and combinations different than those found in Table 18-1 but contained within the experimental region in Figure 18-2. This analysis (data not presented) supports the analysis, results, and conclusions reported in this chapter. It will require additional work and analysis of other drug combinations (some with dissimilar dose response curves) before the degree of usefulness of these procedures can be decided in these types of studies.

Finally, it should be noted that these procedures also have applicability in clinical paradigms and therapeutic scenarios that could greatly benefit the clinician's use of drug combination as well as clinical outcomes (14, 25, 26, 31). This last point clearly offers the clinician innovative opportunities in designing studies and in patient treatment that will require new ways of looking at these problems.

Acknowledgment: Portions of this research work were supported by NIH Contract No. NO1-NS-4-3261, awarded by the Epilepsy Branch, National Institute of Neurological and Communicative Disorders and Stroke.

REFERENCES

1. Swinyard EA. Assay of antiepileptic drug activity in experimental animals: standard tests. In: Mercier J, ed. *International Encyclopedia of Pharmacology and Therapeutics* vol 1. New York: Pergamon Press, 1972:47–75.
2. Swinyard EA, Woodhead JH. Experimental detection, quantitation and evaluation of antiepileptics. In: Woodbury DM, Penry JK, Pippenger CE, eds. *Antiepileptic Drugs.* New York: Raven Press, 1982:111–26.
3. Krall RL, Penry JK, White BG, Kupferberg HJ, Swinyard EA. Anticonvulsant drug screening. *Epilepsia* 1979;19:408–28.
4. Weaver LC, Swinyard EA, Goodman LS. Anticonvulsant drug combinations: diphenylhy-dantoin combined with other Antiepileptics. *J Am Pharm Assoc* 1958;47:645–8.
5. Weaver LC, Swinyard EA, Woodbury LA, Goodman LS. Studies on anticonvulsant drug combinations: phenobarbital and diphenylhydantoin. *J Pharm Exp Ther* 1955;113:359–70.
6. Berenbaum MC. Criteria for analyzing interactions between biologically active agents. *Adv Cancer Res* 1981;35:269–335.
7. Gessner PK. The isobolographic method applied to drug interactions. In: Morsellik PL, Garanttini S, Cohen S, eds. *Drug Interactions.*
8. Gessner PK, Cabana BE. Chloral alcoholate: reevaluation of its role in the intervention between the hypnotic effects of chloral hydrate and ethanol. *J Pharmacol Exp Ther* 1967;156:602–5.
9. Loewe S. The problem of synergism and antagonism of combined drugs. *Arzneimittelforsch* 1953;3:285.
10. Loewe S. Antagonisms and antagonists. *Pharmacol Rev* 1957;9:237–42.

11. Wessinger WD. Approaches to the study of drug interactions in behavioral pharmacology. *Neurosci Behav Rev* 1986;10:103–13.

12. Carter WH, Gennings C, Staniswalis JG, Campbell ED, White KL. A statistical approach to the construction and analysis of isobolograms. *J Am Coll Toxicol* 1988;7:963–73.

13. Mead R, Pike DJ. A review of response surface methodology from a biometric viewpoint. *Biometrics* 1975;31:803–51.

14. Carter WH Jr, Wampler GL, Stablein DM, Campbell ED. Drug activity and therapeutic synergism in cancer treatment. *Cancer Res* 1982;42:2963–71.

15. Carter WH Jr, Jones DE, Carchman RA. Application of response surface methods for evaluating the interactions of soman, atropine and pralidoxine chloride. *Fundam Appl Toxicol* 1985;5:232–41.

16. Jones DE, Carter WH JR, Carchman RA. Evaluation of interaction of soman (GD), atropine sulfate (ATR), pralidoxine chloride (2-PAM), and pyridostygmine bromide (PYR) pretreatment of guinea pigs. *Fundam Appl Toxicol* 5:242–51.

17. Carter WH Jr, Wampler GL, Stablein DM. *Regression Analysis of Survival Data in Cancer Chemotherapy*. New York: Marcel Dekker, 1983.

18. Solana RP, Chinchilli V, Wilson JD, Carter WH Jr, Carchman RA. The evaluation of the interaction of three genotoxic agents in eliciting SCEs using response surface methodology. *Fundam Appl Toxicol* 1987;9:541–9.

19. Finney DJ, *Probit Analysis*. 2nd ed. Cambridge: Cambridge University Press, 1952.

20. Berkson J. A statistically precise and relatively simple method of estimating the bio-assay quantal response, based on the logistic function. *J Am Stat Assoc* 1953;48:565–99.

21. Gennings C, Campbell ED, Staniswalis JD, Boyle RM, Carter WH Jr, Carchman RA, Koplovitz I. Evaluating response surface methods with a reduced sample size based on a study of soman, atropine and pralidoxime chloride. In: Proceedings of the Sixth Medical Chemical Defense Bioscience Review, Columbia, Maryland, August 1987.

22. Gennings C, Staniswalis JG, Campbell ED, Boyle RM, Carchman RA, Carter WH Jr, Koplovitz I. Application of response surface methods for comparing the interactions of soman, atropine and pralidoxime chloride when modeling agent-induced lethality. Proceedings of the Sixth Medical Chemical Defense Bioscience Review, Columbia, Maryland, August 1987.

23. Gennings C, Carchman RA, Carter WH Jr, et al. Assessing physostigmine efficacy by response surface modeling: a comparison to pyridostigmine efficacy. *J Am Coll Toxicol* 1988;7:1013–30.

24. Stablein DM, Carter WH, Wampler GL. Confidence regions for constrained optima in response surface experiments. *Biometrics* 1983;39:759–63.

25. Carter WH, Chinchilli VM, Campbell ED, Wampler GL. Confidence interval about the response at the stationary point of a response surface with an application to preclinical cancer therapy. *Biometrics* 1984;40:1125–30.

26. Wampler GL, Carter WH, Williams VR. Combination chemotherapy: arriving at optimal treatment levels by incorporating side effect constraints. *Cancer Treat Rep* 1978;62:333–40.

27. Clement JG, Shiloff JD, Gennings C. Efficacy of a combination of acetylcholinesterase reactivators, HL-6 and obidoxime against tabun and soman poisoning of mice. *Arch Toxicol* 1987;61:70–5.
28. Solana RP, Chinchilli V, Carter WH Jr, Wilson JD, Carchman RA. The evaluation of biological interactions using response surface methodology. *Cell Biol Toxicol* 1987;3:263–77.
29. Solana RP, Carter WH Jr, Wilson JD, Chinchilli VM, Carchman RA. Qualitative evaluation of sister chromatid exchanges elicited by combinations of genotoxic compounds *J Am Coll Toxicol* 1988;7:975–86.
30. Staniswalis JG, McCrady CW. The use of kernel estimators in describing human T-lymphocyte proliferation induced by phorol esters and Ca^{++} ionophore *J Amer Coll Toxicol* 1988;7:939–51.
31. Myers RH, Carter WH Jr. Response surface techniques for dual response sytems. *Technometrics* 1973;15:301–17.

19

Use of Isobolograms in Predicting Drug Interactions

Ewart A. Swinyard, Jose H. Woodhead, and Harold H. Wolf

Department of Pharmacology and Toxicology, College of Pharmacy, University of Utah, Salt Lake City, Utah, U.S.A.

Despite the trend toward monotherapy, many epileptic patients have multiple seizure types that may require two or more therapeutic agents. Moreover, a considerable number of patients with only one seizure type are not adequately controlled by any one antiepileptic drug. These and many other patients are subjected to polytherapy during the several days required to change from one drug to another drug. More importantly, perhaps, is the fact that when new agents are subjected to Phase II clinical studies, the physician is faced with the problem of adding the new agent to the medication already prescribed for the patient. Therefore, some form of multiple drug therapy is a common practice. As a result, the combined action of anticonvulsant drugs has become a subject of major importance, not only for the prevention and/or control of the seizure, but also from the standpoint of avoiding untoward effects. Nevertheless, comparatively little laboratory research has been devoted to the effect of antiepileptic drug combinations on either toxicity or anticonvulsant potency (1–9).

Relatively few well-controlled clinical combination studies have been reported (10–12). The available antiepileptic drugs, so carefully studied in the laboratory for potency, spectrum of action, and toxicity, are used in combination, even by the expert epileptologist, without the benefit of basic information on their pharmacodynamic interaction. However, as the deleterious aspects of polypharmacy become increasingly recognized by the clinician (13–15), the careful laboratory evaluation of the neurotoxicity and anticonvulsant potency of antiepileptic combinations becomes more important. The isobologram provides a graphic procedure for selecting the doses of two or more similarly acting drugs to be used in combination; it is also used to determine whether the pharmacodynamic interaction of the components results in simple addition, potentiation, or antagonism of the activity evaluated. The primary objective of this presentation is to show how isobolograms may be used for predicting the pharmacodynamic interaction of two or more anticonvulsant drugs tested in combination and to review the advantages and limitations of this procedure.

MATERIALS AND METHODS

Male albino mice (CF #1 strain, 18–25 g) obtained from Charles River, Wilmington, MA, and maintained in their home cage, were allowed free access to both food (Wayne Rodent Blox) and water, except for the brief time they were removed for injection of the drug or drug combination or to be subjected to the test procedure. Felbamate (FBT), phenytoin (PHT), carbamazepine (CBZ), and the various combinations of these drugs were suspended in 0.5% methylcellulose; ethosuximide, valproate, and combinations of these drugs were dissolved in 0.9% saline. All drugs and drug combinations were administered intraperitoneally in a volume of 0.01 ml/g body weight and tested at the previously determined time of peak effect (TPE). Anticonvulsant potency was determined by two well-established tests (16–18): the maximal electroshock seizure (MES) test (50 mA, delivered for 0.2 s via corneal electrodes) or the subcutaneous Metrazol seizure threshold (sc Met) test (85 mg/kg). Prevention of the hindlimb tonic extension was taken as the endpoint for the MES test, whereas prevention of even a minimal seizure was taken as the endpoint for the sc Met test. Minimal neurotoxicity was determined by the rotorod (19) test. Neurological deficit is indicated by inability of the mouse to maintain its equilibrium on the rotating rod for 1 min in each of three trials. The dose of each drug or combination required to produce the desired endpoint in 50% of animals (ED_{50}) in each test, the dose eliciting evidence of minimal neurotoxicity in 50% of animals (TD_{50}), and the standard error (S.E.) were then calculated by means of a computer program based on the method described by Finney (20) and written by NINCDS. These data were then compared with the expected data estimated by means of the isobologram and subjected to the same statistical procedure.

EXPERIMENTAL DESIGN

The first step is to establish a log-probit regression line for each of the two component drugs by the same procedure as that to be used for the combination. The quantal response data obtained by testing the component drugs must yield regression lines that are not *significantly different from parallel*. Likewise, the drug combinations must yield regression lines that are not significantly different from parallel with those of the component drugs. Otherwise, the statistical evaluation of the combination is only valid at the 50% level of response. With these requirements fulfilled, the observed and the expected results (anticonvulsant potency or toxicity) may be compared and the interaction of the two drugs evaluated. This interaction may reflect simple addition, potentiation (supra-additive), or antagonism (infra-additive) of the effects of the individual components. The basic hypothesis is that the less potent (or toxic) drug is merely a diluted form of the more potent (or toxic) drug and that their pharmacodynamic interaction is simply additive.

Regression lines for each of the two drugs to be used in combination are determined by testing eight animals with various doses of the drug at the previously determined TPE until at least four points are established between complete response (protection or toxicity) and no response. The observed points are plotted on logarithmic probability paper, and a regression line is visually fitted to the data. The dose of the drug producing the desired endpoint in 50% of animals (ED_{50} or TD_{50}) is then calculated by a computer program, the regression line is redrawn so as to be statistically correct, and the parallelism of the two regression lines is established. These two regression lines are then used to determine the *component of effectiveness* of each drug so that, when used in combination, the sum of their effectiveness equals the desired level of response, conventionally the 50% level.

Figure 19-1 shows the regression lines for PHT (A) and FBT (B) obtained by the MES test in mice and illustrates the procedure whereby one can select a dose of one drug and add to it a calculated amount of a second drug, so that the predetermined dose of the mixture will produce approximately a 50% response, assuming that the hypothesis of simple addition is operative. The basic procedure may be expressed by the equation shown in Fig. 19-1:

$$ED_x \text{ of drug A} + (ED_{50} \text{ of drug B} - ED_x \text{ of drug B}) = \text{expected } ED_{50} \text{ of the combination}$$

The two regression lines shown in Fig. 19-1 are intersected by two horizontal lines representing the 50% and (in this example arbitrarily) the 25% level of response. By substituting PHT for A and FBT for B in the above equation, and by letting x = 25 (as shown in Fig. 19-1), the estimated ED_{50} of the mixture will be equal to the ED_{25} of PHT (4.3 mg/kg) plus the ED_{50} of FBT minus the ED_{25} of FBT (31 mg/kg − 23.5 mg/kg, or 7.5 mg/kg). The component of effectiveness contributed by the 4.3 mg/kg of PHT is depicted in Fig. 19-1 by the large lined rectangle. It is evident that the remaining component necessary to reach the desired level of 50% response can be contributed either by 1.5 mg/kg of PHT, depicted by the small lined rectangle, or by the calculated 7.5 mg/kg of FBT portrayed by the small dotted rectangle. Therefore, the sum of these two doses (4.3

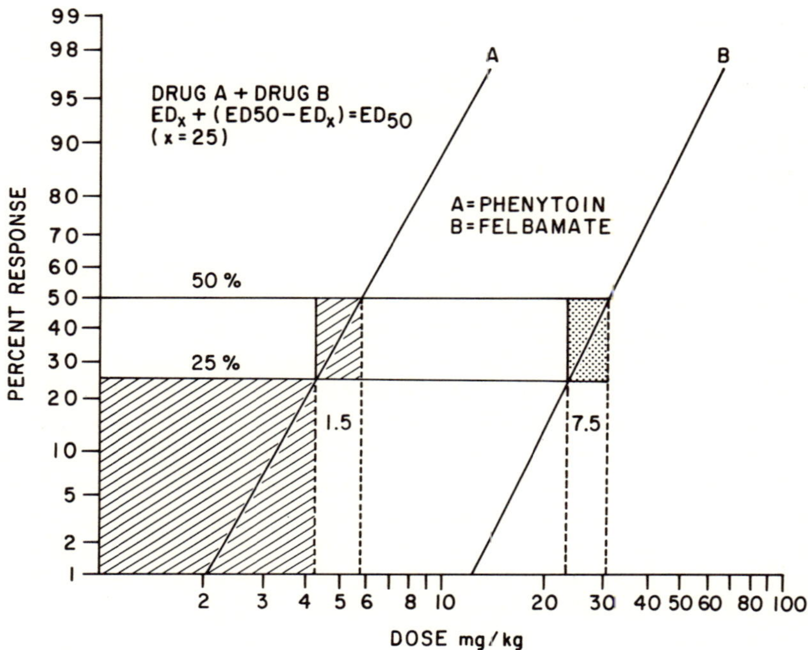

FIG. 19-1. Graphic computation of mixtures of two drugs and of the estimated dose of the combination for 50% anticonvulsant response (MES test).

mg/kg of PHT plus 7.5 mg/kg of FBT; total, 11.8 mg/kg) represents the expected ED$_{50}$ of the combination. Based on this graphic computation, the two drugs are mixed in a ratio of 4.3 parts PHT to 7.5 parts FBT; this mixture is then assayed as a new unknown drug.

The isobologram can also be used for evaluating anticonvulsant drug combinations, or other types of drug combinations, in which more than two components of a mixture are active when measured by the same test. When three drugs (A, B, and C) in a mixture are active, the following formula would apply:

$$ED_x A + (ED_y - ED_x)B + (ED_{50} - ED_y)C = \text{expected } ED_{50}$$

where x and y represent selected levels of response. Obviously, there is no limit to the number of drugs that can be combined. It should be emphasized that with this procedure, the expected response, as estimated graphically, invariably falls within a few mg/kg of the observed response determined experimentally, assuming the two drugs interact additively.

Thus, by comparing the expected response of the combination with the observed response, any striking difference can be seen without the necessity of quantitative calculations.

APPLICATIONS OF ISOBOLOGRAMS

Isobolograms may be effectively used in at least three ways: (a) to evaluate the results of combination studies in which the component doses were *arbitrarily* selected, (b) to select component doses and rapidly screen anticonvulsant drug combinations, and (c) to select a sufficient number of component doses to cover the entire anticonvulsant profile, complete a regression line for each selected combination, and statistically compare the expected ED_{50} (or TD_{50}) with the observed ED_{50} (or TD_{50}). The examples that follow illustrate these applications.

Evaluation of Arbitrary Combination Data

Suppose an investigator reports that after the administration of 4.3 mg/kg of drug A to eight mice, two were protected when subjected to the MES test. Likewise, after the administration of 23.5 mg/kg of drug B to eight mice, two were protected. However, when a combination of 4.3 mg/kg of drug A and 23.5 mg/kg of drug B were given to eight mice, six of the eight were protected. Therefore, according to the investigator, a supra-additive (potentiation) effect was observed. Figure 19-2 illustrates how an isobologram may be used to evaluate the validity of such claims. As shown in Fig. 19-2, 4.3 mg/kg of drug A would be expected to protect 25% of mice subjected to the MES test, and 23.5 mg/kg of drug B would also be expected to protect 25% of the animals. However, when these two doses are combined, the expected response would be at least 75%, as shown by either

$$ED_{25} \text{ of } A + 4.3 \text{ mg/kg drug } A = ED_{82} \qquad \text{or}$$

$$ED_{25} \text{ of } B + 23.5 \text{ mg/kg of drug } B = ED_{85}.$$

Therefore, the six of eight protected represents only an additive effect of the two drugs. This example emphasizes the fact that more drug is required to go from 0 to 25% (4.3 mg/kg, drug A; 23.5 mg/kg, drug B) than to go from 25 to 50% (1.5 mg/kg, drug A; 7.5 mg/kg, drug B). Therefore, one *cannot arbitrarily* combine doses and anticipate that the expected response will be equal to the sum of the response of the individual components.

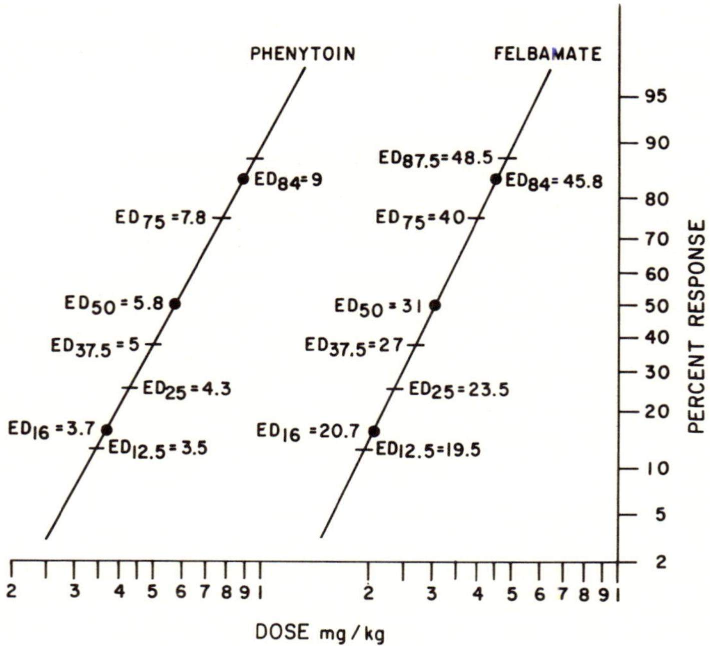

FIG. 19-2. Graphic representation of the response to various doses of either phenytoin or felbamate in mice (MES test).

Screening Anticonvulsant Combinations

The isobologram procedure for selecting combinations of two active drugs on the basis of components of effectiveness is a valuable procedure for rapidly screening potentially useful antiepileptic drug combinations. This procedure is applicable only when the dose-response lines for the component drugs are parallel. With the isobologram procedure, the expected ED_{50}, estimated graphically, invariably falls within a few mg/kg of the observed ED_{50} mathematically determined. Thus, a comparison of the graphically estimated ED_{50} of the combination with the results obtained in a single experiment (eight mice/group) provides an insight as to the direction of the pharmacodynamic interaction. Promising combinations can then be further evaluated, sufficient data accumulated to establish a regression line, and the data analyzed statistically.

The anticonvulsant activity and minimal neurotoxicity of PHT, CBZ, and four combinations of these two drugs are shown in Table 19-1. These data suggest that combinations I and II may have an infra-additive effect on anticonvulsant activity, whereas combination IV perhaps has a supra-additive effect. With respect to neurotoxicity, combinations I and II seem

Table 19-1. Anticonvulsant Activity and Minimal Neurotoxicity of Four Combinations of Phenytoin and Carbamazepine as Estimated by the MES and Rotorod Tests in Mice

Combination no.	Components and combinations	Dose (mg/kg) PHT + CBZ	Estimated ED_{50} or TD_{50} (mg/kg)	Observed response (r/n)[a]
Anticonvulsant activity				
	Phenytoin (PHT)	—	5.8^{b}	—
I	PHT ED_{25} + (CBZ $ED_{50} - ED_{25}$)	4.3 + 1.0	5.3	2/8
II	PHT $ED_{12.5}$ + (CBZ $ED_{50} - ED_{12.5}$)	3.5 + 1.6	5.1	0/8
III	CBZ $ED_{12.5}$ + (PHT $ED_{50} - ED_{12.5}$)	2.3 + 6.2	8.5	4/8
IV	CBZ ED_{25} + (PHT $ED_{50} - ED_{25}$)	1.5 + 6.8	8.3	8/8
	Carbamazepine (CBZ)	—	7.8^{b}	—
Minimal neurotoxicity				
	Phenytoin (PHT)	—	60.4^{b}	—
I	PHT TD_{25} + (CBZ $TD_{50} - TD_{25}$)	55.0 + 5.5	60.5	4/8
II	PHT $TD_{12.5}$ + (CBZ $TD_{50} - TD_{12.5}$)	52.0 + 8.5	60.5	3/8
III	CBZ $TD_{12.5}$ + (PHT $TD_{50} - TD_{12.5}$)	8.0 + 37.5	45.5	8/8
IV	CBZ TD_{25} + (PHT $TD_{50} - TD_{25}$)	5.0 + 40.5	45.5	8/8
	Carbamazepine (CBZ)	—	45.5^{b}	—

[a] (r)Response/(n)number tested.
[b] Calculated ED_{50} or TD_{50}.

Table 19-2. Anticonvulsant Activity and Minimal Neurotoxicity of Six Combinations of Ethosuximide and Valproate as Estimated by the sc Metrazol Threshold and Rotorod Tests in Mice

Combination no.	Components and combinations	Dose (mg/kg) ETH + VPA	Estimated ED_{50} or TD_{50} (mg/kg)	Observed response (r/n)[a]
Anticonvulsant activity				
	Ethosuximide (ETH)	—	103[b]	—
I	ETH $ED_{37.5}$ + (VPA $ED_{50} - ED_{37.5}$)	94 + 25	119	0/8
II	ETH ED_{25} + (VPA $ED_{50} - ED_{25}$)	86 + 49	135	5/8
III	ETH $ED_{12.5}$ + (VPA $ED_{50} - ED_{12.5}$)	75 + 75	150	6/8
IV	VPA $ED_{12.5}$ + (ETH $ED_{50} - ED_{12.5}$)	28 + 134	162	3/8
V	VPA ED_{25} + (ETH $ED_{50} - ED_{25}$)	17 + 160	177	1/8
VI	VPA $ED_{37.5}$ + (ETH $ED_{50} - ED_{37.5}$)	9 + 184	193	3/8
	Valproate (VPA)	—	209[b]	—
Minimal neurotoxicity				
	Ethosuximide (ETH)	—	384[b]	—
I	ETH $TD_{37.5}$ + (VPA $TD_{50} - TD_{37.5}$)	370 + 11	381	1/8
II	ETH TD_{25} + (VPA $TD_{50} - TD_{25}$)	350 + 31	381	2/8
III	ETH $TD_{12.5}$ + (VPA $TD_{50} - TD_{12.5}$)	330 + 46	376	1/8
IV	VPA $TD_{12.5}$ + (ETH $TD_{50} - TD_{12.5}$)	375 + 54	429	5/8
V	VPA TD_{25} + (ETH $TD_{50} - TD_{25}$)	390 + 34	424	4/8
VI	VPA $TD_{37.5}$ + (ETH $TD_{50} - TD_{37.5}$)	410 + 14	424	5/8
	Valproate (VPA)	—	421[b]	—

[a] (r)Response/(n)number tested.
[b] Calculated ED_{50} or TD_{50}.

Table 19-3. Combinations and Doses of Felbamate (FBT) and Phenytoin (PHT) Selected for Anticonvulsant (MES) Studies in Mice

Comb. no.	Drug combinations	Dose (mg/kg) FBT + PHT	Estimated ED_{50} (mg/kg)
I	FBT $ED_{37.5}$ + (PHT $ED_{50} - ED_{37.5}$)	27.0 + 0.8	27.8
II	FBT ED_{25} + (PHT $ED_{50} - ED_{25}$)	23.5 + 1.5	25.0
III	FBT $ED_{12.5}$ + (PHT $ED_{50} - ED_{12.5}$)	19.5 + 2.3	21.8
IV	PHT $ED_{12.5}$ + (FBT $ED_{50} - ED_{12.5}$)	3.5 + 11.5	15.0
V	PHT ED_{25} + (FBT $ED_{50} - ED_{25}$)	4.3 + 7.5	11.8
VI	PHT $ED_{37.5}$ + (FBT $ED_{50} - ED_{37.5}$)	5.0 + 4.0	9.0

to have an additive effect, whereas combinations III and IV may have a supra-additive effect. Therefore, combinations III and IV may be somewhat more potent, but may also be somewhat more toxic. In either case, these two combinations are worthy of further study.

The above screening procedure is especially useful when the anticonvulsant test involves a time-consuming procedure such as the sc Met test. Table 19-2 shows the anticonvulsant potency and minimal neurotoxicity of ethosuximide, valproate, and six combinations of these two drugs as estimated in mice by the sc Met seizure threshold and rotorod tests. These data suggest that combination III may have some supra-additive anticonvulsant action. Therefore, this combination should be subjected to further study. Also, combinations I and V should perhaps be repeated in order to rule out possible antagonism by these combinations. Otherwise, it would appear that the other three combinations reflect similar joint action. With respect to minimal neurotoxicity, it would appear that combinations I, II, and III interact infra-additively, whereas combinations IV, V, and VI interact additively. Thus, combinations II and III are worthy of further study, since the data suggest that these two combinations may have a somewhat wider margin of safety.

Isobolograms and the Evaluation of Combination Data

The isobologram shown in Fig. 19-1 was also used to select the component doses of six combinations of PHT and FBT. Table 19-3 shows the identification number (I through VI), the isobologram formula for each combination, the dose of FBT to PHT in each combination, and the estimated ED_{50}s. The combination number (Roman numerals) identifies the drug combination, i.e., Combination I: FBT $ED_{37.5}$ + (PHT $ED_{50} - ED_{37.5}$). The same combination numbers will be used to identify all subsequent combination data presented. It may be seen from Table 19-3 that the

Table 19-4. Anticonvulsant Potency of Six Combinations of Felbamate (FBT) and Phenytoin (PHT) as Estimated by the MES Test in Mice

Drug or drug combination	Dose (mg/kg)		Expected $ED_{50} \pm SE$ (mg/kg)	Observed $ED_{50} \pm SE$ (mg/kg)	Potency ratio $\pm$ SE	p
	FBT	PHT				
Felbamate	—	—	—	30.96 ± 3.17	—	—
Combination I	27	0.8	27.8 ± 2.41	26.05 ± 0.92	1.07 ± 0.10	>0.50
Combination II	23.5	1.5	25.0 ± 1.91	21.82 ± 0.98	1.15 ± 0.10	>0.10
Combination III	19.5	2.3	21.8 ± 1.49	20.27 ± 2.88	1.08 ± 0.17	>0.50
Combination IV	11.5	3.5	15.0 ± 2.49	13.68 ± 0.72	1.10 ± 0.19	>0.50
Combination V	7.5	4.3	11.8 ± 2.06	10.53 ± 0.37	1.12 ± 0.20	>0.50
Combination VI	4.5	5.0	9.0 ± 1.58	8.40 ± 0.49	1.07 ± 0.20	>0.70
Phenytoin	—	—	—	5.80 ± 0.66	—	—

estimated ED_{50} of these six combinations ranged from 9.0 to 27.8 mg/kg. Thus, the dose range between the ED_{50}s for FBT and PHT was uniformly covered.

The anticonvulsant potency of FBT, PHT, and six combinations of these two antiepileptics are determined by the MES test in mice are shown in Table 19-4. In Table 19-4 and those to follow, the *expected* ED_{50} (or TD_{50}) represents the value *estimated* from the isobologram and subjected to statistical analysis, whereas the *observed* ED_{50} (or TD_{50}) indicates the values calculated from the laboratory data. Comparison of the expected ED_{50} (or TD_{50}) and (S.E. with the observed ED_{50} (or TD_{50}) and S.E. provides a means for testing the significance of the departure from the prediction of simple addition. The potency (or toxicity) ratio reveals the magnitude of this departure; values of 1.00 indicate *simple addition;* values less than 1.00, *antagonism;* values greater than 1.00, *potentiation.* The p value denotes the significance of this departure.

Obviously, the most desirable result obtainable by the interaction of drugs is a significant increase in potency concomitant with a decrease in toxicity. Nevertheless, when either of the above occurs without the other, an increase in margin of safety is still possible. The ultimate objective is to find a combination with a protective index greater than that for either component of the mixture.

The anticonvulsant potency of these six combinations of FBT and PHT, as estimated by the MES test in mice, is shown in Table 19-4. The observed ED_{50}s were somewhat lower than the expected ED_{50}s. The observed ED_{50}s range from 8.40 to 26.05 mg/kg, whereas the expected ED_{50}s range from 9.0 to 27.8 mg/kg. Thus, the potency ratios (expected ED_{50} divided by the observed ED_{50}) were 1.07, 1.15, 1.08, 1.10, 1.12, and 1.07 for combinations I, II, III, IV, V, and VI, respectively. The most marked

Table 19-5. The Incidence and Time of Peak Minimal Neurotoxicity of Selected Doses of Six Combinations of Felbamate (FBT) and Phenytoin (PHT) in Mice

Combination	Dose (mg/kg)		No. toxic/No. tested				
	FBT	PHT	$\frac{1}{4}$ h	$\frac{1}{2}$ h	1 h	2 h	4 h
Combination I: FBT $TD_{37.5}$ + PHT($TD_{50} - TD_{37.5}$)	299	1.3	0/8	1/8	1/8	(1/8)[a]	0/8
	345	1.5	0/8	0/8	1/8	(2/8)	0/8
	460[b]	2.0	0/8	0/8	2/8	(5/8)	1/8
	598	2.6	1/8	5/8	7/8	(7/8)	7/8
Combination II: FBT TD_{25} + PHT($TD_{50} - TD_{25}$)	286	3.4	0/8	0/8	0/8	(1/8)	0/8
	315	3.8	0/8	0/8	1/8	(2/8)	1/8
	420[b]	5	0/8	0/8	2/8	(4/8)	1/8
	588	7	0/8	0/8	4/8	(7/8)	6/8
Combination III: FBT $TD_{12.5}$ + PHT($TD_{50} - TD_{12.5}$)	192.5	4	0/8	0/8	0/8	(1/8)	0/8
	289	6	0/8	0/8	2/8	(4/8)	0/8
	337	7	0/8	0/8	0/8	(4/8)	0/8
	385[b]	8	0/8	0/8	2/8	(7/8)	4/8
Combination IV: PHT $TD_{12.5}$ + FBT($TD_{50} - TD_{12.5}$)	74.3	39	0/8	1/8	(2/8)	1/8	0/8
	81	42.5	0/8	4/8	(5/8)	3/8	1/8
	87	46	0/8	4/8	(7/8)	6/8	4/8
	99[b]	52	0/8	7/8	(8/8)	8/8	8/8
Combination V: PHT TD_{25} + FBT($TD_{50} - TD_{25}$)	32	27.5	0/8	0/8	(1/8)	0/8	0/8
	48	41.3	0/8	1/8	(3/8)	1/8	1/8
	64[b]	55	2/8	5/8	(6/8)	5/8	5/8
	81	70	4/8	7/8	(7/8)	7/8	7/8
Combination VI: PHT $TD_{37.5}$ + FBT($TD_{50} - TD_{37.5}$)	12	29	0/8	0/8	(1/8)	0/8	0/8
	18	43.5	0/8	1/8	(4/8)	2/8	0/8
	21	50.8	1/8	5/8	(6/8)	4/8	1/8
	24[b]	58	2/8	6/8	(8/8)	6/8	7/8

[a] Time of peak neurotoxicity is in parentheses.
[b] FBT + PHT = expected TD_{50}.

increase in potency was observed in combination II; the observed ED_{50} was 21.82 mg/kg as compared to an expected value of 25.0 mg/kg. Although this represents a 12.7% increase in anticonvulsant potency, the potency ratio and S.E. indicate that there is no significant difference between the expected ED_{50} and the observed ED_{50} of this combination. Likewise, the potency ratios indicate that all of these combinations exhibit similar joint action.

The profile, TPE, and incidence of minimal neurotoxicity induced by six combinations of FBT and PHT are shown in Table 19-5. This table indicates the doses of each component employed in the various combina-

Table 19.6 The Minimal Neurotoxicity of Six Combinations of Felbamate (FBT) and Phenytoin (PHT) as Estimated by the Rotorod Test in Mice

Drug or drug combination	Dose (mg/kg)		Expected $TD_{50} \pm SE$ (mg/kg)	Observed $TD_{50} \pm SE$ (mg/kg)	Toxicity ratio $\pm$ SE	p
	FBT	PHT				
Felbamate	—	—	—	484 ± 25.64	—	—
Combination I	460	2	462 ± 18.83	424 ± 32.47	1.09 ± 0.10	>0.30
Combination II	420	5	425 ± 17.03	401 ± 32.46	1.06 ± 0.10	>0.50
Combination III	385	8	393 ± 12.59	303 ± 25.71	1.30 ± 0.12	<0.01[a]
Combination IV	99	52	151 ± 17.52	120 ± 3.01	1.26 ± 0.15	>0.05
Combination V	64	55	119 ± 13.03	96 ± 9.51	1.24 ± 0.18	>0.10
Combination VI	24	58	82 ± 11.34	58 ± 4.17	1.41 ± 0.22	>0.05
Phenytoin	—	—	—	60 ± 3.04	—	—

[a] Significantly different.

tions, reveals the time of onset and time of peak neurotoxicity of each combination, and identifies the expected TD_{50}. It also shows in parentheses the data used to calculate the observed TD_{50}. It may be seen that the TPE for combinations I, II, and III is 2 h, whereas that for combinations IV, V, and VI is 1 h. Thus, the TPE in which PHT provides the initial ED_x in the selection of doses is 1 h, whereas the TPE of combinations selected on the basis of FBT ED_x is 2 h. These observations emphasize the importance of determining the TPE prior to evaluating the pharmacodynamic interaction.

The minimal neurotoxicity of FBT, PHT, and these six combinations in mice is shown in Table 19-6. As indicated in Table 19-6, the observed TD_{50}s are all lower than the expected TD_{50}s. The observed ED_{50}s range from 58 to 424 mg/kg, whereas the expected ED_{50}s range from 82 to 462 mg/kg. Thus, the toxicity ratios were 1.09, 1.06, 1.30, 1.26, 1.24, and 1.41 for combinations I, II, III, IV, V, and VI, respectively. However, combinations III, IV, V, and VI increased the median minimal neurotoxicity 22.9, 20.5, 19.3, and 29.3%, respectively, over the expected TD_{50}. However, this increase was significant only for combination III. Overall, it would appear that combinations I and II interact additively, whereas combination III, and perhaps to some extent combinations IV, V, and VI, interact supra-additively.

The minimal neurotoxicity of FBT and CBZ and six combinations of these two antiepileptic drugs as determined by the rotorod test in mice is shown in Table 19-7. It may be seen that the observed ED_{50}s range from 121 to 347 mg/kg, whereas the expected TD_{50}s range from 127 to 324 mg/kg. Except for combination V, the toxicity ratios vary from 0.92 to

Table 19-7. The Minimal Neurotoxicity of Six Combinations of Felbamate (FBT) and Carbamazepine (CBZ) as Estimated by the Rotorod Test in Mice

Drug or drug combination	Dose (mg/kg)		Expected $TD_{50} \pm SE$ (mg/kg)	Observed $TD_{50} \pm SE$ (mg/kg)	Toxicity ratio $\pm$ SE	p
	FBT	CBZ				
Felbamate	—	—	—	372 ± 35.44	—	—
Combination I	315	9	324 ± 33.66	347 ± 30.20	0.93 ± 0.13	>0.50
Combination II	265	16	281 ± 25.12	280 ± 8.82	1.00 ± 0.10	>0.90
Combination III	208	25	233 ± 18.05	254 ± 14.33	0.92 ± 0.09	>0.30
Combination IV	164	54	218 ± 37.00	212 ± 12.92	1.03 ± 0.19	>0.70
Combination V	107	63	170 ± 29.94	142 ± 6.54	1.20 ± 0.22	>0.30
Combination VI	57	70	127 ± 23.89	121 ± 3.53	1.05 ± 0.20	>0.70
Carbamazepine	—	—	—	79 ± 7.26	—	—

1.05. The toxicity ratio for combination V is 1.20. Thus, combinations I and III decrease neurotoxicity by 7.1 and 9.0%, respectively, whereas combination V increases neurotoxicity by 16.4%. However, the p values indicate that there is no significant difference in the neurotoxicity of the expected and observed TD_{50}s. Thus, it would appear that with respect to neurotoxicity, FBT and CBZ interact additively.

CONCLUSIONS

The isobologram procedure for selecting combinations of two active drugs on the basis of components of effectiveness provides a method for checking the results obtained when the doses in a combination are arbitrarily selected. It is also useful for selecting component doses and *rapidly screening* antiepileptic drug combinations. With this procedure, the graphically estimated ED_{50} (assuming simple addition) would be expected to produce a 50% response in a single group of animals. It is also useful for the determination and comparison of the ED_{50}s, TD_{50}s, and margins of safety of various drugs and their combinations. The isobologram method, however, is limited to drugs and their combinations that yield parallel regression lines by the test employed. The evaluation of combinations yielding regression lines that are not parallel with those of the component drugs is only valid at the 50% level of response. Nevertheless, laboratory studies on anticonvulsant drug combinations should provide valuable information for the practicing epileptologist.

Acknowledgment: The authors express their gratitude to Lloyd Bush for the computer program used in the statistical evaluation of the combination data. This research was supported by NIH contract No. N01-NS-4-2361 awarded by the Epilepsy Branch, National Institute of Neurological and Communicative Disorders and Stroke.

REFERENCES

1. Loewe S. Anticonvulsant actions of trimethadione-phenobarbital and trimethadione-diphenylhydantoin combinations. *Fed Proc* 1948;7:240–1.
2. Weaver LC, Swinyard EA, Goodman LS. Potency of anticonvulsant drug combinations vs Metrazol seizures in mice; dilantin combined with other antiepileptics. *Fed Proc* 1953;12:379.
3. Weaver LC, Swinyard EA, Goodman LS. Potency of anticonvulsant drug combinations as determined by the maximal electroshock seizure pattern test in rats; mephobarbital combined with diphenylhydantoin sodium and phenobarbital sodium combined with phethenylate sodium. *J Pharmacol Exp Ther* 1954;110:52.
4. Chen G, Ensor CR. The combined anticonvulsant activity and toxicity of Dilantin and N-methyl-5-phenyl-succinimide. *J Lab Clin Med* 1953;41:78–83.
5. Chen G, Ensor CR. A study of the anticonvulsant properties of phenobarbital and Dilantin. *Arch Int Pharmacodyn Ther* 1954;100:234–48.
6. Weaver LC, Swinyard EA, Woodbury LA, Goodman LS. Studies on anticonvulsant drug combinations: phenobarbital and diphenylhydantoin. *J Pharmacol Exp Ther* 1955;113:359–70.
7. Weaver LC, Swinyard EA, Goodman LS. Anticonvulsant drug combinations: diphenylhydantoin combined with other antiepileptics. *J Am Pharm Assoc (Sci Ed)* 1958;47:645–8.
8. Leppick IE, Sherwin AL. Anticonvulsant activity of phenobarbital and phenytoin in combination. *J Pharmacol Exp Ther* 1977;200:570–5.
9. Morris JC, Dodson WE, Hatlelid JM, Ferrendelli JA. Phenytoin and carbamazepine, alone and in combination: anticonvulsants and neurotoxic effects. *Neurology* 1987;37:1111–8.
10. Merritt HH, Brenner C. Treatment of patients with epilepsy with sodium diphenylhydantoinate and phenobarbital combined. *J Nerv Ment Dis* 1942;96:245–50.
11. Cereghino JJ, Brock JT, Van Meter JC, Penry JK, Smith LD, White BG. The efficacy of carbamazepine combinations in epilepsy. *Clin Pharmacol Ther* 1975;18:733–41.
12. Hakkerainen H. Carbamazepine vs diphenylhydantoin vs their combination in adult epilepsy. *Neurology* 1980;30:354.
13. Trimble MR, Thompson PJ. Anticonvulsant drugs, cognitive function, and behavior. *Epilepsia* 1983;24(suppl 1):555–63.
14. Theodore WH, Porter RJ. Removal of sedative-hypnotic antiepileptic drugs from regimens of patients with intractable epilepsy. *Ann Neurol* 1983;13:320–4.
15. Albright PS, Bruni J. Reduction of polypharmacy in epileptic patients. *Arch Neurol* 1985;42:797–9.
16. Swinyard EA. Assay of antiepileptic drug activity in experimental animals:

standard tests. In: Mercier J, ed. *International Encyclopedia of Pharmacology and Therapeutics*. New York: Pergamon Press, 1972:47–65.

17. Swinyard EA, Woodhead JH. Experimental detection, quantitation and evaluation of antiepileptics. In: Woodbury DM, Penry JK, Pippenger CE, eds. *Antiepileptic Drugs*. New York: Raven Press, 1982:111–26.

18. Krall RL, Penry JK, White BG, Kupferberg HJ, Swinyard EA. Anticonvulsant drug screening. *Epilepsia* 1978;19:409–28.

19. Dunham NW, Miya TS. A note on a simple apparatus for detecting neurological deficit in rats and mice. *J Am Pharm Assoc* 1957;46:208–9.

20. Finney DJ. *Probit Analysis*. 3rd ed. London: Cambridge University Press, 1971.

Stable Isotope Breath Tests: A Simple, Safe, and Noninvasive Procedure for Identifying Potential Pharmacokinetic Drug Interactions in Man

[1]Alvin N. Kotake, [2]Steven K. Kuwahara, [3]George H. Lambert, and [4]Dale A. Schoeller

[1]CIBA-GEIGY Corporation, Pharmaceuticals Division, Summit, New Jersey; [2]Division of Clinical Pharmacology, Johns Hopkins Hospital, Baltimore, Maryland; [3]Department of Pediatrics, Loyola University, School of Medicine, Maywood, Illinois; and [4]Department of Medicine, The University of Chicago, Chicago, Illinois, U.S.A.

Combination drug therapy is an accepted practice in the treatment of epilepsy and is an origin for numerous recorded drug interactions (1–3). The most frequent are pharmacokinetic interactions, where combination therapy may alter the pharmacokinetic profile of one or both agents. These include changes in absorption, bioavailability, clearance, and volume of distribution. Therapeutically, alterations in these parameters may lead to a decrease in efficacy or an increase in toxicity. Thus, it is important to identify potential drug interactions and to utilize this information in the management of epilepsy.

As an example, phenytoin, the drug of choice for the treatment of all types of epilepsy except absence seizures, has a narrow therapeutic range and a small margin of safety (4) and exhibits nonlinear pharmacokinetics resulting in a disproportionate increase in plasma drug levels relative to the increase in dose. Since alterations in the steady-state drug levels result in a loss of seizure control or toxicity, it is, therefore, important to identify those drugs that when co-administered with phenytoin may alter its clearance. Phenytoin is also an inducer of the hepatic microsomal enzymes responsible for its own metabolism and the metabolism of other drugs used in the treatment of epilepsy. Thus, it is equally important to identify those effects of phenytoin therapy that alter the disposition of other drugs.

Standard procedures to identify potential drug interactions in humans typically involve monitoring changes in the pharmacokinetic profile of drugs from blood, saliva, or urine. Methods used to examine drug interactions identify changes in the steady-state drug level and the drug concentration–time profile. These procedures typically monitor differences in substrate disappearance from the systemic circulation, which may result from alterations in drug absorption, metabolism, volume of distribution, and plasma protein binding. The mechanisms responsible for alterations in a drug's pharmacokinetic profile are difficult to identify by these procedures. Further disadvantages of these procedures are that they may often be invasive, require studying subjects for longer periods of time, require highly trained personnel to perform the study, are time consuming, the analyses are technically difficult to perform), and are not conducive to performing sequential tests in the same individual. For these reasons, few studies are specifically designed in early drug development to identify changes in a drug's pharmacokinetic profile resulting from the simultaneous administration with other drugs.

The CO_2 breath test is an alternative procedure for identifying drug–drug interactions. The metabolism of many drugs are catalyzed by cytochrome P-450–dependent mono-oxygenase, which are primarily responsible for controlling their rate of elimination from the body. A common route of metabolism is dealkylation. The cleaved alkyl group is oxidized to fomaldehyde, which then undergoes further oxidation to formate and then bicarbonate and is then partially exhaled as CO_2. If dealkylation is the rate-determining step in the conversion to CO_2, then the appearance of the labeled CO_2 in the breath should reflect the rate of dealkylation. Aminopyrine, in which the N-methyl groups were labeled with ^{14}C or ^{13}C, was the first CO_2 breath test substrate tested for assessing hepatic microsomal function. Aminopyrine has many of the characteristics required for an ideal breath test substrate: (a) rapid and consistent absorption, (b) high water solubility, (c) distribution in total body water, (d) negligible binding to plasma proteins, (e) low hepatic extraction, (f) metabolism primarily by the liver, (g) little pharmacological effect, and (h) safety at doses used in the breath test (5–7). In addition, preparation of a labeled compound with a stable isotope is relatively inexpensive and has sufficient rates of expiration of label in the breath to permit its measurement by mass spectroscopy or infrared spectroscopy.

AMINOPYRINE AND CAFFEINE BREATH TESTS

The aminopyrine breath test (ABT) and caffeine breath test (CBT) have been under development for the past 10 years and are reported to be capable of monitoring in vivo hepatic cytochrome P-450 metabolizing capacity in both animals (8–12) and humans (13–16). These tests are simple to perform, noninvasive, and relatively safe, and they overcome many of the limitations of the test procedures described above. When administered intraperitoneally or intravenously, changes in the labeled aminopyrine and caffeine CO_2 expiration profile result primarily from alterations in hepatic cytochrome P-450 metabolic capacity. Following the oral administration of these substrates, changes can occur by increasing or decreasing cytochrome P-450 level, resulting in inverse changes in the rates of metabolism, or by altering substrate concentration delivered to the liver due to changes in rates of gastric emptying or drug absorption. The major disadvantage of this procedure is that several biochemical transformations are required before the labeled carbon derived from the drug appears in the breath as labeled CO_2. Alterations in these pathways can invalidate interpretation of the breath test results. The history of the development of breath test, an indepth description of its validity, and advantages and disadvantages of this test are beyond the scope of this discussion and are described elsewhere (5, 17–21). The objective of this article is to describe potential applications of breath tests for identifying pharmacokinetic drug interactions.

INDUCTION AND INHIBITION OF METABOLISM

Increasing numbers of reports have appeared that have utilized the breath test to assess the potential of a drug to inhibit or induce hepatic cytochrome P-450 systems. Lambert et al. (21) list 31 agents that induce or inhibit the ABT and CBT in animals and humans. Phenobarbital, phenytoin, and rifampicin have been reported to increase the ABT relative to untreated control subjects. Conversely, disulfiram, oral contraceptives, norethinedrone, and cimetidine have been reported to attenuate the ABT. The following study illustrates the use of the breath test for studies ex-

Table 20-1. Effects of Cimetidine on the Aminopyrine and Caffeine Breath Tests

Subject	Breath test	Basal % dose/h	Post-cimetidine[a] % dose/h	% of basal
CB	ABT	7.03	3.82	54
	CBT	2.29	1.15	50
WS	ABT	6.38	4.24	34
	CBT	2.67	1.64	39

[a]Cimetidine, 300 mg four times daily for 5 days; ABT and CBT administered on the morning of day 5 and day 6, respectively.

Table 20-2.   Effect of Rifampicin on the Aminopyrine and Caffeine Breath Tests

Subject	Breath test	Basal % dose/h	Post-rifampicin[a] % dose/h	% of basal
CB	ABT	6.90	9.10	134
	CBT	2.60	5.30	204
WS	ABT	7.10	8.60	121
	CBT	2.40	3.20	133

[a]Rifampicin, 300 mg three times daily for 5 days; ABT and CBT administered on the morning of day 5 and day 6, respectively.

amining induction and inhibition. Two normal subjects, having a 2-h cumulative ABT value of 6–8%/dose, were selected to participate in this study. These values are midrange for the breath test values and were chosen to permit the identification of induction (14–17% dose/2 h) or inhibition. The effects of cimetidine and rifampicin treatment on the ABT and CBT were examined (Tables 20-1 and 20-2). Basal breath tests were performed 2 days prior to the administration of cimetidine (200 mg q.i.d.) or rifampicin (300 mg t.i.d.) for 4 days. ABT and CBT were performed 1 h after the last dose of cimetidine and 8 h after the last dose of rifampicin. Cimetidine and rifampicin protocols were separated by a 2-week wash-out period. In this study, rifampicin induced both the ABT and CBT, and cimetidine attenuated the ABT and CBT. The utility of breath tests to identify potential agents that induce or inhibit hepatic cytochrome P-450 activity has clearly been established.

In a second study, we measured the effect of rifampicin on subjects exhibiting a wider range of basal ABT and CBT values (22). We observed that rifampicin at a dose of 300 mg t.i.d. for 4 days increased rates of exhaled $^{13}CO_2$ following the administration of labeled aminopyrine, and the magnitude of the induction was inversely proportional to their basal rates (Fig. 20-1). In contrast, rifampicin treatment in the same subjects had variable effects on the CBT. Moderate inductions in the CBT were observed in the low and moderate metabolizers of caffeine. However, rifampicin treatment of rapid metabolizers resulted in decreases in the CBT (Fig. 20-2). Although an excellent correlation existed between basal ABT and CBT values before treatment with rifampicin, no correlation was noted between the ABT and CBT after treatment. In addition, there was no correlation in the magnitude of induction of the ABT and CBT. These findings suggest that, prior to treatment, the metabolism of aminopyrine and caffeine was mediated by the same isoenzyme(s) of cytochrome P-450, but, after treatment, their metabolism may be mediated by different cytochrome P-450s. Alternatively, an alteration in the aminopyrine or caf-

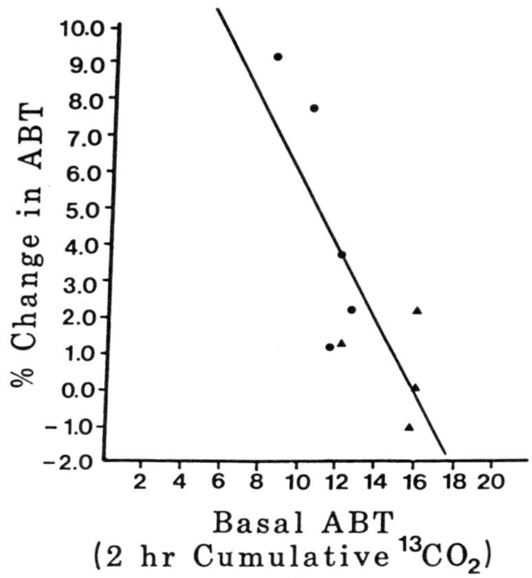

FIG. 20-1. Correlation between the basal ABT and the magnitude of induction of the ABT following the administration of rifampicin. Points represent individual subjects (triangles, smokers; circles, nonsmokers).

feine metabolic pathways had occurred. More detailed metabolic studies are required to resolve this issue.

SEQUENTIAL BREATH TEST STUDIES

The ability to safely perform sequential breath tests in a single subject is another advantage of the breath test. This permits evaluation of the time course of the drug interaction. For example, the time course of the effects of influenza vaccination (23), chemo-immunotherapy (24) and diet (25) have been examined using this procedure. The time course of the depression of the ABT was monitored before and after a single dose of influenza vaccine (23) or before and during a prolonged treatment with bacillus Calmette-Guérin or *Corynebacterium parvum* alone or in combination with cyclophosphamide (26). Juan et al. (25) used a similar design to profile the effects of dietary changes. In this study, the effect of low- and high-protein diets on the ABT and CBT were followed for several weeks. Eight days of low-protein diet were required to demonstrate significant changes in the ABT, whereas 16 days of low-protein diet were required to demonstrate significant changes in the CBT. On terminating the diet, the ABT returned to baseline values more rapidly than the CBT. The same subjects were then placed on a high-protein diet, and no statistically significant changes in the ABT or CBT were observed. There was a tendency, however, for the CBT to increase on this diet, with no changes in the ABT. From these studies, it becomes obvious that performing a single test following an intervention may provide only partial information

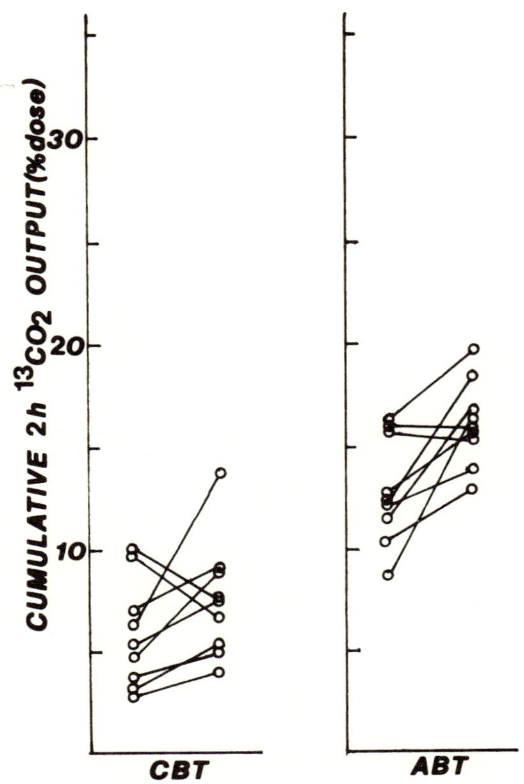

FIG. 20-2. The effects of rifampicin treatment on the ABT and CBT in volunteers. The points represent the ABT or CBT in individual subjects prior to and after treatment with rifampicin.

and that multiple tests are required to fully evaluate the effect of any treatment on hepatic mono-oxygenase activity.

BREATH TEST STUDIES IN PREGNANT FEMALES AND CHILDREN

Potentially, the most exciting uses of the stable isotope breath test are for examining drug pharmacokinetic interactions in pregnant females, neonates, and children where other invasive procedures are more difficult to perform. Kotake et al. (27) and Lambert et al. (28) have confirmed the feasibility of such studies in animal models. Rating et al. (29) have recently applied the ABT to evaluate the effect of transplacental exposure to various anticonvulsants on human neonatal cytochrome P-450 activity. The ABT in 12 newborns exposed in utero to anticonvulsants was compared to newborns not exposed to anticonvulsants. The cumulative 2-h expiration of $^{13}CO_2$ for three newborns not exposed in utero to anticonvulsants was 0–2%/dose, whereas in three newborns exposed to primodone alone or primodone in combination with diphenylhydantoin, the range was 20.8–

29.3%/dose. Data from five newborns exposed to valproic acid or valproic acid in combination with primidone showed a range of 0.9–5.3%/dose, and data from three newborns exposed to diphenylhydantoin indicated 3.6–13.7%/dose. For reference, the normal adult range is 12.2 ± 2.1%/dose, suggesting that in humans newborns, prenatal exposure to inducing agents may increase cytochrome P-450 activity beyond adult ranges. These findings contrast with similar studies in rodents, where the expression of drug metabolism activity and inducing capacity are expressed only after birth (30).

Relative to the adult population, children can be considered an orphan group on subjects related to drug pharmacokinetic and drug interactions. Nontherapeutic research has been limited in these populations due to the higher risk:benefit ratio and the legality of obtaining a valid informed consent from the patient. The use of the ABT to monitor hepatic drug metabolizing capacity in the developing rat and pregnant mouse has been reported (28). Safety, however, is of paramount concern in nontherapeutic research, especially when dealing with pediatric and pregnant patients, and procedures developed for use in these populations should be safe, noninvasive, and simple. Aminopyrine has been reported to produce agranulocytosis in patients at a frequency between 1 in 10,000 to 1 in 40,000 (31) and has been shown to be teratogenic in the mouse (32). The use of aminopyrine in pregnant women, neonates, and children is thus still subject to risk:benefit evaluation. In contrast, caffeine is an ubiquitous substrate in our diet with well-documented pharmacological effects. In the human CBT, the dose of caffeine (3 mg/kg) is at the lower limits of the pharmacological dose and is equivalent in the adult to one or two cups of coffee; in a 20-kg child, the dose is equivalent to a 12-oz can of caffeinated soda. The CBT meets the safety criteria for its use in pregnant females and children.

Using the CBT, Lambert et al. (24) evaluated the role of chronological age, maturation, and gender on caffeine 3-N-demethylase activity in 62 subjects (3–20 years of age) and the feasibility of performing this test in children. This study demonstrated that the CBT can be safely and easily conducted in children. The CBT generally decreased in children with increasing chronological age (Table 20-3). When subjects were grouped according to their pubertal stage, a general decrease in CBT was observed with maturation (Table 20-4). When the subjects were further subdivided according to their pubertal stage and gender, only the CBT values of females in pubertal stage I differed significantly from adult females. In males, the CBT values of the subjects of pubertal stages I, II, III, and IV were significantly higher than the values for adult males. These data also indicated that a gender difference occurs during pubertal stage III, and this sex difference is related to an earlier onset of sexual maturation of the CBT in females.

Table 20-3. The Caffeine Breath Test in Children According to Age and Gender

	Age, years		
	3–9	9–15	15–20
Total subjects			
Number	18	33	11
CBT 2-h CO_2[a]			
Median value	6.7[b]	5.0	4.3
Range	4.0–10.8	2.3–12.8	2.1–11.4
Male subjects			
Number	12	17	7
CBT 2-h CO_2			
Median value	7.3[c]	5.6	5.05
Range	5.7–10.8	2.3–12.8	2.1–11.4
Female subjects			
Number	6	16	4
CBT 2-h CO_2			
Median value	6.0	4.1	3.5
Range	4–6.9	2.6–10.7	2.4–5.2

Data reproduced from Lambert et al. (24) with permission.
[a] Percent dose exhaled over 2 h.
[b] $p < 0.01$, versus subjects 15–20 years old.
[c] $p < 0.05$, versus females of same age group.

INFUSION BREATH TEST STUDIES

Although drug inhibition interactions can easily be ascertained in animals and humans, it is extremely difficult to determine the effect of increasing dose on the time of onset and time to reach maximum inhibition. With standard procedures, the pharmacokinetic profile of a model drug is determined alone and in the presence of an inhibitor. Under the conditions when two substrates are administered together, plasma concentrations of the agents vary independently of each other, and only qualitative information regarding their potential pharmacokinetic interactions are derived from these studies. To attain information on the time of onset, magnitude, and duration of inhibition, it is necessary to infuse the model drug to a steady-state level and to monitor changes in the steady-state drug level in the presence of the inhibitor. As stated previously, procedures that monitor substrate disappearance are subject to misinterpretation. An example is the study performed by Schary et al. (33) who examined the mechanism by which phenylbutazone administration results in the decrease in warfarin plasma steady-state concentrations. This study

Table 20-4. The Caffeine Breath Test in Children According to Pubertal Stage and Gender

	Pubertal stage					
	I	II	III	IV	V	Adult[a]
Total subjects						
Number	23	6	11	11	11	21
CBT 2-h CO_2[b]						
Median value	6.7[c,d]	5.1[d,e]	5.5[c]	5.0[c]	4.2	3.4
Range	2.6–10.8	3.6–12.8	3.4–8.4	3.4–11.4	2.1–7.8	1.9–6.4
Male subjects						
Number	14	3	5	7	7	11
CBT 2-h CO_2						
Median value	6.9[d,e]	6.5[e,f]	7.1[g,d,e]	5.4[f]	4.3	3.5
Range	4.1–10.8	4.6–12.8	3.9–8.4	3.4–11.4	2.1–7.8	2.3–6.4
Female subjects						
Number	9	3	6	4	4	10
CBT 2-h CO_2						
Median value	6.3[d,e]	3.8	4.3	4.1	3.5	3.4
Range	2.6–10.7	3.6–5.6	3.4–6.0	3.5–7.0	2.4–5.2	1.9–6.3

Data reproduced from Lambert et al. (24) with permission.
[a] Healthy nonsmoking adults.
[b] Percent dose exhaled over 2 h.
[c] $p < 0.01$ versus pubertal stage V.
[d] $p < 0.01$ versus adult.
[e] $p < 0.05$ versus pubertal stage V.
[f] $p < 0.05$ versus adult.
[g] $p < 0.05$ versus same pubertal stage females.

supports the hypothesis that the decrease in warfarin plasma steady-state levels resulted from an increase in plasma-free fraction of warfarin by displacement of warfarin binding by phenylbutazone accompanied by a decrease in warfarin metabolism. The examination of substrate disappearance thus may be misleading and interpreted incorrectly.

Teunissen et al. (34) have demonstrated the advantage of not only using a steady-state model but using the change in metabolite production to examine alterations in drug metabolism resulting from drug interactions. In this study, osmotic minipumps containing antipyrine were used to achieve steady-state plasma levels of antipyrine and metabolites in humans. These investigators demonstrated that cimetidine administration increased antipyrine levels and decreased metabolite production, indicating that cimetidine inhibits the metabolism of antipyrine. Kuwahara et al. (6) described

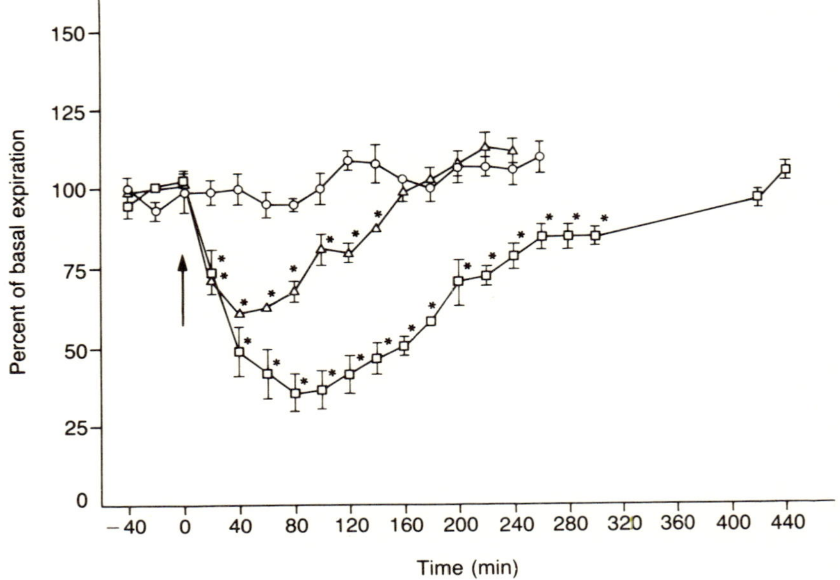

FIG. 20-3. Effect of cimetidine treatment on the aminopyrine infusion breath test. An osmotic minipump containing ^{14}C-aminopyrine was implanted sc into rats. The rats were treated with saline (○) 24 h later. The same rats were treated 48 h and 96 h later with cimetidine, 75 mg/kg (△) and 160 mg/kg (□), respectively. Points represent the mean ± SE of four rats. * indicates points significantly different from the basal rate of expiration determined 60 min before treatment. The arrow indicates the time of treatment.

a simple procedure capable of assessing the onset, magnitude, and duration of inhibition in small animals. Radiolabeled aminopyrine was constantly infused into a rat using an Alza osmotic minipump implanted subcutaneously. After implanting the minipump, a constant rate of expiration of ^{14}CO$_2$ was achieved in 24 h, and this rate was maintained for 6 days. The effects of cimetidine, an inhibitor of cytochrome P-450 mono-oxygenase activity, on the expiration of ^{14}CO$_2$ from aminopyrine were studied. Rats were administered 75 or 160 mg/kg of cimetidine intraperitoneally. Expired ^{14}CO$_2$ was collected continuously in 20-min intervals over the period of the study. Cimetidine administration resulted in a dose-related decrease in the time of onset of inhibition and resulted in an increase in the magnitude and duration of inhibition (Fig. 20-3). The rate of recovery from inhibition was similar at both doses. These findings suggest that the rates of absorption and elimination of cimetidine are similar at the two doses of cimetidine tested. This study demonstrates the potential of performing similar types of studies in humans using ^{13}C breath test substrates in humans.

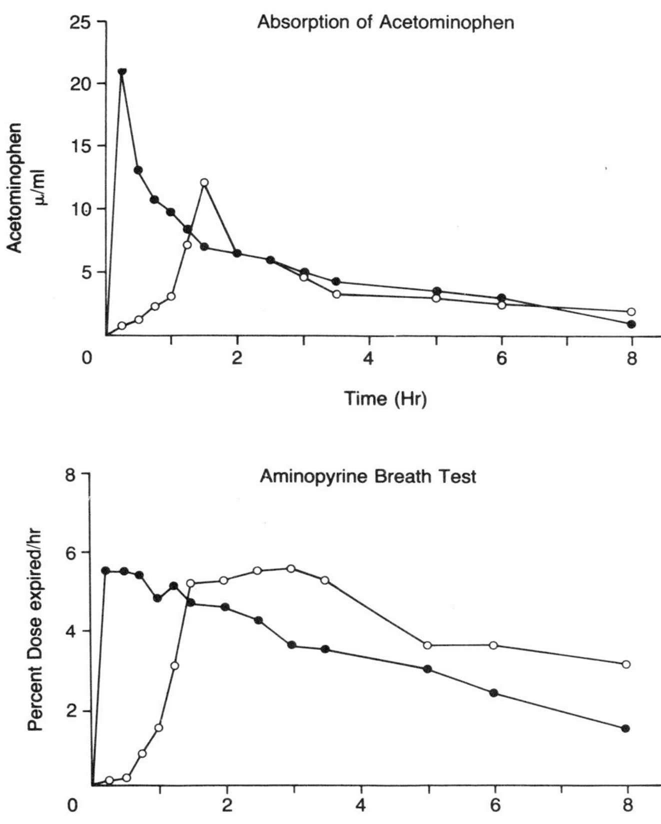

FIG. 20-4. Effect of codeine on the ABT and plasma levels of acetaminophen. A volunteer received a combination of ^{13}C-aminopyrine (2 mg/kg) and acetaminophen (600 mg), and samples of breath and plasma were taken for analysis of $^{13}CO_2$ and acetaminophen, respectively (●). Following a 1-week wash-out period, the same subject received 50 mg of codeine 60 min before receiving the test drugs (○).

CHANGES IN GASTRIC EMPTYING AND DRUG ABSORPTION

Nimmo et al. (35) have demonstrated that drug plasma-time profiles can be affected with the co-administration of drugs that effect gastric emptying. These studies were validated by examining the blood pharmacokinetic profiles of test drug alone and in the presence of an inhibitor of gastric emptying. To test the hypothesis that breath tests are amenable to identifying the effects of gastric emptying on drug absorption, a study combining the ABT with measurements of acetaminophen pharmacokinetic determination was performed alone and 1 h after the oral adminis-

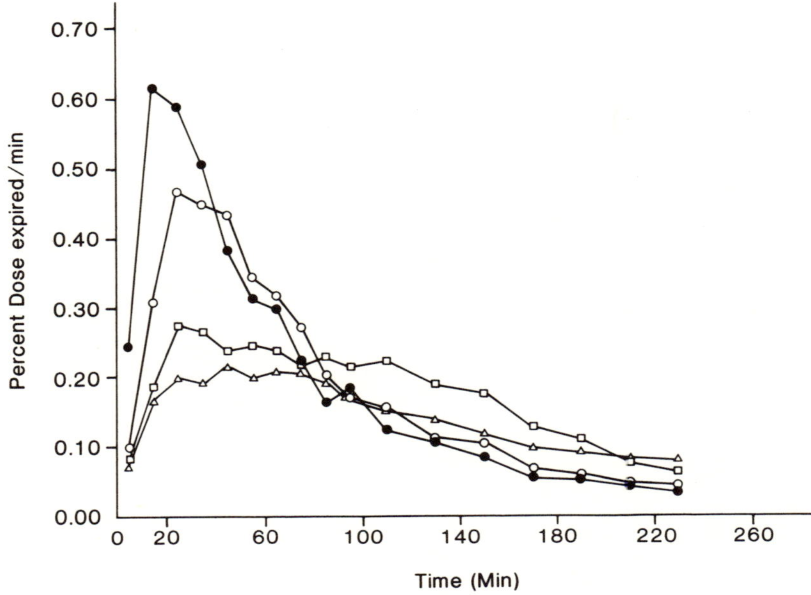

FIG. 20-5. Typical $^{14}CO_2$ expiration profiles following the oral administration of ^{14}C-aminopyrine dissolved in various combinations of water and PEG 400. Rats were treated with ^{14}C-aminopyrine (10 mg/kg) dissolved in 0% (●), 25% (○), 50% (□), or 100% (△) solutions of PEG 400. The volume administered was the same to each rat (10 ml/kg).

tration of 50 mg of codeine, a known inhibitor of gastric emptying (Fig. 20-4). Following the administration of ^{13}C aminopyrine and acetaminophen, breath $^{13}CO_2$ and plasma acetaminophen level peaked within 15 min of the administration, suggesting that gastric emptying and absorption of both agents were rapid. In contrast, pretreatment with codeine 1 h before the test resulted in delaying both the peak expiration of $^{13}CO_2$ and peak plasma levels of acetaminophen to 1.5 h after the administration of the test solution. Codeine had no discernible effects on the plasma acetaminophen and ABT elimination phases, which indicates that the metabolism of aminopyrine and acetaminophen was not affected by the co-administration of the three test agents.

It is generally assumed that the absorption of drugs following oral administration is more rapid and constant when administered as a solution. Thus, the biological effects of drugs with low water solubility are often studied by administering them dissolved in an aqueous mixture of propylene glycol-400 (PEG 400) or other excipients. We used the aminopyrine breath test to determine if PEG 400 affected the absorption and bioavailability of aminopyrine. The ABT was performed by administering aminopyrine in water, or in a solution of 25%, 50%, or 100% PEG 400 (10 ml/kg). Increasing the percentage of PEG 400 in the solution resulted in a concentration-related decrease in peak $^{14}CO_2$ expiration rate and the area under the curve (Fig. 20-5). If the PEG 400 solution was administered orally and the aminopyrine administered intraperitoneally, no decrease in peak rates or areas occurred compared to the oral administration of an equal volume of water. This study demonstrates that the decrease in peak rate is due to inhibition of the absorption of aminopyrine and not due to the inhibition of metabolism of aminopyrine by PEG 400. Thus, PEG 400 affects the absorption and bioavailability of aminopyrine and probably other drugs.

CONCLUSIONS

Premarketing studies designed to identify clinical drug interactions are costly and time consuming. The inclusion of such studies often delays marketing of the drug. Drug–drug interactions are usually identified only after a drug is marketed, and the absence of such studies to identify these interactions prior to marketing often results in unanticipated fatalities. Breath tests could be employed to identify these pharmacokinetic interactions, eliminating many of the objections to performing these studies. The advantages of the breath tests over classic methods are that they are safe, simple, rapid, and amenable to repetitive administration. Of secondary importance, these tests are adaptable to field use, since elaborate equipment is not required and samples are stable at room temperature for at least 6 months (36). At present, the major disadvantage of this test is the high technology required for the analysis of $^{13}CO_2$. However, recent advances in infrared spectroscopy now permit rapid and cost-effective analysis of $^{13}CO_2$ breath samples. The removal of this last obstacle may accelerate progress to develop additional stable isotope breath tests and to validate other applications.

REFERENCES

1. Hansten PD. Harmful drug-drug interactions. In: Maronde RF, ed. *Topics in Clinical Pharmacology and Therapeutics*. New York: Schatlauer-Verlag, 1986:382–96.
2. Hansten PD, Horn JR. The assessment of risk in the clinical outcome of drug interactions. *Drug Interactions Newsletter* 1986;6:21–6.
3. Medical letter. In: Abramowicz M., *et al.*, eds. *Drugs for Epilepsy*. New Rochelle: Medical Letter, Inc., 28:91–4.
4. Kutt H, Winters W, Kokenge R, McKowell F. Diphenylhydantoin metabolism, blood levels and toxicity. *Arch Neurol* 1964;11:642–8.
5. Baker AL, Kotake AN, Schoeller DA. Clinical utility of breath tests for assessment of hepatic function. *Semin Liver Dis* 1983;3:330–40.

6. Kuwahara SK, Schreider BD, Kotake AN. The aminopyrine (AP) infusion breath test (AIBT): a method for monitoring the inhibition profile of AP N-demethylation (APD) by SKF 525-A and cimetidine in rats. *Pharmacologist* 1986;28:136.

7. Lane EA, Parashos I. Drug pharmacokinetics and the carbon dioxide breath test. *J Pharmacokinet Biopharm* 1986;14:29–49.

8. Desmond PV, Patwardhan R, Parker S, Schenker S, Speeg KV. Effect of cimetidine and other antihistamines on the elimination of aminopyrine, phenacetin and caffeine. *Life Sci* 1980;26:1261–8.

9. Houston JB, Lockwood GF, Taylor G. Aminopyrine demethylation kinetics: use of metabolite exhalation rates as an index of enhanced mixed-function oxidase activity *in vivo*. *Drug Metab Dispos* 1981;9:449–55.

10. Kotake AN, Schreider BD, Latts J. The *in vivo* measurement of expired $^{14}CO_2$ derived from the N-demethylation of aminopyrine as a reflection of the *in vitro* hepatic cytochrome P-450 drug metabolism activity in rats. *Drug Metab Dispos* 1982;10:251–8.

11. Lauterburg BH, Bircher J. Expiratory measurement of maximal aminopyrine demethylation *in vivo:* effect of phenobarbital, partial hepatectomy, portocaval shunt and bile duct ligation in the rat. *J Pharmacol Exp Ther* 1976;196:501–9.

12. Speeg KV, Patwardhan RV, Avant GR, Mitchell MC, Schenker S. Inhibition of microsomal drug metabolism by histamine H_2-receptor antagonists studies *in vivo* and *in vitro* in rodents. *Gastroenterology* 1982;82:89–96.

13. Hepner GW, Vesell ES. Assessment of aminopyrine metabolism in man by breath analysis after administration of ^{14}C-aminopyrine. *N Engl J Med* 1974;291:1384–8.

14. Hepner GW, Vesell ES. Quantitative assessment of hepatic function by breath analysis after oral administration of [^{14}C]-aminopyrine. *Ann Intern Med* 1975;83:632–8.

15. Kotake AN, Scholler DA, Lambert GH, Baker AL, Schaffer DD, Josephs H. The caffeine CO_2 breath test: dose response and route of N-demethylation in smokers and nonsmokers. *Clin Pharmacol Ther* 1982;32:261–9.

16. Schoeller DA, Kotake AN, Lambert GH, Krager PS, Baker AL. Comparison of the phenacetin and aminopyrine breath tests: effect of liver disease, inducers and cobaltous chloride. *Hepatology* 1985;5:276–81.

17. Bruch M, Kling L, Legrum W, Maser E. The $^{14}CO_2$ breath test: facilities and limitations of a rapid and noninvasive method for *in vivo* evaluation of a modified hepatic cytochrome P-450—a critique. *Arch Toxicol* 1987;60:81–85.

18. Farag MM, Volicer L. Aminopyrine breath test and zonal hepatic damage in rats. *Pharmacology* 1985;31:309–17.

19. Hepner GW. Breath test in gastroenterology. *Adv Intern Med* 1978;18:25–45.

20. Hildebrandt AG, Roots I, Heinemeyer G, Nigram S, Helge H. Aminopyrine as one of the parameters to measure *in vivo* drug metabolism activity in man and animals. In: Estabrook RW, Lindenlaub E, eds. *The Induction of Drug Metabolism,* New York: Schatlauer Verlag, 1979:615–27.

21. Lambert GH, Kotake AN, Schoeller DA. The CO_2 breath test as a monitor of cytochrome P-450 dependent mix-function oxidase system. In: MacLeod SM, et al., eds. *Developmental Pharmacology,* New York: Alan R. List Inc., 1983:119–45.

22. Kotake AN, Lambert G, Schoeller DA, Baker AL. Differences in the response of cytochrome P-450 mediated caffeine and aminopyrine N-demethylation to rifampcin treatment in humans. II World Conference on *Clin Pharmacol Ther* 1983;109.

23. Kramer P, McClain CJ. Depression of aminopyrine metabolism by influenza vaccination. *N Engl J Med* 1981;305:1262–4.

24. Lambert GH, Schoeller DA, Kotake AN, Flores C, Hay D. The effect of age, gender and sexual maturation on the caffeine breath test. *Dev Pharmacol Ther* 1986;9:375–88.

25. Juan D, Worwag EM, Schoeller DA, Kotake AN, Hughes RL, Frederiksen MC. Effects of dietary protein on theophylline pharmacokinetics and caffeine and aminopyrine breath tests. *Clin Pharmacol Ther* 1986;40:187–94.

26. Lipton A, Hepner GW, White DS, Harvey HA. Decreased hepatic drug demethylation in patients receiving chemo-immunotherapy. *Cancer* 1978;41: 1680–4.

27. Kotake AN, Starr RM. The *in vivo* evaluation of the effect of age and sex on the developmental profile of aminopyrine N-demethylase activity in the newborn rat. *Drug Metab Dispos* 1982;10:259–63.

28. Lambert GH, Lietz H, Kotake AN. The effect of pregnancy on the P-450 system. *Biochem Pharmacol* 1987;36:1965–71.

29. Rating D, Jager-Roman E, Koch S, Nau H, Klein PD, Helge H. Enzymes induction in neonates due to antiepileptic therapy during pregnancy. In: Jantz D, et al., eds. *Epilepsy, Pregnancy and the Child.* New York: Raven Press, 1982: 349–55.

30. Guenther TM, Mannering GJ. Induction of hepatic mono-oxygenase systems fetal and neonatal rats with phenobarbital, polycyclic hydrocarbons and other xenobiotics. *Biochem Pharmacol* 1977;26:567–75.

31. Dameshek W, Colmes A. Aminopyrine hypersensitivity, with particular references to effect of drugs on production of agranulocytes. *J Clin Invest* 1936;15:85–97.

32. Saito H, Namenohur S, Kitagawa H, Ueno K, Sabai T. Induction of drug metabolizing enzymes by phenobarbital and embryotoxicity and teratogenicity of aminopyrine. *Res Commun Subst Abuse* 1980;1:63–277.

33. Schary WL, Lewis RJ, Rowland M. Warfarin-phenylbutazone interactions in man: a long term multiple dose study. *Res Commun Chem Pathol Pharmacol* 1975;10:663–72.

34. Teunissen MWE, Kleinbloesem CH, deLeede LGJ, Breimer PD. Influence of cimetidine on steady state concentrations on metabolite formation from antipyrine infused with a rectal osmotic minipump. *Eur J Clin Pharmacol* 1985;28:681–4.

35. Nimmo WS, Heading RC, Wilson J, Tothill P, Prescott LF. Inhibition of gastric emptying and drug absorption by narcotic analgesic. *Br J Clin Pharmacol* 1975;2:509–13.

36. Schoeller DA, Schneider JF, Solomon NW, Watkins JB, Klein PD. Clinical diagnosis with the stable isotope ^{13}C in CO_2 breath test: methodology and fundamental considerations. *J Lab Clin Med* 1977;90:412–21.

21

Alternative Approaches to the Prediction of Antiepileptic, Idiosyncratic, or Drug–drug Interactions

C. E. Pippenger, [1]Xianzhong Meng, and Frederick Van Lente

Department of Biochemistry, The Cleveland Clinic Foundation, Cleveland Ohio, U.S.A. and [1]Kashan Disease Institute, Harbin Medical College, Harbin, Peoples Republic of China

For decades there has been a continuous search for diagnostic test procedures capable of accurately predicting the potential adverse drug reaction index (ADRI) in any individual. Ideally, any ADRI procedure would be noninvasive, inexpensive, have a rapid analytical turnaround time, and have a high predictive value. The general topic of adverse drug reactions has been extensively reviewed (1–4). Antiepileptic drug interactions have also been extensively reviewed (5). For the purpose of this discussion, it is necessary to divide drug interactions into two categories.

DRUG–DRUG OR PHARMACOKINETIC INTERACTIONS

These interactions occur with the concomitant administration of two or more drugs. The most common drug–drug interactions are associated with decreased clearance rates and increased plasma concentrations of the drug whose clearance is being inhibited as a consequence of the drug–drug interaction. The elevated drug concentrations are usually associated with a change in the patient's clinical status, e.g., the development of clinical signs of drug intoxication. (Classic examples of a drug–drug interaction include the development of clinical phenytoin or carbamazepine drug intoxication following the administration of erythromycin or cimetidine.) Conversely, it is also possible that the simultaneous administration of multiple drugs may result in a decrease in total plasma drug concentrations rather than an increase. This phenomenon is usually associated with enhanced drug clearance rates that occur either by (a) a direct induction of microsomal enzymes responsible for a drug or (b) the displacement of a drug from its protein-binding site, which increases the free drug concentrations and causes an enhanced drug clearance.

The distinguishing feature between these two enhanced drug clearance interactions is the time course required for the development of the interaction. If the decreased plasma drug concentration is secondary to the induction of microsomal drug metabolizing enzymes, the change in plasma drug concentrations of the drug whose clearance rate is being enhanced is gradual. Drug concentration changes are dependent on the synthesis rate of additional microsomal drug-metabolizing enzymes, which takes place gradually over a period of weeks. This phenomenon is commonly referred to as induction or as autoinduction when a drug induces its own metabolism. Autoinduction is more pronounced with some drugs than others. Carbamazepine induces its own metabolism. Often within 1 week of carbamazepine therapy, plasma concentrations are optimal and seizure control is usually achieved in most patients. If the patient is maintained on the same mg/kg dose for 1 month, reanalysis of carbamazepine concentrations will be 40–50% lower than the original values. This decrease is secondary to the synthesis of additional carbamazepine metabolizing enzymes within the microsomal P-450 drug-metabolizing system. Since more enzyme is now available to metabolize the drug, the carbamazepine clearance rate increases and the plasma and tissue concentrations fall. Clinically, the previously well-controlled patient may experience breakthrough seizures as the plasma concentrations become suboptimal. Multiple drug therapy even with drugs that are not of the same class can also induce drug metabolizing enzyme concentrations and enhance drug clearance rates.

In contrast, if the drug interaction is the result of a drug's displacement from its protein-binding sites, the fall in the total plasma concentrations can be extremely rapid (within hours) as the displaced free drug is cleared. Under these circumstances, a new total and free steady-state drug concentration will be reached within five drug half-lives. The classic example of a protein-binding displacement interaction is observed following administration of valproic acid (VPA) to patients stabilized on phenytoin. VPA has greater affinity for the drug-binding sites on albumin than does phenytoin. VPA displaces phenytoin from its protein-binding sites, thus increasing the free plasma phenytoin concentrations. The displaced (free) phenytoin is now available to enter the heptocyte, where it is rapidly metabolized. Thus, the clearance rate of phenytoin is enhanced, and a new equilibrium between total and free phenytoin is established at lower total drug concentrations. Clinically, it is quite common to encounter a 30–50% drop in a patient's total phenytoin concentration within 24 h following the addition of VPA to the therapeutic regimen. VPA also displaces carbamazepine from its protein-binding sites, with a resultant increase in free carbamazepine concentrations to concentrations that may precipitate clinical carbamazepine toxicity in the patient.

Clinically, drug–drug interactions of any type may be characterized by either a dramatic or subtle change in the patient's clinical status. If the plasma concentration of an antiepileptic drug has increased, the end result will usually be the development of clinical signs of drug toxicity; conversely, if the antiepileptic drug concentration has decreased, one expects to see an exacerbation of seizures. Our clinical experience has taught us that when new antiepileptic drugs that inhibit drug metabolism or displace a drug from its protein-binding sites are added to a patient's therapeutic regimen, clinical signs of the drug–drug interaction are usually apparent within three to five half-lives of the drug whose clearance has been altered. Thus, patients who have erythromycin added to their carbamazepine therapy will begin to exhibit carbamazepine toxicity within 2–3 days following the institution of erythromycin therapy. In contrast, following the addition of a new antiepileptic drug that induces drug metabolism, we would not expect to see the clinical signs of induction until 3–4 weeks following the institution of the new drug therapy. At that time the patient may experience breakthrough seizures.

In summary, drug–drug interactions are easily identified, because there is usually a clear-cut clinical marker (the development of adverse side-effects or an exacerbation of the disease process) that indicates that a drug–drug interaction is occurring. Therefore, many drug–drug interactions can be identified simply by carefully monitoring a patient's clinical status before and after any change in their therapeutic regimen. Quantitation of the patient's drug concentrations identifies which drugs are interacting.

Once a drug–drug interaction has been identified, appropriate alteration of the patient's therapeutic regimen will eliminate the interaction, and the patient's clinical status will return to its previous level as the drug concentrations return to their previous values over a finite time interval. Ideally, one should be searching for ways to identify those drugs that are apt to precipitate drug–drug interactions prior to their addition to the patient's therapeutic regimen. Clearly, any new antiepileptic drug whose chemical structure and properties assure that its protein binding, hepatic metabolic pathways, or renal excretion patterns are similar to those of the currently marketed antiepileptic drugs would have the potential to precipitate a drug–drug interaction.

Let us assume that a new antiepileptic drug (Nosiez) was about to undergo a clinical trial. Nosiez is 90% protein-bound and has an aromatic ring that is hydroxylated during its metabolism. Nosiez has a greater affinity for the microsomal drug-metabolizing enzyme than phenytoin. When Nosiez is administered to a patient already receiving phenytoin, one would anticipate a Noisez-phenytoin interaction in which the patient would develop toxicity secondary to elevated phenytoin concentrations. In addition, one would anticipate that the addition of any co-medication known to interact with phenytoin (macrolide antibiotics, cimetidine, etc.) will also inhibit the metabolism of Nosiez, with the subsequent development of Nosiez toxicity. It is for this reason that patients' therapeutic regimens are kept constant during clinical trials. If during a clinical trial the patient becomes acutely ill and requires some other medication, that medication is always administered with the clinician's understanding that the potential for a drug–drug interaction occurrence is very high. The routine monitoring of drugs administered during a clinical trial is essential to identify which drugs are precipitating adverse drug effects.

IDIOSYNCRATIC DRUG INTERACTIONS

One of the major concerns about any new drug entering into a clinical trial is the investigator's constant fear that the drug will produce a severe idiosyncratic drug interaction. The clinical hallmark of idiosyncratic drug reactions is that they usually occur without any warning. There is no correlation between the patient's prior clinical status, drug dose, or plasma drug concentrations and the adverse reaction. It is generally accepted that idiosyncratic reactions are most likely to occur early during the course of new drug therapy. Therefore, the clinician is taught to be especially vigilant during the first few weeks or months following introduction of a new drug into the patient's regimen. However, an idiosyncratic reaction can occur at any time during the course of therapy. The hepatotoxicity or acute pancreatitis associated with VPA therapy has been reported to occur 1 month to 4.5 years after a patient has been placed on therapy. Thus, the potential for any drug to present with an adverse idiosyncratic reaction at any time must always be remembered.

One of the most common idiosyncratic reactions is the appearance of "drug rashes." However, different types of idiosyncratic drug interactions can occur at different times in the same patient. We are all aware of the VPA idiosyncratic interactions, which range from the undesirable but nonlife-threatening alopecia to fatal hepatotoxicity. These interactions are concisely summarized in the report of Dreifuss et al. (6).

It is possible for a patient to experience multiple idiosyncratic reactions simultaneously or sequentially. The underlying mechanisms of each idiosyncratic reaction can be strikingly variable, depending on the physiological or biochemical system involved in the reaction. Thus, the VPA-produced hyperammonemia, alopecia, and acute pancreatitis or hepatotoxicity are all idiosyncratic drug reactions, each initiated by alterations of different physiological and/or biochemical systems. It is generally believed that the increased blood ammonia concentrations following valproate therapy are related to an alteration of carnitine catabolism, whereas the mechanisms for the development of acute pancreatitis or hepatotoxicity appear to be unrelated to elevated blood ammonia concentrations. Valproate-induced alopecia is probably related to a marginal zinc deficiency that occurs in some patients during valproate therapy.

For decades we have been searching for analytical techniques that would allow identification of those patients who are at risk to develop idiosyncratic drug reactions while receiving any drug therapy. Ideally, one would like to be in a position where a series of biochemical or physiological tests could establish whether or not patients are at risk to develop an idiosyncratic reaction prior to the time they are placed on a specific therapeutic regimen. To date, the achievement of this goal has remained elusive, because our understanding of the mechanisms that precipitate idiosyncratic reactions remains obscure. Clearly, we must search for new and unique techniques that will allow us to identify those patients who are at risk to develop idiosyncratic and/or drug–drug interactions. The following sections present approaches to predict adverse drug reactions before they occur.

WAYS TO IDENTIFY POTENTIAL DRUG–DRUG INTERACTIONS INCLUDING PHENOTYPING

The marked individual variability in both the pharmacokinetic and pharmacodynamic response to drugs is well established (1–4). There is a multimodal distribution of drug clearance rates across the general population. Genetic influences can modify the drug responses observed in a given patient. Extensive population studies have clearly demonstrated that the marked interindividual variability in drug clearance rates is under genetic control. Genetic differences in drug clearance occur not only between individuals, but also between different ethnic groups (7). (For example, Orientals are rapid acetylators, whereas blacks and Caucasians are slow acetylators.)

One approach to identifying those individuals who are at risk to develop adverse drug–drug interactions following the administration of a new drug is to phenotype drug clearance patterns in individual patients. The distinct advantage in phenotyping individuals, particularly prior to their entrance into a new drug clinical trial, is the ability to predict where within the general population that patient's drug clearance pattern falls. If that patient is a slow drug metabolizer and the trial drug is cleared through a metabolic pathway similar to that of other administered drugs, it should be possible to optimize the trial drug dosage to maintain optimum drug concentrations. Identification of a slow drug metabolizer allows the clinical investigator to initiate new drug therapy at a lower dose while still maintaining optimal drug concentrations. Thus, the potential for the precipitation of a drug–drug interaction or development of toxic drug concentrations and clinical toxicity in the slow drug metabolizer is reduced.

Identification of the patient who phenotypically is a fast drug metabolizer allows the clinical investigator to quickly increase the trial drug dose to achieve optimal concentrations. A fast drug metabolizer who is placed on standard doses of a trial drug and fails to achieve the desired therapeutic response will be classified a therapeutic failure. Too often fast metabolism is unrecognized; thus, the trial drug fails its efficacy trials. In clinical trials where fast metabolizers are placed on an appropriate (increased) maintenance dose of the trial drug, the patient may very well become a therapeutic success.

Clearly, the ability to phenotype patients prior to their entry into a new drug clinical trial allows the clinical investigator to provide better medical management of patients with altered drug clearance rates. Phenotyping also insures that the experimental drug receives a fair clinical evaluation. Unfortunately, the routine phenotyping of patients prior to the administration of an experimental drug is not standard practice today.

There are two approaches to phenotyping patients prior to the administration of a new antiepileptic drug. The most logical and least expensive approach is determining the pharmacokinetic profiles of the antiepileptic drugs that the patient is currently receiving so as to establish the patient's phenotype. Today, numerous computer programs exist that calculate the various pharmacokinetic parameters (elimination constants, half-life, volume of distribution, etc.) based on the quantitation of 2–3 drug concentrations within a dosing interval. The advantages to phenotyping individual patients prior to their clinical trial entry include: (a) the development of baseline pharmacokinetic data that can be compared to pharmacokinetic data for the same drugs while the patient is receiving the trial drug; if changes in the pharmacokinetic profile occur, the direction of the change is easily identified; (b) dosages of the trial drug can be individualized to compensate for individual variability in drug clearance; (c) the pharmacokinetic profiling does not require specialized informed consent; and (d) the cost of the phenotyping is minimal.

An alternative but less desirable approach would be to administer a test compound (antipyrine, debrisoquine, dapsone, or mephenytoin) that has been classically utilized to phenotype individuals in various pharmacokinetic population studies. For example, numerous phenotyping studies of hydroxylation capacity have been performed utilizing a test dose of debrisoquine. The disadvantages of utilizing test doses of phenotyping drugs include: (a) they are limited to specific metabolic pathways (e.g., dapsone to acetylation and debrisoquine to hydroxylation, mephenytoin to demethylation and hydroxylation); (b) the quantitation of plasma concentrations of the phenotyping drugs require special analytical procedures that are not readily available in most medical centers; specialized analytical techniques are expensive; (c) specific protocols for phenotyping usually require 5–6 serial drug concentrations and are considered experimental; thus, specialized informed consent is required; and (d) the correlation between the kinetics of a test compound may not necessarily agree with those of administered drugs if the test compound is metabolized by a different isoenzyme of the cytochrome P-450 system.

There are, however, some novel approaches to phenotyping individuals that would be readily applicable in most medical centers. Recent evidence suggests that administration of a test dose of an over-the-counter drug can be utilized to phenotype drug metabolism (8). Phenotyping with these compounds is certainly worth further study in the epileptic patient receiving antiepileptic drug therapy or any patient about to enter a new drug clinical trial. The commonly prescribed analgesic, phenacetin, has the distinct advantage of being metabolized through multiple pathways. It is acetylated to acetaminophen, which is then hydroxylated. Therefore, administration of a standard analgesic dose of phenacetin with monitoring of the plasma concentrations may provide a unique approach to the phenotyping of an individual with respect to both their hydroxylation and acetylation capacity. High-pressure liquid chromatography is utilized to quantitate phenacetin and its metabolites. The advantage of phenacetin phenotyping lies in its ready recognition by all patients as a safe drug.

Alternatively, caffeine is another drug whose potential application as a diagnostic tool is just beginning to be recognized (9–12). A number of studies have demonstrated its value in assessing hepatic function. Caffeine has the distinct advantage of being metabolized through a series of demethylation steps via the xanthine oxidase pathways that is a cytochrome P-448 enzyme. It has been suggested that changes in P-448 enzyme activity parallel changes in P-450 enzyme activity. Caffeine clearance can be assessed simply by giving a patient a fixed caffeine dose in the form of a caffeine beverage (Pepsi-Cola, Coca-Cola, or coffee).

The major advantage of caffeine phenotyping lies in the potential to perform caffeine clearance tests in a noninvasive format (12). In brief, a test dose of caffeine as Pepsi-Cola, Coca-Cola, or coffee is administered to the patient at time zero. Three and 6 h after the test dose, the patient provides a salivary specimen by chewing a disposable collection device for quantitation of caffeine concentrations. The availability of an enzyme mediated immunoassay technique EMIT (Syva Co., Palo Alto, Calif.) for quantitative caffeine determination makes this procedure applicable in any laboratory. Since this procedure is noninvasive, is inexpensive, and utilizes a common over-the-counter preparation at safe doses, informed consent is not required. We would suggest that routine monitoring of caffeine clearance at regular intervals throughout any new drug clinical trial could serve as a marker for altered hepatic drug metabolism.

In summary, there are clear advantages to phenotyping the drug clearance pattern of any patient who is entering a new drug clinical trial during the baseline period. The easiest and most cost-effective method is to phenotype the individual patient by establishing the clearance rates of the patient's currently administered antiepileptic drugs. In addition, there are distinct advantages to determining the patient's caffeine clearance rate as a phenotype for those drugs where a direct relationship between the plasma drug concentration and its pharmacodynamic effects exist. Phenotyping has the distinct and clinically relevant advantage of allowing the clinical investigator to identify patients who are at risk to fail a clinical trial secondary to altered pharmacokinetic profiles. Slow drug metabolizers, who are apt to develop clinical side-effects, and fast drug metabolizers, who may fail to achieve a therapeutic response following the administration of standard doses of that drug, can be easily identified. Unfortunately, patient phenotyping has no clinical utility in predicting which patients are going to develop idiosyncratic drug reactions.

BIOCHEMICAL PHENOTYPING TO PREDICT IDIOSYNCRATIC DRUG REACTIONS

Recently, we have witnessed significant advances in our understanding of both the physiological and pathophysiological role of oxygen free radicals in the maintenance of cellular integrity. While the bulk of this work has been performed in relation to cardiac myopathies, myocardial ischemia, and reperfusion injury, there is evidence suggesting free radicals play a role in producing the cellular damage associated with certain types of antiepileptic drug toxicity. Spielberg et al. (13) demonstrated membrane tissue damage to leukocyte cell cultures exposed to phenytoin. They attributed the damage to the binding of a postulated phenytoin epoxide intermediate, which is formed during the metabolism of phenytoin to p-hydroxyphenytoin, to the cell membrane. Recent evidence suggests the cellular damage associated with VPA-induced hepatotoxicity may be directly related to the enhanced microsomal metabolism of VPA to a series of -ene- compounds (14). The synthesis of valproate -ene- metabolites requires an unstable epoxide intermediate whose decomposition is associated with the release of free radicals.

We believe that an increase in cellular free radical concentrations can precipitate irreversible cellular damage that presents clinically as an idiosyncratic drug reaction. It follows that the mechanisms that normally protect the body against the accumulation of excessive free radical concentrations may be deficient in those patients who develop an idiosyncratic drug reaction. Under these circumstances, a patient would not develop an idiosyncratic drug reaction until the total body (or cellular) burden of free radical production exceeds the capacity of the body (or cells) to inactivate the free radicals.

Oxidation and reduction are fundamental chemical reactions in all mammalian cells. Oxygen is absolutely necessary for cell survival. However, oxygen has two faces, one benign and the other malignant. Some reduced oxygen intermediates (free radicals), produced through univalent and trivalent reduction of molecular oxygen, are highly toxic to mammalian cells as well as other life forms (1–2).

Recent reviews of those enzymes involved in the maintenance of cellular integrity by preventing the excessive accumulation of free radicals are available (15–20).

There are two pathways for the reduction of oxygen to water in mammalian cells: (a) Mitochondrial enzymes are capable of reducing oxygen to water by tetravalent reduction without the production of oxygen intermediates. (b) Under physiological conditions, 59% of the cellular oxygen consumption proceeds by a univalent pathway resulting in the formation of several oxygen intermediates (20). Toxic oxygen intermediates include the superoxide ion ($.O_2^-$), hydrogen peroxide (H_2O_2), and the hydroxyl radical ($.OH$). Hess and Manson (21) have outlined the pathways for the production of oxygen free radicals as follows:

	$2e^-$	$2e^- + 2H + 2H^+$		$e^- + H^+$	
$2O_2$	$2 \cdot O_2^-$		H_2O_2	H_2O	$\cdot OH$

Molecular oxygen has two unpaired electrons in its ground state. Therefore, the univalent reduction pathway is preferred. With the acceptance of the first electron, molecular oxygen is reduced to $.O_2^-$. ($.O_2^-$ is commonly referred to as the superoxide ion.) This free radical readily undergoes spontaneous or enzymatic degradation dismutation, forming H_2O_2. The production of $.OH$ can result from the further reduction of H_2O_2 by glutathione peroxidase to water.

It is known that oxygen intermediates, especially $.OH$, can quickly react with a variety of organic compounds present in cells. Oxygen-free radicals can bind to unsaturated fatty acid side-chains in biomembranes, initiating a chain reaction that results in the peroxidation of membrane lipids. (22, 23). Oxygen free radicals can oxidize sulfhydryl (SH) groups present in membrane proteins. This oxidation of SH groups changes the protein's three-dimensional conformation, resulting in an increase in membrane fluidity and permeability. Thus, free radicals damage cells by destroying their structural and functional integrity. The toxic effects of oxygen free radicals on membrane proteins has been reviewed by Kato (24).

Under normal physiological conditions, there is no opportunity for oxygen free radicals to accumulate, because cells possess specific defense systems against oxygen toxicity. Among these defenses, the free radical scavenging enzymes (antioxidant enzymes) are the most important.

In 1969, McCord and Fridovich (25) identified the enzymatic activity of superoxide dismutase (SOD) in bovine erythrocytes. SOD catalyzes the dismutation of $.0_2{}^-$ at a rate that is 10^9 times faster than the spontaneous dismutation of oxygen (26). To date, two SOD isoenzymes have been identified in mammalian cells: (a) an SOD enzyme containing copper–zinc is present in the cytosol, and (b) an SOD enzyme containing manganese is present in mitochondria (27). SOD is responsible for scavenging superoxide radicals. Therefore, SOD serves as the first line of defense against the formation and accumulation of toxic, oxygen free radicals by converting them to H_2O_2.

The H_2O_2 (a cellular toxin) produced by the dismutation of superoxide radicals is converted to water by the enzymes catalase and glutathione peroxidase. Catalase, a cytoplasmic heme-enzyme, catalyzes the divalent reduction of H_2O_2 to water (28). Since cellular catalase concentrations are a thousand times higher than any other free radical scavenging enzyme, it may be visualized as the first-line defense against H_2O. Glutathione peroxidase (GSH-PX) may represent the backup (fail-safe) defense line against H_2O_2 in case the catalase fails.

GSH-PX is a selenium-dependent enzyme (29) present in cytosol. GSH-PX metabolizes H_2O_2 to water through the oxidation of reduced glutathione. The cellular supply of reduced glutathione, the substrate necessary for GSH-PX activity, is supplied by another enzyme, glutathione reductase (30), which, by converting oxidized glutathione to reduced glutathione, assures that a constant supply of substrate is available to maintain GSH-PX activity at its maximum level.

Therefore, glutathione reductase may play a more important role than catalase in the protection of cells against oxygen-free, radical-mediated injury. Recently, a GSH-PX enzyme that does not require selenium as a co-factor has been identified (31). This enzyme selectively scavenges organic peroxides (rather than H_2O_2) (32). Some evidence suggests this enzyme may actually be glutathione-S-transferase (33).

There is no direct enzymatic defense system specific for scavenging hydroxyl radicals, the most toxic oxygen intermediates. In cells, the other free radical defense systems are present in sufficient excess to scavenge free radicals prior to their conversion to hydroxyl radicals. Thus, cellular damage initiated by hydroxyl radicals is prevented by scavenging the precursors necessary for hydroxyl radical generation.

The balance between the production and catabolism of oxygen-free radicals in cells is critical for the maintenance of cellular integrity. A pathophysiological process would be induced if the defense systems against oxygen toxicity were defective or overwhelmed. Recently, much attention has been paid to the potential role of oxygen free radicals and antioxidant enzymes in some pathological processes, especially those related to myocardial ischemia and reperfusion cellular injuries. Increasing evidence has implicated oxygen free radicals in the development and progression of ischemia and reperfusion injury in myocardium. This subject has been extensively reviewed (21, 34).

As indicated above, there are numerous factors that regulate the activity of free radical scavenging enzymes. Of particular importance to the normal functioning of the free radical system is the presence of trace elements as co-factors for the enzymes glutathione, peroxidase, and superoxide dismutase. GSH-PX is dependent on selenium as the major activating co-factor for its enzymatic activity. Cytoplasmic SOD is dependent on both copper and zinc as co-factors. Mitochondrial SOD is dependent on manganese for its activity. Any factor that depletes cellular trace element concentrations will ultimately result in a decreased activity of the free radical enzyme scavenging systems.

It is also important to recognize that the absolute concentration of free radical scavenging enzymes in any given patient within the general population is genetically controlled. Each cell has an excess of free radical scavenging enzymes. However, the degree of excess varies within the population. The free radical scavenging enzyme activity in children is less than it is in adults.

Based on the above observations, we decided to investigate the interrelationships between free radical scavenging enzyme activity and antiepileptic drug therapy. To our knowledge, this is the first study describing these interrelationships.

We have compared the trace element concentrations and free radical enzyme system activity in a group of epileptic patients receiving various combinations of antiepileptic drug therapy to controls who were not receiving antiepileptic drugs. The enzymatic activities of GSH-PX, SOD, catalase, glutathione reductase, and glutathione transferase were measured by previously described techniques (25, 28, 30, 33). The whole blood concentrations of selenium, copper, zinc, and manganese were quantitated by atomic absorption spectroscopy. The results of this pilot study are preliminary. However, it is of particular interest to note that those patients receiving VPA had decreased GSH-PX activity when compared to normal controls and to those patients receiving other antiepileptic drugs. Valproate-treated patients also had lower whole blood selenium, copper, and zinc concentrations but higher manganese concentrations. There is a direct correlation between whole blood selenium concentration and GSH-PX activity. The higher the selenium concentration, the greater the glutathione peroxidase activity. In addition, all of the patients who were receiving VPA monotherapy had selenium concentrations that were below or at the lower limits of the general population mean. In contrast, those patients receiving carbamazepine had higher than normal glutathione transferase activity.

We recently had the opportunity to investigate the free radical enzyme scavenging activity in a 5-year-old female who had been treated over the past 2-year period with VPA for intractable myoclonic seizures. Throughout the course of her therapy, she has had intermittent acute pancreatitis attacks at 4–6 month intervals. No other antiepileptic therapy was successful in controlling her seizures; therefore, she was maintained on VPA. Whenever she had an acute pancreatitis attack, VPA was discontinued until the pancreatitis resolved. Valproate therapy was reinstituted when her seizures recurred.

During a recent acute pancreatitis attack, the following laboratory values were obtained: Total VPA concentration was 123.7 μg/ml, free VPA concentration was 22.3 μg/ml. Serum amylase was 220 IU/L (normal = 10–135 IU/L) and lipase was 511 IU/L (normal = 20–85 IU/L). A second series of blood specimens was drawn 21 days later, when the acute pancreatitis had subsided, and valproate therapy had been reinstituted. Total valproic concentration was 75.9 μg/ml, and free VPA concentration was 9.4 μg/ml. Amylase was 110 IU/L, and lipase was 106 IU/ml. On a whole blood specimen obtained at the same time, we analyzed the free radical scavenging enzyme activity with the following results: GSH-PX was 30.2 IU/g Hb (normal = 34.6 ± 3.5 IU/g Hb), catalase was 14.6×10^3 U/g Hb (normal = $15.4 ± 1.8 \times 10^3$ U/g Hb), superoxide dismutase was 1708 U/g Hb (normal = 2465 + 352 U/g Hb), glutathione reductase was 6.3 IU/g Hb (normal = 6.6 ± 1.0 IU/g Hb), and glutathione transferase was 0.93 IU/g Hb (normal = 1.44 ± 0.57 IU/g Hb). In addition, we measured her serum lipid peroxide concentration, which was 1.3 nmol MDA/ml (normal = 1.1 ± 0.3 nmol MDA/ml). Serum lipid peroxide concentration is considered to be an index of tissue damage secondary to binding of free radicals to cell membranes and the induction of lipid peroxidation associated with free radical interaction with cell membranes.

To our knowledge, this is the first reported case of the free radical scavenging enzyme activity in a patient following valproate-induced acute pancreatitis.

Based on a series of studies carried out in the isolated perfused rabbit pancreas preparation, Sanfey et al. (35) have proposed a mechanism for the generation of acute pancreatitis. Utilizing an isolated perfused canine pancreas model, they defined acute pancreatitis as occurring when the perfusing solution contained elevated concentrations of amalyse and lipase released secondary to cellular damage. Regardless of whether the acute pancreatitis was precipitated by either a high fatty acid load, a 2-h period of ischemia, or partial duct obstruction with secretion stimulation, the pancreatitis could be prevented by perfusing the pancreas with a solution containing either catalase, or superoxide dismutase, or both. The authors concluded that the underlying mechanism for the initiation of the acute pancreatitis was the generation of an excessive free radical burden on the pancreas, regardless of the technique utilized to initiate pancreatitis in their model.

Further support for the importance of free radical scavenging enzyme activity is provided by the studies dealing with the generation of postperfusion ischemic damage and reperfusion injury associated with coronary bypass surgery. In experimental dogs, Rao et al. (22) established that the addition of superoxide dismutase to the cardiac perfusion solution decreased the amount of ischemic damage that occurred following reperfusion. These studies support the concept that a given level of enzyme activity is necessary to scavenge free radicals in order to prevent their interaction with tissue membranes to produce cellular damage.

The availability of free radical scavenging enzyme systems throughout every cell in the body is a defense mechanism to assure the stabilization and integrity of cell membranes. Generally, these enzymatic systems are present in large excessive concentrations in order to assure that the cell is in a stable environment. The absolute concentration of free radical scavenging enzymes present in cells is genetically determined and varies from individual to individual. Free radical scavenging enzyme activity in an individual can be altered by various factors, some of which remain to be elucidated. We do know that age and nutritional status play a major role in regulating free radical scavenging enzyme activity. GSH-PX activity is age-dependent. The younger the individual, the less free radical scavenging systems present in proportion to body size. The role of nutritional status in regulating free radical scavenging enzyme activity has been demonstrated. The decreased GSH-PX activity in residents of New Zealand has been linked to their selenium-deficient diet. Patients with Keshan's disease, a fatal cardiac myopathy, is limited to certain areas of China, where the population is selenium-deficient, and GSH-PX activity is also decreased. Zinc and copper deficiencies have been associated with decreased SOD activity in experimental animals. Unfortunately, population studies of SOD and other free radical scavenging enzyme activity in relation to nutritional status are not available.

Failure of the free radical scavenging system is dependent on a combination of factors occurring together. These factors include (a) a genetically determined low absolute concentration of free radical scavenging enzymes, (b) an increased amount of free radical production with the cells, and (c) a cellular lack of sufficient enzymatic activity within the free radical scavenging system that prevents the cell from compensating for the increased free radical burden. When all of these factors are present in a given patient at any time, the probability that the patient will develop an idiosyncratic drug reaction increases significantly. Fortunately, these factors rarely occur at the same time in a given patient. It is for this reason that idiosyncratic drug reactions rarely occur in the general population.

REFERENCES

1. Gilman AG, Goodman LS, Rall TW, Murand F, eds. *The Pharmalogical Basis of Therapeutics.* 7th ed. New York: Macmillan, 1985.
2. Speight TM (ed). *Avery's Drug Treatment.* Auckland, New Zealand: Adis Press, 1987.
3. Katcher BS, Young LY, Koda-Kimble MA, eds. *Applied Therapeutics.* 3rd ed. Spokane, WA: Applied Therapeutics, 1983.
4. Evans WE, Schentag JJ, Jusko WJ, eds. *Applied Pharmacokinetics.* 2nd ed. Spokane, WA: Applied Therapeutics, 1986.
5. Woodbury DM, Perry JK, Pippenger CE, eds. *Antiepileptic Drugs.* 2nd ed. New York: Raven Press, 1982.
6. Dreifuss FE, Santilli N, Langer DH, Sweeney KP, Moline KA, Menandez KB. Valproic acid hepatic fatalities: a retrospective review. *Neurology* 1987;37:379–85.
7. Kalow W, Goedde HW, Agarwal DP, eds. *Ethic Differences in Reactions to Drugs and Xenobiotics.* New York: Alan R. Liss, 1986.
8. Clark DWJ. Genetically determined variability in acetylation and oxidation. *Drugs* 1985;29:342–75.
9. Renner E, Wietholz H, Huguenin P, Arnaud MK, Presig R. Caffeine: a model compound for measuring liver function. *Hepatology* 1984;4:38–46.
10. Desmond PV, Patwardhan RV, Johnson RF, Schenker S. Impaired elimination of caffeine in cirrhosis. *Dig Dis Sci* 1980;25:193–7.
11. Wahllander A, Renner E, Presig R. Fasting plasma caffeine concentration: a guide to the severity of chronic liver disease. *Scand J Gastroenterol* 1985;20:1133–41.
12. Jost G, Wahllander A, von Mandach U, Presig R. Overnight salivary caffeine clearance: a liver function test suitable for routine use. *Hepatology* 1987;7:338–44.
13. Spielberg SP, Gordon GB, Blake DA, Mellits BE, Bross DS. Anticonvulsant in vitro: possible role of arene oxides. *J Pharmacol Exp Ther* 1981;217:386–9.
14. Rettie AE, Rettenmeir AW, Howland WN, Baillie TA. Cytochrome P-450-catalyzed formation of delta-4-VPA. A toxic metabolite of valproic acid. *Science* 1987;235:890–3.
15. Singal PK, ed. *Oxygen Radicals in the Pathophysiology of Heart Disease.* Boston: Kluwer Academic Publishers, 1988.
16. Halliwell B, ed. *Oxygen Radicals and Tissue Injury.* Proceedings of a Brook Lodge Symposium, Augusta, Michigan, April 1987. Kalamazoo, MI: The Upjohn Company, 1988.
17. Southorn PA, Powis G. Free radicals in medicine I. Chemical nature and biologic reactions. *Mayo Clin Proc* 1988;63:381–389.
18. Southorn PA and Powis G. Free radicals in medicine II. Involvement in Husman disease. *Mayo Clin Proc* 1988;63:390–408.

19. McCord JM, Fridovich I. The biology and pathology of oxygen radicals. *Ann Intern Med* 1978;89:122–7.
20. Fridovich I. The biology of oxygen radicals. *Science* 1978;201:875–80.
21. Hess ML, Manson NH. Molecular oxygen: friend and foe. The role of the oxygen free radical system in the calcium paradox, the oxygen paradox and ischemia/reperfusion injury. *J Mol Cell Cardiol* 1984;16:969–85.
22. Rao PS, Cohen MV, Mueller HS. Production of free radicals and lipid peroxides in early experimental myocardial ischemia. *J Mol Cell Cardiol* 1963;15:713–6.
23. Thomas MJ, Mehl KS, Pryor WA. The role of the superoxide anion in the xanthine oxidase-induced autoxidation of linoleic acid. *Biochem Biophys Res Commun* 1978;83:927–32.
24. Kako KJ. Free radical effects on membrane protein in myocardial ischemia/reperfusion injury. *J Mol Cell Cardiol* 1987;19:209–11.
25. McCord JM, Fridovich I. Superoxide dismutase. *J Biol Chem* 1969;244:6049–55.
26. Fridovich I. Superoxide dismutases. *Ann Rev Biochem* 1975;44:147–55.
27. Weisiger RA, Fridovich I. Superoxide dismutase. *J Biol Chem* 1973;248:3582–92.
28. Aviram I, Shaklai N. The association of human erythrocyte catalase with the cell membrane. *Arch Biochem Biophys* 1981;212:329–37.
29. Rotruck JT. Selenium: biochemical role as a component of glutathione peroxidase. *Science* 1973;179:588–90.
30. Chang JC, Van Der Hoevan LH, Haddox CH. Glutathione reductase in the red blood cells. *Ann Clin Lab Sci* 1978;8:23–9.
31. Ursini F, Maiorino M, Gregolin C. The selenoenzyme phospholipid hydroperoxide glutathione peroxidase. *Biochim Biophys Acta* 1985;839:62–70.
32. Shreve MR, Morrissey PG, O'Brien PJ. Lipid and steroid hydroperoxides as substrates for the non-selenium-dependent glutathione peroxidase. *Biochem J* 1979;177:761–3.
33. Chasseaud LF. The role of glutathione and glutathione s-transferases in the metabolism of chemical carcinogens and other electrophilic agents. *Adv Cancer Res* 1979;29:175–244.
34. Thompson JA, Hess ML. The oxygen free radical system: a fundamental mechanism in the production of myocardial necrosis. *Prog Cardiovasc Dis* 1986;28:449–62.
35. Sanfey H, Bulkley GB, Cameron JL. The role of oxygen derived free radicals in the pathogenesis of acute pancreatitis. *Ann Surg* 1984;200:405–13.

22

Development of Anticonvulsant Drugs: Extrapolation of Dispositional Profiles from Animals to Man

Richard M. Welch, [1]Derrick N. Parsons, and James B. Hubbell

The Wellcome Research Laboratories, Research Triangle Park, North Carolina, U.S.A.; and [1]Wellcome Research Laboratories, Langley Court, Beckenham, Kent, U.K.

Although considerable effort is spent on the design and screening of new therapeutic agents, many promising compounds become identified as failures too late in their clinical development because of incomplete information on disposition in animals early in their discovery. Experience indicates that information regarding metabolism and disposition is essential for a complete pharmacological and toxicological evaluation. In fact, the absence of such information often results in misleading or inaccurate conclusions regarding safety and efficacy. This is particularly evident when developing antiepileptic drugs (AEDs). This communication describes past experiences with a few pharmacologically active anticonvulsants that were not clinically useful because they were metabolized too rapidly, or because they provided an unacceptable pharmacokinetic profile in man. In most cases, more comprehensive disposition studies in animals might have uncovered these deficiencies prior to their clinical evaluation in man.

Cinromide was shown to have a wide spectrum of anticonvulsant activity in animals (1) but failed to show efficacy as an anticonvulsant in man. In rats, cinromide was shown to be metabolized to 3-bromocinnamic acid and 3-bromocinnamamide (Fig. 22-1). These metabolites appeared as ma-

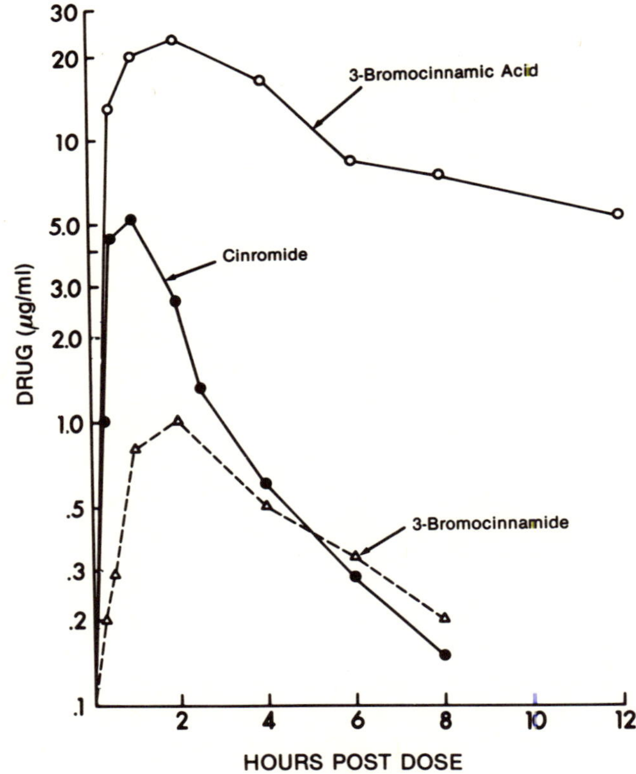

FIG. 22-1. Plasma metabolites of cinromide in animals and man.

FIG. 22-2. Mean plasma levels of cinromide and its major metabolites in rats after an oral dose of 26 mg/kg (ED$_{50}$).

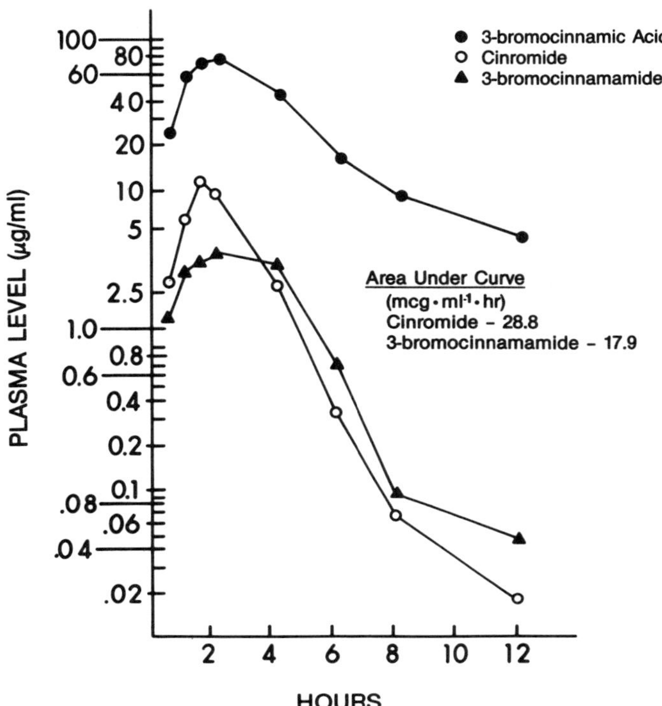

FIG. 22-3. Mean plasma levels of cinromide and its major metabolites in beagle dogs after an oral dose of 100 mg/kg of cinromide.

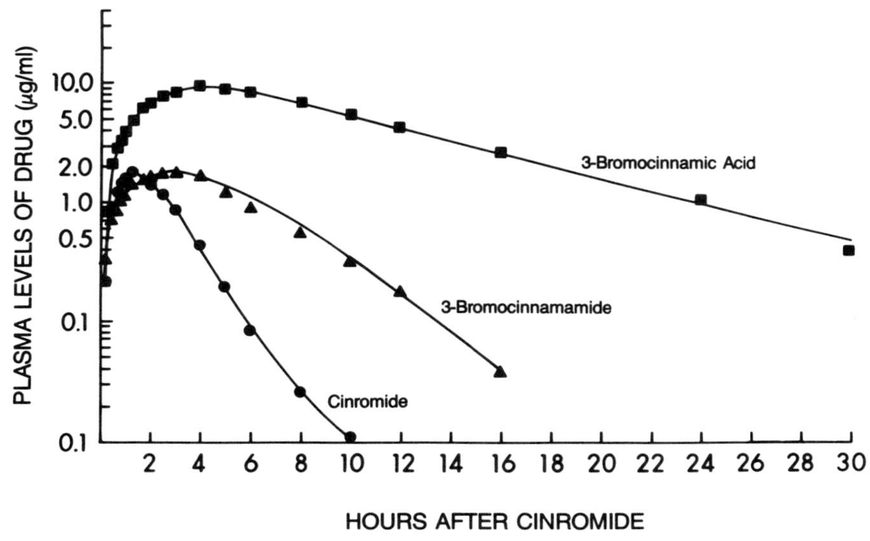

FIG. 22-4. Mean plasma levels of cinromide and its major metabolites in man after an oral dose of 300 mg of cinromide.

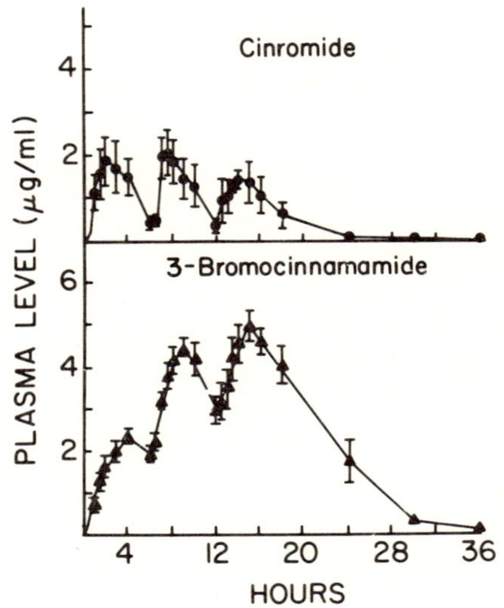

FIG. 22-5. Mean plasma levels of cinromide and its metabolite (3-bromocinnamamide) in human volunteers following the oral administration of 600 mg of cinromide three times a day (mean ± SE).

FIG. 22-6. BW233U [(+)threo-2-tert-butylamino-1-(3-trifluoromethyl phenyl)-propanol hydrochloride].

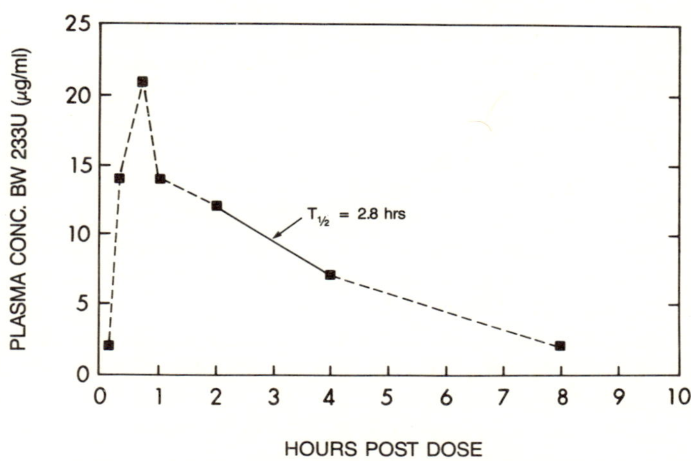

FIG. 22-7. Mean plasma levels of BW233U in rats after an oral dose of 25 mg/kg.

jor constituents in rat plasma, along with the parent drug (2). The relative concentrations of these metabolites following an oral ED_{50} dose of 26 mg/kg to rats are shown in Fig. 22-2. The major plasma metabolite was 3-bromocinnamic acid, a product formed by hydrolysis of the amide bonds in cinromide and 3-bromocinnamamide, and this metabolite had no pharmacological activity. Lower concentrations of 3-bromocinnamamide were also present in rat plasma, but they generally remained low relative to cinromide.

Interestingly, the 3-bromocinnamamide metabolite also showed anticonvulsant activity with an ED_{50} of about 55 mg/kg, but, unfortunately, this metabolite also produced sedation and at slightly higher doses caused ataxia in rats. The significance of the formation of this metabolite became more important during the clinical development of cinromide. However, in the rat, cinromide was the most active species, and plasma levels of the parent drug usually exceeded the 3-bromocinnamamide metabolite by a factor of four based on relative plasma concentration under the curve (AUC).

As the preclinical development of cinromide proceeded to studies in dogs, it was observed that plasma levels of 3-bromocinnamamide were similar to cinromide. As shown in Fig. 22-3, the AUC for cinromide was 28.8 units, whereas 3-bromocinnamamide achieved 18 units. The relatively high concentrations of the amide metabolite in the dog suggested that sedation associated with 3-bromocinnamamide might become more of a problem in man than anticipated from the rat studies. Indeed, in a single oral dose study of cinromide in man, 3-bromocinnamamide was found to be a major metabolite achieving plasma concentrations as high as cinromide. As shown in Fig. 22-4, after a single oral dose of cinromide (300 mg), the AUC of plasma concentration for 3-bromocinnamamide exceeded that for cinromide, and the plasma half-life of 3-bromocinnamamide appeared to be significantly longer than cinromide. In addition, the plasma half-life of cinromide in man was slightly over an hour. This combination of kinetics would suggest that after frequent dosing with cinromide in man, the 3-bromocinnamamide metabolite might accumulate to high concentrations, causing excessive side-effects. In a 30-day, multiple oral dose study of cinromide in man (Fig 22-5), significantly higher plasma concentrations of 3-bromocinnamamide were achieved than for cinromide, and eventually the development of the compound was discontinued because of the lack of efficacy and the appearance of significant side-effects. In retrospect, the short half-life of cinromide in animals and man along with the appearance of a major metabolite with significant side-effects eventually led to the failure of cinromide. Another important aspect to consider was that cinromide was a very insoluble compound that resulted in slow absorption characteristics; this property, coupled with high hepatic extraction and metabolism, markedly reduced the bioavailability

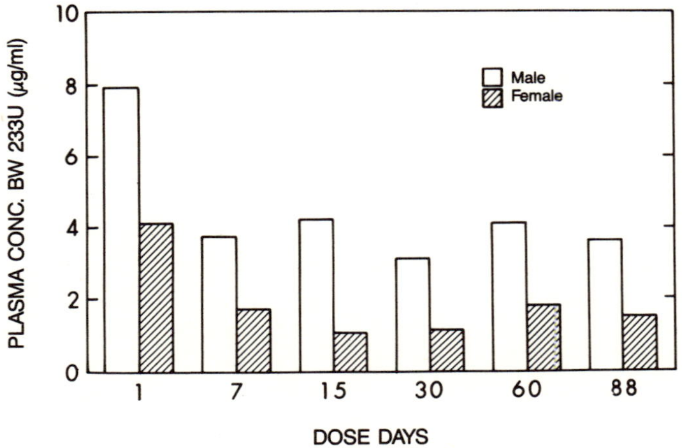

FIG. 22-8. Mean plasma levels of BW233U in dogs on various days 1 h after the first of two daily oral doses of 12.5 mg/kg.

of the compound. In man, very large doses had to be administered frequently to maintain reasonable plasma levels of cinromide. Perhaps a closer examination of the metabolism and pharmacokinetics of cinromide during preclinical and early clinical development might have discouraged further development much earlier.

Attempts to find a potent anticonvulsant with a long duration of action led to the discovery of a phenylpropanolamine series, and specifically to compound (BW233U) with a structure shown in Fig. 22-6. This particular compound possessed potent phenytoin-like activity in rats, with an oral ED_{50} against maximal electroshock (MES) of about 5 mg/kg and a duration of action greater than 8 h. Similar activity against MES was also observed in mice, and the compound blocked audiogenic induced seizures in this species. The compound was freely soluble in water and was rapidly absorbed. Plasma levels of the drug in rats after 25 mg/kg orally indicated a plasma half-life of about 3 h (Fig. 22-7). Because of the unusual potency and long duration of action of BW233U in rodents, attempts to develop the compound proceeded rapidly. During a 90-day toxicity study in male and female beagle dogs given 12.5 mg/kg twice daily, single plasma concentrations were determined on specific days during the study. By day 7, it was noted that plasma concentrations taken 1 h after the first daily dose had already declined to one-half the initial values observed on day 1 (Fig. 22-8). These data suggested that BW233U was inducing its own metabolism during the chronic administration of high doses to the dog, and the metabolism of such compounds are usually increased by other anticonvulsants that cause liver enzyme induction, such as phenobarbital and phenytoin. However, the magnitude of the change in apparent steady-

Table 22-1. Comparative Pharmacokinetic Parameters of BW233U in Normal and Epileptic Subjects

Group	Subject no.	Dose (mg)	AUC $(ng/h/ml^{-1})$	C_{max} (ng/ml)	Approximately plasma $t_{1/2}$ (oral)	Clearance $(L/h^{-1}/F)$
Control	103		9,267	658	18	21.6
	105	200	16,404	1,186	24	12.2
	109		16,607	1,204	33	12.0
	110		9,547	658	13	20.9
Mean ± SEM			12,956 ± 2,051	927 ± 155	22 ± 4.3	16.7 ± 2.6
Epileptic	106		1,708	284	3.2	117.1
	109	200	912	234	3.4	219.3
	105		1,031	394	4.5	194.0
Mean ± SEM			1,217 ± 247	304 ± 47	3.7 ± 0.4	176.8 ± 30.7
Control	102	400	26,873	1,294	10.6	14.9
	104		33,489	1,548	12.2	11.9
Mean ± SEM			30,181 ± 3,308	1,421 ± 127	11.4 ± 0.8	13.4
Epileptic	101	400	7,143	812	6.2	56.0
	104		8,595	1,468	4.0	46.5
	108		11,410	910	6.0	35.0
Mean ± SEM			9,049 ± 1,252	1,063 ± 204	5.4 ± 0.70	45.8 ± 6.0

Table 22-2. Some Ideal Characteristics For the Development of
Anticonvulsant Drugs

1. Predictable oral bioavailability
2. Long-duration action ($t_{\frac{1}{2}}$)
3. Absence of enzyme induction
4. Absence of drug interactions
5. Renal clearance preferred over hepatic clearance
6. Display dose-independent pharmacokinetics
7. Broad spectrum of activity
8. Water solubility

state plasma concentrations observed in dogs was not appreciated until further studies were initiated in human epileptic subjects. As shown in Table 22-1, very marked alterations in the pharmacokinetics of BW233U were observed between normal human subjects and epileptic subjects. After a single oral dose of 200 mg of BW233U, the plasma half-life in normal subjects was 22 h and the clearance was 16.7 L/h. In epileptic subjects, the plasma half-life declined to only 3.7 h and the clearance increased tenfold to 176.8 L/h. Similar changes were observed after a higher dose of BW233U. This dramatic alteration in the pharmacokinetics of BW233U in epileptic subjects was most likely caused by marked increases in hepatic clearance in epileptic subjects. Such subjects are known to have the activity of their liver microsomal enzymes increased, a phenomenon that precipitates a variety of drug interactions (3). In retrospect, this phenomenon could have been identified earlier in animals during the preclinical development of BW233U. Pretreatment of rats with other anticonvulsants such as phenytoin and phenobarbital, followed by a pharmacokinetic study of BW233U, would have identified the potential for the metabolism of BW233U to be increased by long-term exposure to these other anticonvulsants. Also, during the dog toxicity study (Fig. 22-8), it would have been better if the AUC for BW233U were monitored, rather than measuring single time points, since AUC provides a better index for determining changes occurring in metabolism during subchronic drug administration.

From the experiences derived with cinromide and BW233U, as well as with other compounds that had the wrong physiochemical properties, some general concepts regarding metabolism and disposition might be considered for the development of anticonvulsant drugs. These are shown in Table 22-2. For instance, from a clinical viewpoint, reproducible oral bioavailability is a very important parameter in controlling seizures and avoiding unnecessary side-effects. This may be best achieved by avoiding the development of very insoluble compounds that are absorbed slowly

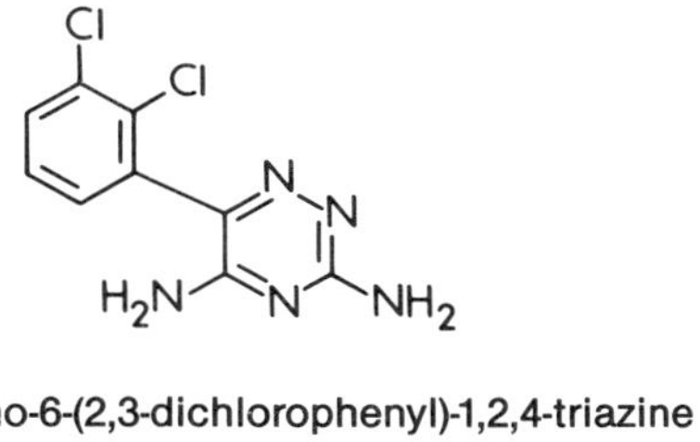

FIG. 22-9. Lamotrigine—3,5-diamino-6-(2,3-dichlorophenyl)-1,2,4-triazine.

3,5-Diamino-6-(2,3-dichlorophenyl)-1,2,4-triazine

and have a high potential for metabolism. Such characteristics usually result in high first-pass metabolism, poor bioavailability, and marked variability in plasma concentrations.

With respect to hepatic clearance, compounds with a high propensity for metabolism are more apt to cause liver enzyme induction and increase their own metabolism or increase the metabolism of other drugs. Drugs that are cleared principally by hepatic metabolism may also inhibit the metabolism of other drugs, and the therapeutic problems associated with enzyme inhibition are numerous (4). In addition, hepatic clearance is subject to greater individual variation than renal clearance (5). Therefore, to avoid drug interactions related to metabolism, it would be best for an anticonvulsant to be eliminated by renal clearance. This is a very important consideration, since anticonvulsant drugs are usually administered to epileptic subjects who have a high capacity to metabolize drugs. Another advantage of renal clearance is that it is less subject to saturation than hepatic clearance, and compounds excreted by this process would be more apt to exhibit dose-independent pharmacokinetics. Indeed, a major problem with phenytoin is that it displays dose-dependent Michaelis-Menten type kinetics (6), which leads to a significant number of side-effects (7) and individual variations in therapeutic responses (8).

Many of the above criteria were met fortuitously by a new anticonvul-

Table 22-3. Plasma Levels of Lamotrigme, Phenytoin, and Phenobarbital After Administration of a Single Oral Dose to Rats at Multiples of the MES Anticonvulsant ED$_{50}$[a]

Dose (ED$_{50}$ X)	Plasma level (μg/ml)		
	1X	2X	4X
Lamotrigine	1.55 ± 0.45	1.99 ± 0.18	3.11 ± 0.59
Phenytoin	3.54 ± 1.72	5.58 ± 2.5	8.7 ± 3.6
Phenobarbital	7.5 ± 2.9	14.1 ± 2.7	25.9 ± 2.9

[a]Male rats were dosed orally with multiples of the maximal electroshock ED$_{50}$ and killed 2 h after the dose.

Table 22-4. Effect of Pretreatment of Male Marmosets for 30 Days with Lamotrigine on Liver Microsomal Metabolism

Lamotrigine daily dose (mg/kg)	Cytochrome P-450[a]	Aminopyrine demethylation[b]	Nitrophenol glucuronidation[b]	Ethoxyresorufin dealkylation[b]	Aniline hydroxylation[b]
0	0.48 ± 0.05	3.07 ± 1.1	14.0 ± 2.1	0.48 ± 0.12	0.85 ± 0.34
10	0.42 ± 0.14	3.46 ± 0.22	13.5 ± 1.4	0.45 ± 0.17	1.14 ± 0.50
22.5	0.48 ± 0.13	3.24 ± 0.42	13.4 ± 3.7	0.30 ± 0.14	1.0 ± 0.43
50.0	0.44 ± 0.03	3.91 ± 1.58	13.4 ± 2.4	0.50 ± 0.23	1.1 ± 0.21

Results are expressed as mean ± SD.
[a] Expressed as nmoles of P-450/mg protein.
[b] Expressed as nmoles of product formed/min/mg protein.

Table 22-5. Lamotrigine Single-Dose Study: Mean Pharmacokinetic Parameters (SD)

Parameter	Lamotrigine dose (mg)			
	120 (n = 9)	240 (n = 9)	360 (n = 4)	480 (n = 4)
$t_{1/2}$ (h)	22.6 (9.0)	19.4 (8.0)	20.6 (6.8)	19.2 (8.1)
AUC (h × μg/ml)	47.1 (29.2)	72.5 (32.5)	130.7 (60.8)	168.7 (98.4)
C_{max} (μg/ml)	1.41 (0.36)	2.66 (0.36)	4.70 (1.05)	5.92 (1.90)
t_{max} (h)	2.89 (1.39)	2.44 (1.26)	1.90 (1.52)	1.50 (1.12)
CL/F (L/h/kg)	0.040 (0.014)	0.050 (0.018)	0.041 (0.015)	0.045 (0.014)
V_d/F (L/kg)	1.16 (0.27)	1.24 (0.20)	1.09 (0.05)	1.08 (0.03)

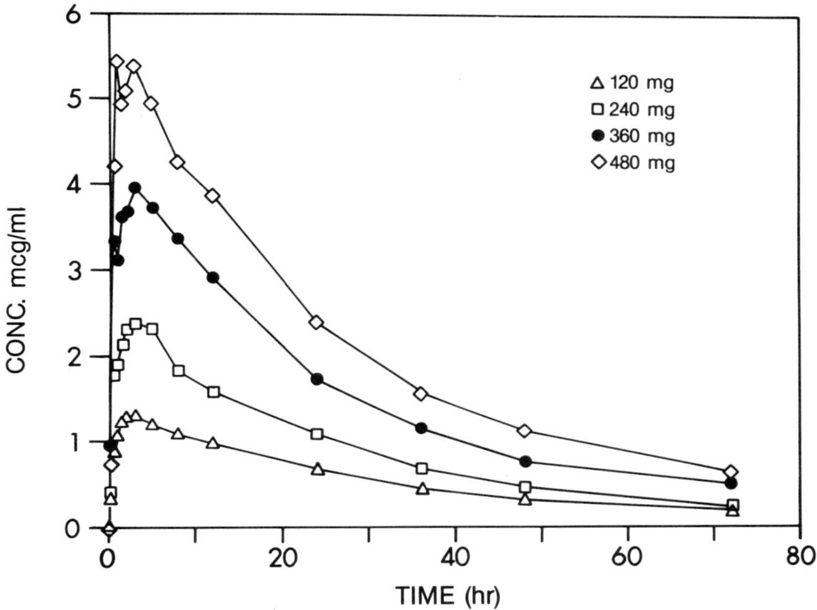

FIG. 22-10. Mean lamotrigine plasma levels in normal human volunteers.

sant, lamotrigine, presently in advanced stages of clinical development (9). Lamotrigine is a water soluble compound with a chemical structure shown in Fig. 22-9. It exhibited high potency against MES in both mice and rats with oral ED_{50}s in the range of 2–4 mg/kg, and its peak activity lasted for up to 8 h (10). Peak plasma levels of lamotrigine, phenobarbital, and phenytoin at multiples of their ED_{50}s are shown in Table 22-3. At 4 times the ED_{50} the peak plasma levels of lamotrigine were only 3.1 μg/ml, whereas the same values for phenytoin and phenobarbital were as high as 8.7 μg/ ml and 25.9 μg/ml, respectively.

As discussed above, the importance of enzyme induction in epilepsy cannot be underestimated. Therefore, the ability of lamotrigine to cause this phenomenon in marmosets after pretreatment for 30 days was investigated, and the results are shown in Table 22-4. Measurements of standard indicators showed no changes from controls after 30 days of treatment at doses of lamotrigine ranging from 10 to 50 mg/kg. Thus, unlike many other clinically used antiepileptic drugs, lamotrigine appears not to cause liver enzyme induction in a mammalian species and would not be expected to participate in a number of drug interactions associated with this phenomenon.

Based on favorable preclinical studies with this anticonvulsant, clinical studies of lamotrigine in normal human subjects were initiated. The plasma

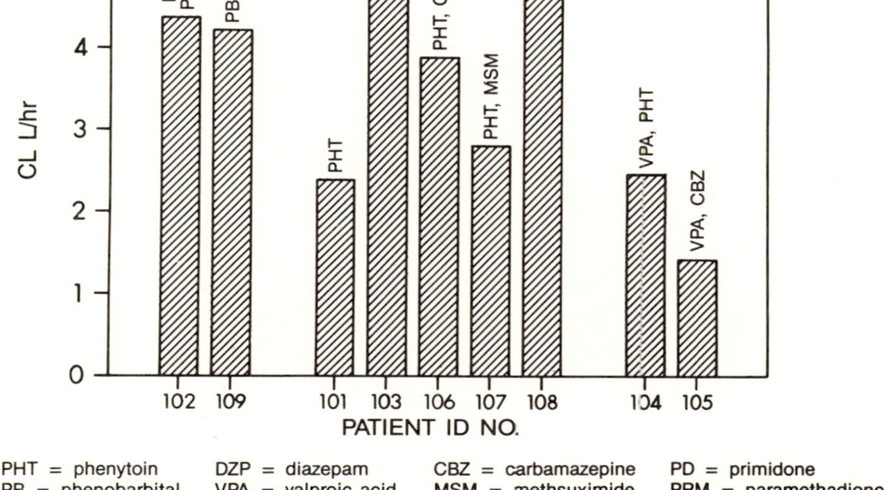

FIG. 22-11. Average clearances of lamotrigine in epileptic patients after a single dose of lamotrigine.

levels of lamotrigine during a rising single dose tolerance study in normal subjects are shown in Fig. 22-10, and the various pharmacokinetic parameters are listed in Table 22-5. The plasma half-lives in these subjects ranged between 19.2 and 22.6 h, and the C_{max} and plasma concentration AUCs were linear over a range of doses of 120–480 mg. The renal clearance of the drug was constant over the dose range studied at 0.045 L/h/kg, and the V_d/F was small, averaging about 1.2 L/kg. The urine contained mostly lamotrigine glucuronide and some parent drug. This encouraging profile in phase I clinical studies, coupled with the favorable preclinical profile, encouraged further development. Thus, lamotrigine, unlike cinromide and BW233U, is not subject to significant phase 1 metabolism in human liver. Since lamotrigine will usually be administered in combination with other anticonvulsants, it was important to examine the clearance of lamotrigine in epileptic subjects being treated with other anticonvulsants. As shown in Fig. 22-11, only valproic acid caused a significant change in the clearance of lamotrigine. This interaction appears to be based on a competition for glucuronidation between valproic acid and lamotrigine, resulting in a decrease in the clearance and prolongation in the plasma half-life of lamotrigine. Removal of the vaporate from the treatment regimen restores the clearance of lamotrigine to normal values. Although lamotrigine is not subject to extensive phase I metabolism, it does undergo significant conjugation by N-glucuronidation in normal subjects, and this conjugation is increased in epileptic patients. In epileptics the increased N-glucuronidation appears to account for a decrease in the plasma half-life of lamotrigine. In a series of subjects co-medicated with carbamazepine and/or phenytoin, the plasma half-life of lamotrigine was reduced to an average value of 15 h (9) compared to an average value of 20.4 h, shown in Table 22-5.

The above report describes the development of three anticonvulsant drugs, all with excellent pharmacological properties in early screens in animals but with marked differences in their metabolic and dispositional characteristics. The metabolic and dispositional characteristics can be identified early in preclinical development when the profiles are less than ideal, and appropriate changes can be made in the chemical series to eliminate these problems. The potential value of a comprehensive preclinical profile that includes complete dispositional data as well as pharmacological and safety assessment information is particularly important in the process of developing potentially useful anticonvulsant drugs. The present report summarizes several of the physical, metabolic, and dispositional factors found most useful in the development of an effective anticonvulsant.

REFERENCES

1. Chiu P, Lipnowski S, Bruni J, Burnham M. Effects of cinromide, a new anticonvulsant on cortex and amygdala kindled seizures in the rat. *Can J Neurol Sci* 1981;8:193.
2. DeAngelis RL, Robinson MM, Brown AR, Johnson TE, Welch RM. Quantitation of the anticonvulsant cinromide (3-Bromo-N-Ethylcinnamamide) and its major plasma metabolites by thin-layer chromotography. *J Chromatogr* 1980;221:353–60.
3. Conney AH. Pharmacological implications of microsomal enzyme induction. *Pharmacol Rev* 1967;19:317–66.
4. Park BK, Breckenridge AM. Clinical implications of enzyme induction and inhibition. *Clin Pharmacokinet* 1981;6:1–24.
5. Gibaldi M. Pharmacokinetic variability—body weight, age, sex, and genetic factors. In: Gibaldi M *Biopharmaceutics and Clinical Pharmacokinetics*. Philadelphia: Lea & Febiger, 1984:206–27.
6. Mawer GE, et al. Phenytoin dose adjustment in epileptic patients. *Br J Clin Pharmacol* 1974;1:163–8.
7. Kutt H, et al. Diphenylhydantoin metabolism, blood levels and toxicity. *Arch Neurol* 1964;11:642–8.
8. Lund L. Effects of phenytoin in patients with epilepsy in relation to its concentration in plasma. In: Davies DS, Prichard BNC, eds. *Biological Effects of*

Drugs in Relation to their Plasma Concentrations. New York: Macmillan, 1973:227–38.

9. Binnie CD, et al. Acute effects of lamotrigine (BW430C) in persons with epilepsy. *Epilepsia* 1986;27:248–54.

10. Miller AA, et al. Lamotrigine. In: Meldrum BS, Porter RJ, eds. *New Anticonvulsant Drugs.* London: John Libbey and Company Ltd, 1986:165–77.

23

Drug Interactions: Can They Be Predicted?

Harvey J. Kupferberg

*Preclinical Pharmacology Section, Epilepsy Branch,
National Institute of Neurological Disorders and Stroke, National
Institutes of Health, Bethesda, Maryland, U.S.A.*

When two or more drugs are used simultaneously, the pharmacological or toxicological response is not always predictable. This is because one drug may interact with the action of another drug. There are many mechanisms of drug interactions; some are chemical, some biochemical. The chances for interactions increase as the search for more potent pharmacological agents continues to be combined with the practice of polypharmacy. Some of the mechanisms for the interactions are easily understood as they act by altering absorption, distribution, metabolism, excretion, and action at receptor sites.

Examples of drug interactions are numerous in the field of anticonvulsant therapy. Most anticonvulsants have narrow therapeutic indices, and clinicians practice polypharmacy. The mechanism for these interactions are mainly due to changes in protein binding or inhibition of drug metabolism. Most of these interactions are clinically important; others are more a pharmacokinetic curiosity. Not all drug interactions produce harmful effects, nor can all be used in a beneficial way.

Several methods are used to identify and investigate drug interactions: (a) spontaneous reporting or fortuitous observation, (b) retrospective or prospective studies, and (c) experimental studies in human and animals. Most of the drug interactions in anticonvulsant therapy are found fortuitously. The interaction of isoniazid and primidone was discovered in this manner. A patient's plasma sample was analyzed by chance for primidone and its major metabolites, phenobarbital and phenylethylmalonamide (PEMA) (1). The medication provided poor seizure control with no side-effects. Primidone and phenobarbital plasma levels were found to be 45 μg/ml and 15 μg/ml, respectively. These values were inconsistent with other patients' plasma levels for the dose of primidone (250 mg four times a day). A review of the patient's medical history indicates that she had tuberculosis and was receiving isoniazid (100 mg three times a day). The patient was admitted to the hospital and isoniazid was discontinued. The primidone levels decreased, and phenobarbital and PEMA levels rose to expected values.

This interaction is not surprising, since isoniazid inhibits the metabolism of phenytoin (2). Isoniazid is a known inhibitor of phenytoin metabolism in epileptic patients (3). Kutt demonstrated isoniazid's noncompetitive inhibition of phenytoin metabolism using rat liver microsomes. The concentration of isoniazid in the incubation mixture was similar to the concentration in the plasma of patients taking isoniazid (4).

Some of the drug interactions with antiepileptic therapy are found from retrospective studies. Fincham and Schottelius (5) showed that the phenobarbital/primidone ratio is less in a patient population receiving primidone alone than in a patient population receiving phenytoin and primidone. They hypothesized that phenytoin induced the conversion of primidone to phenobarbital. They also speculated that phenytoin interfered with the hydroxylation or excretion of phenobarbital. In a prospective study, Porro and co-workers (6) studied the same interaction in an epileptic patient treated with primidone alone, as well as primidone and phenytoin for 3 months. The addition of phenytoin to the regimen increased the steady-state phenobarbital and PEMA plasma levels and decreased the levels of primidone and parahydroxyphenobarbital, the major metabolite of phenobarbital. When phenytoin was discontinued, the plasma phenobarbital levels decreased and primidone levels increased. The hydroxyphenobarbital levels also rose rapidly. They concluded from the plasma and urinary data that phenytoin initially induces the conversion of primidone to phenobarbital and PEMA and inhibits the hydroxylation of phenobarbital. Although these phenomena appear to be contradictory, they clearly explain the changes observed by Fincham and Schottelius in their retrospective study. Demonstration of this interaction in experimental animals has not been reported. However, Kutt (3) showed that phenobarbital competitively inhibits phenytoin metabolism in rat liver microsomes.

Valproic acid has been shown to interact with other antiepileptic drugs, either by inhibiting metabolism or altering protein binding. Valproic acid inhibits the metabolism of phenobarbital (7). The addition of valproic acid can cause increases in phenobarbital levels of 28 to 67%. The rise in plasma phenobarbital levels was paralleled by lengthening the phenobarbital elimination half–life.

The above study was followed by an in vitro demonstration of the inhibition (8). Valproic acid was shown to inhibit the microsomal metabolism of phenobarbital in a competitive manner. The in vitro decrease in the velocity of phenobarbital's p-hydroxylation is similar to that found in epileptic patients. These studies supported the idea that the in vivo interaction was metabolic in nature.

More dramatic interactions in epileptic patients occur with nafimidone (9) and denzimol (10). Both compounds are 1-imidazoles and are potent inhibitors of microsomal metabolism of phenytoin and carbamazepine (11). 1-imidazoles are known to be potent inhibitors of microsomal metabolism (12, 13). Unfortunately, the animal data was not taken into account prior to clinical trials in epileptic patients.

The extrapolation of data between humans and animals may not always be as impressive as noted in the example above. Felbamate (2-phenyl-1,3-propanediol dicarbamate), a new antiepileptic agent, is presently under clinical efficacy evaluation. In early clinical studies, felbamate was shown to increase phenytoin plasma levels and to slightly reduce carbamazepine plasma levels (14). The increase in phenytoin levels was moderate, approximately 20%. The increase appears to be related to the dose of phenytoin and the V_{max} of phenytoin for the patient.

Interaction studies using rat liver microsomes could not confirm this observation, even though the concentrations of felbamate in the incubation mixture was equal to or greater than the concentrations found in patient's plasma. The mechanism of this interaction can be explained on the basis that both phenytoin and felbamate both undergo phenyl ring hydroxylation.

The most difficult interactions to evaluate in man are those that occur at the receptor site. These types of interactions lead to antagonism, addition, or potentiation of pharmacodynamic effects and cannot be explained by pharmacokinetic mechanisms. Weaver and co-workers (15) evaluated the pharmacodynamic interactions of phenytoin and phenobarbital in rats using the maximal electroshock test. Their results indicated that, depending on the combination ratio of anticonvulsants, the observed anticonvulsant activity was greater than could be predicted from the estimated activity from the dose response curves of each anticonvulsant.

This type of interaction would be extremely important in developing new therapeutic agents. Data from animal experiments could be used in designing the protocols for the early clinical efficacy trials of new drugs. Most clinical trials are carried out in therapy-resistant patients, and the experimental drug is added to the existing therapy. If animal experiments indicated that the new compound interacted with one of the clinically used drugs to produce a potentiated or supra-additive effect, then the clinical trial could then use this combination. The supra-additive effects might occur if the experimental drug worked by a mechanism different from the existing medication. In theory, this type of interaction would be of benefit to the patient.

In summary, most drug interactions observed in patients can either be explained by existing knowledge or can be duplicated in animal experiments. The major problem facing the clinician is the wide variety of drugs that are given to patients. It becomes an impossible task to predict whether a drug used for other indications will interact with the antiepileptic therapy. An excellent example of the problem is the interaction of carbamazepine and triacetyloleandomycin, an antibiotic (16).

In some instances, controlled experimental studies in humans have failed to confirm drug interactions in anecdotal clinical reports. In a case report, Garrettson and co-workers (17) showed that methylphenidate caused increases in serum levels of primidone, phenytoin, and phenobarbital in a child suffering from attention deficit disorder and general tonic–clonic seizures. Kupferberg and co-workers (18) were unable to duplicate this interaction in 11 adult epileptic patients who were given methylphenidate (30 mg) for 6 weeks and then discontinued. The reason for the differences in results is not clear, but the incidence of the interaction most likely is small.

The advantage of experimental human studies is that they can predict the clinical significance of the interaction by establishing its degree, time course, and dosage aspects. These factors cannot be precisely determined from animal experimentation. Goodman (16) states "At best, animal pharmacology provides only paradigms and analogies, the clinical predictive value of which remains to be demonstrated. The best model for a cat is another cat. The best model for man is man himself."

REFERENCES

1. Sutton G, Kupferberg HJ. Isoniazid as an inhibitor of primidone metabolism. *Neurology (Minneap)* 1975;25:1179–81.
2. Kutt H, Winters W, McDowell F. Depression of parahydroxylation of diphenylhydantoin by antituberculosis chemotherapy. *Neurology (Minneap)* 1969;19:611–6.
3. Kutt H. Interactions with antiepileptic drugs involving multiple mechanisms. In: Morselli PL, Garattini S, Cohen SN, eds. *Drug Interactions* New York: Raven Press, 1974:211–22.
4. Kutt H, Verebely K. Metabolism of diphenylhydantoin by rat liver microsomes. I. Characteristics of the reaction. *Biochem Pharamcol* 1970;19:675–86.
5. Fincham FW, Schottelius DD. Primidone: interactions with other drugs. In: Woodbury DM, Penry JK, Pippenger CE, eds. *Antiepileptic Drugs.* New York: Raven Press, 1982:421–40.
6. Porro MG, Kupferberg HJ, Porter RJ, Theodore WH, Newark ME. Phenyt-

oin: an inhibitor and inducer of primidone metabolism in an epileptic patient. *Br J Clin Pharmacol* 14:294–7.

7. Kapetanovic IM, Kupferberg HJ, Porter RJ, Theodore W, Schulman E, Penry JK. Mechanism of valproate-phenobarbital interaction in epileptic patients. *Clin Pharmacol* 1981;29:480–6.

8. Kapetanovic IM, Kupferberg HJ. Inhibition of microsomal phenobarbital metabolism by valproic acid. *Biochem Pharmacol* 1981;30:1361–3.

9. Treiman DM, Ben-Menachem E, Barber KD, Chelberg R. Inhibition of carbamazepine and phenytoin metabolism by nafimidone, a new antiepileptic drug. *Neurology (Minneap)* 1984;34:213.

10. Patsalos PN, Shorvon SD, Elyas AA, Smith G. The interaction of denzimol (a new anticonvulsant) with carbamazepine and phenytoin. *J Neurol Neurosurg Psychiatry* 1985;48:374–7.

11. Kapetanovic IM, Kupferberg HJ. Nafimidone, an imidazole anticonvulsant, and its metabolite as potent inhibitors of microsomal metabolism of phenytoin and carbamazepine. *Drug Metab* 1984;12:560–4.

12. Wilkinson CF, Hetnarski K, Cantwell GP, DiCarlo FJ. Structure-activity relationships in the effects of 1-alkylimidazoles on microsomal oxidation in vitro and in vivo. *Biochem Pharmacol* 1974;23:2377–86.

13. Testa B, Jenner P. Inhibitors of cytochrome P-450s and their mechanism of action. *Drug Metab Rev* 1981;12:1–117.

14. Wilensky AJ, Friel PN, Ojemann LM, Kupferberg HJ, and Levy RH. Pharmacokinetics of W-544 (ADD03055) in epileptic patients. *Epilepsia* 1985;26:602–6.

15. Weaver LC, Swinyard EA, Woodbury LA, Goodman LS. Studies on anticonvulsant drug combinations: phenobarbital and diphenylhydantoin. *J Pharmacol* 1955;113:359–70.

16. Mesdjian E, Dravet C, Cenraud B, Roger J. Carbamazepine intoxication due to triaceyloleandomycin administration in epileptic patients. Epilepsia 1980;21:489–96.

17. Garrettson LK, Perel JM, and Dayton PG Methylpenidate interaction with both anticonvulsants and ethyl biscomacetate. *JAMA* 1969;207:2053–6.

18. Kupferberg HJ, Jeffery W, and Hunninghake DB. Effects of methylphenidate on plasma anticonvulsant level. *Clin Pharmacol Ther* 1972;13:201–4.

19. Goodman LS. The problem of drug efficacy: an exercise in dissection. In: Talalay P, ed. *Drugs in Our Society*. Baltimore, Maryland: Johns Hopkins Press, 1964.

Index